The

Entrepreneurial
Nutritionist

3rd edition

Kathy King, RD, LD

Helm Publishing
Lake Dallas, Texas

The Entrepreneurial Nutritionist, 3rd edition

Cover design: Julie Horton
Printing: Sheridan Books
Layout: Pamela Murphy
Copyediting: Dollie Parsons

First edition   Copyright 1987 by Harper & Row
Second edition   Copyright 1991 by Kathy King Helm

For information or to order books or handouts:

Helm Publishing
P.O. Box 2105
Lake Dallas, TX 75065
Toll Free 877-560-6025
www.helmpublishing.com

ISBN 0-9631033-4-2

This book is dedicated to my family and friends who have taken
their time to share their wisdom and life's lessons. Also, to my
daughters, Savannah and Cherokee for their
never ending love and support.

Table of Contents ────────────

Introduction

Section I   The Beginning
1   The Entrepreneurial Spirit 3
2   Is Self-Employment for You? 11

Section II   Building a Strong Foundation
3   Business Strategies and Management 27
4   Building Your Credibility 45
5   Nurturing Your Creativity 53
6   Ethics and Malpractice 61
7   Creating a Good Image 73
8   Counseling Expertise 81

Section III   Managing Your Business
9   Business Plan 95
10   Marketing 103
11   Forms of Business Ownership 123
12   Protecting Your Ideas and Interests 135
13   Choosing Business Advisors 149
14   Finance and Money 157
15   Start-up Decisions and Costs 181
16   Fees and Reimbursement 197
17   Negotiation, Selling and Contracts 207
18   Computers in Nutrition Practice 221
19   Office Policies and Dealing with Clients 225

Section IV Taking Your Ideas to Market
20   Promoting Your Venture 235
21   Using the Internet 259
22   Website Basics 271
23   Promoting Your Website 297

Section V   Developing Your Professional Practice
24   Jobs with Physicians and Other Accounts 325
25   Consulting in Long Term Care 333
26   Communicating with Food 343
27   The "Write" Way to Get Published 367
28   Media Savvy 383
29   Sports and Cardiovascular Nutrition 395
30   The Wellness Movement 407
31   Continued Competency 417

Index 422

Introduction

Entrepreneurship will be one of the most challenging, difficult projects you ever undertake. It may also be one of the most satisfying and exciting. Trial and error, adjusting to market changes and trusting your gut instincts are part of every new venture. Passion for the project is a must. Becoming skilled requires study, action, money, assessment, more action, more time and money.

The mere idea of starting a business venture of some sort was embraced by only a few maverick dietitians in the 1960's and 70's. Self-employment became more popular in the 1980's and 90's. Today, entrepreneurship is in the mainstream of dietetics and worldwide business.

Dietitians are choosing self-employment to make more money per hour, to have more flexible hours, to try new ideas, to work with new client populations or food in a different way. According to ADA's Membership Survey (1), successful self-employment has the potential to generate as much income as top jobs in education and food service management. Some private practitioners make $100,000-200,000 or more per year.

BOILED FROG SYNDROME

Now is not the time to have the boiled frog syndrome. Simply stated, when you put a live frog into a pan of boiling water it will jump out. However, if you put a live frog into lukewarm water and slowly turn up the heat, it will sit there and eventually boil. It is easier to react when you are put in a hostile environment, but many people don't react in time when profound, irreversible change happens more gradually.

The marketplaces where dietitians have traditionally worked are changing. Some practitioners have assessed the new (or lost) opportunities and adjusted their departments and career plans accordingly. Others have denied or fought the changes, fully expecting the former norms to return.

Health care is in a state of flux. In many locations of the U.S., medical care and its availability have never been poorer (2). Patients are slipping through safety nets of managed care programs (3). In a review of studies on deaths from prescriptions taken correctly in the hospital, it was found they account for 137,000 deaths and 2.7 million serious side effects per year. Prescriptions handed out by physicians are the sixth leading cause of death in the U.S. (4). It's no surprise there is a groundswell of interest in the public for alternative therapies and healthy lifestyle choices. Nutrition's "window of opportunity" is wide open, and the field of nutrition will continue to offer new opportunities for some time.

The dietitians who founded our profession were innovative, risk taking individuals. Many were consultants, authors or innovators who created their hospitals' and universities' first dietary departments.

Eloise Treasher began the earliest known clinical private practice in 1949 in Baltimore, Maryland. As Eloise retired from work at The Johns Hopkins Hospital, many physicians wanted to continue sending their patients to her, and her consulting business began. Eloise stated, "Private practice is not for everyone, and not everyone will be good at it. But, if you offer quality service, you will be in demand."

In 1953, Norma MacRae began her counseling business in Seattle, Washington. Her practice included writing successful cookbooks. When asked about her success, Norma stated, "I knew I had 'arrived' when physicians started coming to see me as patients."

Other pioneers include Virginia Bayles, RD, a consulting nutritionist in Houston, Texas, and author, Dorothy Revel, RD, from Fargo, North Dakota. Carol Hunerlach, RD, of Maryland is credited with spearheading the movement to organize the Nutrition Entrepreneurs (formerly Consulting Nutritionists) Dietetic Practice Group of The American Dietetic Association.

Today, there are dietitians who own multi-million dollar companies, restaurants, health food stores, vineyards, publishing houses, home health agency, large long-term care consulting firms, and computer companies. Others offer services on a smaller scale where they consult to cruise lines, act as a chef or personal trainer, or counsel private clients. Entrepreneurial nutritionists write newspaper columns, host television and radio programs, author books, invent products, develop web sites, consult to top athletes, speak professionally, and act as media spokespersons.

The Editor

I graduated in Food Science and Nutrition from Colorado State University, which gave me a good, solid academic background. My internship was at Beth Israel Hospital in Boston, a Harvard teaching hospital, where I discovered my love for outpatient counseling.

After practicing two years as a clinical dietitian, I began my business in 1972 in Denver, Colorado. The lack of prevention and ongoing counseling in the hospital setting frustrated me. I decided to go into the outpatient setting and start my private practice.

My business strategy was easy: Keep my overhead low, work day and night for a year and then reevaluate. This decision was not hard to come by, since I was single and had nothing of value to borrow against--but I had the time and dedication.

My business started at one physician's office two days per week for $5 per hour. I lived on that income while I developed my business, working out of six other physicians' offices. I spent a lot of time in transit, waiting for patients to arrive, and marketing to physicians so they would remember to refer clients.

The first year I charged $7 for the initial visit and $2 for revisits-and some people still complained about my fees! I supported myself from the start, supplementing my income with cleaning houses and sewing. For every hour I generated income in the business, I usually worked three hours on paperwork or marketing with no guarantee of income.

Before one year was up, I knew the concept worked. I decided to borrow $1000 from my grandparents and open a 10'x 13' office in the new medical complex being built next to the suburban hospital where I had last worked. I loved it. Patients came to me and I didn't have to counsel them over the stirrups on an exam table. I furnished my office with antiques and plants. I raised my fees slightly to cover the increased overhead, and it looked like a legitimate business.

To promote my business, I usually gave several free speeches each week. I appeared weekly on NBC TV's "NoonDay" and monthly on KMGH TV's "Blinky's Fun Club," for a total of eight years. I volunteered to the Colorado Dietetic Association so that other dietitians would get to know me and I them. After 3-4 years, over half of my new consultant accounts were referrals from other dietitians.

I learned more about sports nutrition by volunteering for three years to the exercise physiology staff at the University of Denver. I was their "on call" nutritionist for speaking at sports conferences, and counseling athletes. I invented a natural sports drink with the aid of the Herty-Peck Company in Indianapolis, which 7-11 stores wanted to buy, but that is another book.

Sports consulting with the Denver Bronco Football Team, Denver Avalanche Soccer Team, paid media work, media spokesperson jobs, lecturing, and writing started to come my way as my expertise and reputation grew. My approach to nutrition was from a wellness point of view, so when the trend finally hit Denver, I was ready to grow with it. My commitment to the profession grew as I was elected President of the Colorado Dietetic Association, and spent five years in the leadership of the Council on Practice, and two years on ADA's Board of Directors, and House of Delegates.

When I married and moved to Texas in 1983, I didn't want to start over again building a group of clinical offices. Instead, I helped develop a hospital-based wellness program, consulted at The Greenhouse Spa, hosted my own nationally syndicated radio talk show for a year, and traveled giving lectures and seminars. In between, I stayed home with two daughters.

This book has been translated into Japanese by Reiko Hashimoto, an outstanding private practitioner in Tokyo who also counsels sumo wrestlers. I self-published the second edition of this book in 1991. That experience opened doors to more writing and publishing other dietitians' material. Helm Publishing is now a mail-order cataloger with over 50 products, mainly for self-study continuing education for dietitians and dietetic technicians. We started marketing on the web in 1997 at www.helmpublishing.com, which is maintained by chapter authors, Teresa Pangan, PhD, RD, and her partner, Julie Horner, of Puttin'OnTheWeb.

In 1997, I purchased a rundown feed store to hold my publishing company and a gift store less than a mile from my home in Lake Dallas, Texas. I had it renovated into a beautiful peach-colored store with a white front porch, surrounded by an herb garden. It is now called Herb Garden Antiques. In the spring we sell live herb plants. I started selling nutritional and herbal supplements when we opened, but they are too mainstream now to be profitable in a small retail business.

From my experience, I learned that when the tough decisions have to be made, no one can do it better than I. I have stopped looking for that expert on a white horse. I try to learn from each experience and person I meet who knows something I don't. I have learned skills I never wanted to know. I find it still takes time and patience to break into new business arenas where I am unknown. I, and other entrepreneurs I know, continue in business because we love the chance to be creative, to work with people and the freedom. The difficulty of the challenge makes us appreciate the rewards even more.

Innovative practitioners will continue to lead our profession into new, non-traditional job markets. We as a profession need to identify these trailblazers and let them teach us how to find these new career avenues. We should be willing to learn about new areas of practice and act as mentors to our younger members. Or, recognize when someone is willing to take the risk and support that individual with our goodwill and enthusiasm--not the Tall Poppy Syndrome where an innovator is punished by their peers. If you can't give your support then let them pass because we need this type of growth and experimentation to take place worldwide in dietetics today.(5)

This Book

This book was written for dietitians and dietetic technicians to offer practical suggestions and guidelines on the development of business knowledge, skills, and moneymaking ventures. I have included interviews and stories about successful practitioners. Many chapters are written by top consultants and private practitioners.

This third edition is totally updated with new chapters on marketing on the Internet, using the Internet without a website, culinary communication skills, and consulting in long term care. It has numerous practical examples to illustrate points, and answers to questions commonly asked by new and seasoned entrepreneurs. The term "entrepreneur" will be used to identify both self-employed people and employed intrapreneurs.

The opinions are obviously those of the various authors. They should provide you with a starting point for your own research and personal growth.

I have been told by hundreds of dietitians that the first two editions of this book have helped them start and maintain their successful businesses. For others, it has taught skills and strategies that are used daily in their employment setting. Many say they referred to the book over the years as new decisions and hassles arose. I hope you find this book helpful and interesting!

Kathy King, RD, LD

REFERENCES

1. ADA Membership Survey, *J Amer Diet Assoc;* 01:1.
2. Second-Class Medicine. *Consumer Reports;* September 2000.
3. Kleinke JD. *Oxymorons: The Myth of a U.S. Health Care System.* San Francisco: Jossey-Bass; 2001.
4. Posner H. Letters to the Editor. *New Eng J Med;* Feb. 1999.
5. Helm KK. Risk taking isn't risky like it used to be. *J Amer Diet Assoc;* 04:89.

—— The Beginning ——

Words of Wisdom:

"Do not follow where the path may lead. Go instead where there is no path and leave a trail."

"Many of life's failures are men who did not realize how close they were to success when they gave up."

"Choice, not chance determines destiny."

Chapter 1

The Entrepreneurial Spirit

Many dietitians, like a growing number of other Americans, are embracing the entrepreneurial spirit. Their ingenuity, creative verve, aggressiveness, and willingness to handle fear of failure are leading them and the worldwide dietetic profession into new fields of experience.

Dietitians are best selling authors, personal chefs, media spokespersons, and sports nutritionists. They own public relations firms, publishing houses, and nursing homes. A few are inventors of products like fruit-sweetened cookies, diet card games, educational videos, and multi-million dollar computer data companies. Dietitians are culinary and nutrition consultants to movie stars, spas, restaurants, and fast food chains. Others offer consultant management expertise in inventory control and reducing the incidence of malnutrition. A growing number of Nutrition Therapists are pursuing new areas of clinical practice like Integrative Medicine and Functional Nutrition Therapy.

Becoming an entrepreneur fulfills for many people the desire to create their own destinies. Some people say they are more satisfied—financially and personally—than ever before. Others say they have never worked so hard for so little return. It is not an option everyone will want to try.

THE ENTREPRENEURIAL EXPLOSION

Entrepreneurism is thriving in America. Being an entrepreneur has moved from cult status in the 80's to become de rigueur at the turn of the century. Today, there are more than 25 million small businesses in the U.S., and more than 12.3 million Americans are self-employed. (1) According to the Small Business Administration (SBA), these businesses represent: (1,2,3)

- 99 percent of all employers
- 75 percent of the new net jobs
- 51 percent of the private sector output
- 96 percent of all exported goods

Fifty-three percent of these small businesses are home-based, 44 percent have offices, and another 3 percent are franchises.(1) Small firms provide part time jobs for the elderly and first jobs for a large number of young employees (67 percent) where they learn basic job skills. (1)

According to Dun and Bradstreet, the average business owner today has three employees, 1.3 locations of business, and is not a part of a franchise organization. They found owners typically work about 50 hours a week at businesses that generate average revenues of $50,000 to $200,000.(4) In a survey of members of the National Association of the Self-Employed, 24 percent held a bachelor's degree versus 16.5 percent of all Americans over the age of 25 years. (5)

Traditionally, business schools prepared their students for middle management positions in large businesses. However, between 1990 and 1995, the number of entrepreneurial programs in colleges and universities grew from 25 to 60 throughout the U.S. (6)

One of the fears of starting an entrepreneurial venture is the failure rate of new businesses. However, an Advocacy study by the Small Business Administration of employer business starts from 1989 to 1992, found that "66 percent of businesses remained open at least 2 years, 49.6 percent at least 4 years, and 39.5 percent at least 6 years. Not all closures were failures, as 57 percent of owners said their firms were successful at closure."(1) Businesses commonly close because of the owner's desire for less work, poor realized profit, family illness, difficulty finding qualified employees, zoning and local disputes, spouse transfers, or a better opportunity comes along.

In 1999, the latest year of reported figures, there were 9.1 million women-owned businesses in the U.S., which represented 38 percent of all businesses.(7) They employed 27.5 million people (a four-fold increase since 1987), and generated over $3.6 trillion in annual sales—a 436 percent increase over 1987.(7) Women started their own businesses at twice the rate of men. (8)

In a survey of influential Americans completed for Ernst & Young, results showed 78 percent believed entrepreneurship would be the defining trend of the 21st century.(9) People who completed the survey felt the major factors that would contribute to this rise in entrepreneurship were: (9)

- 76 percent new technology (helps small businesses compete)
- 53 percent economic conditions (low inflation)
- 45 percent social conditions (two-incomes, return to family)
- 33 percent global economy

Even before the terrorist activities, more people wanted to stay closer to home and better control their work environments and quality of life.

4

Thomas Petzinger, a Wall Street Journal columnist and author of The New Pioneers, believes, "Everyone will have to be an entrepreneur in the future."(10) This statement comes from the awareness that jobs have changed drastically in the past two decades and entrepreneurship is more mainstream. "Entrepreneurship was really an immigrant activity for many generations."(10) Business life helped immigrants learn English and slowly assimilate into society. Petzinger sees all ages becoming entrepreneurs, and bringing new ideas on social goodwill, creative solutions, and more holistic views on merging their home and business lives. (6)

In his classic book, *Innovation and Entrepreneurship* (11), Peter Drucker, veteran business consultant and management philosopher, says "the entrepreneurial spirit is based on the premise that change is normal, healthy, and desirable, that it sees the major task in society, and especially in the economy, as doing something different rather than doing better what is already being done." Entrepreneurship is a way of thinking where you see the possibilities of an idea before you dwell on its limitations.

Rosabeth Moss Kanter, former editor of the Harvard Business Review and author of *Change Masters,* a book based on her study of fifty corporations, concluded that those companies on a downward slope were there because of "the quiet suffocation of the entrepreneurial spirit."(12) There is a close relationship between entrepreneurship and innovation in meeting new customers' needs, increasing job satisfaction, devising new work methods, and improving quality. (13) New ideas are essential.

In *The Atlantic Monthly*, authors Stephen Pollan and Mark Levine, made observations about small business: (14)

- Small businesses have been so successful that large, hungry corporations have been moving into areas traditionally left to entrepreneurs, like childcare. As big businesses move, entrepreneurs are moving into areas that once were thought beyond their scope, like manufacturing for global markets.
- Creativity and innovation remain the province of the entrepreneur. More than half the major inventions since World War II have come from small business people.
- Technology—in particular computerization and information processing—is lowering the start-up costs associated with small business and helping them seize chances.
- Government at all levels realizes that small businesses are the primary creators of jobs, and is offering incentives encouraging entrepreneurs into their communities.
- The current tax situation makes it clear to Americans that owning one's own business is one of the few opportunities people have to create wealth.

CHANGES IN THE EMPLOYMENT ENVIRONMENT ——

Jobs are changing. Job loyalty is changing. As more companies cut costs, merge, and consolidate, an increasing number of highly educated or experienced people will be let go.(15) Business experts see a trend toward replacing many employees with a staff of subcontractors and consultants who will only be used on an on-call or per-project basis—no fringe benefits and no regular paychecks, but more pay per hour. This will hit the Baby Boomers especially hard, since so many will be vying for the too few good top level positions their years of experience and expertise warrant.

Former President of the American Dietetic Association, Judith Dodd, MS, RD, FADA, agreed when she wrote, "A starting point is recognizing there is no safe place in any health-care-related field. It is difficult to identify a position or a site that remains unaffected by technology, cost containment, takeovers, or mergers."(16)

The average American changes jobs about every four years, due to a better job opportunity, boredom, cutbacks, spouse transfers, or other reasons.(13) Some experts believe we also will change the focus of our careers multiple times. For some, change is unsettling, but others see it as an opportunity to grow, meet new people and try new ideas.

Spencer Johnson, author of *Who Moved My Cheese* (17), stated in an interview, "What's changing is the speed of change; it's accelerating. I think the major challenge will be not only to adapt to change but to enjoy change and view it in such a way that it works to your advantage. The other half of that coin is to keep things in balance, and slow down a bit, and ask ourselves, 'Is this change really necessary?' Knowing when to change and when not to will call for good judgment and those who have it will win in the 21st century."(6)

Working from Home

Four and one half million Americans work in home-based businesses, either full or part time, and another 3.5 million work at home for an employer.(1) Working at home is a growing option, especially for people who consult, write, publish, speak, make client home visits, or use the computer for the bulk of their work. A home office keeps the overhead low, reduces travel time, allows more time with your family, and offers scheduling flexibility. However, unless you are careful, it can overwhelm your personal and family life. Any negative stigma associated with working at home is quickly disappearing.

Global Markets

Global markets will change the competitive environment world-wide. Jobs will be lost to overseas companies if they produce products or services more economically and equal in quality. Products sell well when they are new, innovative and ahead of the market curve. They often own the market until a competitor reproduces them at a much lower cost. To compete, we must continually improve the level of our skills, upgrade the uniqueness of our products, and offer services that are not easily duplicated. Our customer service must be helpful, timely and better than the closest competitor's.

Where Do You Find Nontraditional Jobs?

In the nontraditional job arena communication links are less formal and structured, so self-promotion is a must. People learn about quali-fied practitioners through personal interviews, mutual friends, speaking, writing, networking, and through memberships in organiza-tions and on committees. Most self-employed people will tell you their good jobs come upon referral. In fact, career experts estimate that 70 to 80 percent of employment opportunities actually come from refer-rals.

Consultant and writer, Howard Shenson found the type of marketing strategies used by consultants who make over $110,000 per year are different than those who make less than $55,000 per year. (19) Top earners promoted themselves through:

calling on prospects referred by satisfied clients; lectures to civic, trade or professional audiences; and writing articles, books, and newsletters.

The consultants who earned less marketed themselves primarily through:

cold calling new accounts who had not heard of them before; direct mail brochures and sales letters; and no charge consultations to pre-qualified leads.

These last methods are time-consuming and expensive, but not as effective. By looking at the top-earner list, you can see that people seek consultants with established identities, ones who are accepted and promoted by others. So, it boils down to getting to know people, becoming known for your knowledge and talents, investing in your future while bringing home enough income to live on.

Many new graduates see nutrition's potential in the market-place and want to try something different. They eagerly watch and listen to the role models who are blazing new trails, or they see markets and trails that no one has tapped. This wonderful enthusiasm must be tempered with reality—their business skills may be limited, networking contacts take time to establish, and start-up funds have to be available. Will waiting five to ten years guarantee success? Of course not, it depends what they do while they wait. While employed, they should try new ideas, save money, and meet people.

As many dietitians reach the top of their professional career ladders, they look for new ways to grow. They want to be successful, recognized and well paid for their expertise. Jean Yancey, a former small business consultant from Denver called this their "X-Point," or crossroads, where they arrive at a decisive point where they feel they must do something different. These successful practitioners feel like so many things they used to do need to be left behind (been there, done that). It almost feels like starting over again to pursue new career avenues, but this time on a much higher level of expertise.

For some, the answer is entrepreneurship. This is the chance to be their own boss, schedule their own time, and create new services or products to make a personal profit. It streamlines decision-making, making it more effective. Entrepreneurship stimulates productivity and relieves boredom. It capitalizes on the personal and professional relationships the person has nurtured over the years.

THE FUTURE

Presently, the marketing window of opportunity for nutrition is wide open. Nutrition has never been a "hotter" topic, and it will remain so for some years to come. However, as with all great ideas and trends, it too will fade as our very large target markets become saturated with nutrition information and products. Markets will become segmented and there will be other health professionals ready and willing to answer the needs of those new markets with skills and information dietitians have not yet learned or rejected as unnecessary.

Nonetheless, there always will be an ongoing need for good nutritional information as each new generation goes out for sports, has babies, fights obesity, prevents or recovers from illness, and wants to stay healthy as it grows older.

Career avenues for dietitians who distinguish themselves will abound. Competing successfully in the new markets of the future may require experience and education outside the required nutrition curriculum and traditional career settings. Today, dietitians are learning about Integrative Medicine, Functional Nutrition Therapy, medicine, psychotherapeutic counseling skills, media broadcasting, business management, culinary, pharmaceuticals, exercise physiology, law, marketing and sales, product manufacturing, writing and public speaking. As is often said when faced with so much opportunity, only the person's imagination and energy will limit what she or he can do.

In a speech to undergraduates at Cornell University in 1990, Tom Peters gave sage advice that fits this topic well. He said: (20)

1. **Don't think, do.** You only really know if something works after you try it, so don't spend all your time and energy planning. You will never make all of the right decisions before you start something. Things get better as you apply what you learn.
2. **Fail with flair.** Quoting novelist Tom Robbins: "If you've any sense at all, you must have learned by now that we pay just as dearly for our triumphs as we do for our defeats. Go ahead and fail with wit, fail with grace, fail with style." Sadly, all too many newly minted college grads, and forty-year olds, fear failure—that in the end is to fear living itself.
3. **Listen naively.** Don't just listen, but also "hear." Hearing is about empathy and taking the time to respect others. If you are not empathetic (by this point), I don't know what to tell you—except, don't be the boss.
4. **Ask dumb questions.** You couldn't possibly know all the answers, so ask and improve your ability to solve problems.
5. **Get others involved.** It takes time to listen, hear, trust, and gain commitment but it is time well spent. Others come to us with motivation and then we go about destroying it with demeaning attitudes and humiliating rules instead of enthusiasm for new ideas.
6. **Go where the action is.** The best, most successful chiefs and generals spend their most time at the firing line, and the least in the office.
7. **Make it fun.** All human endeavor is about emotion—zest, joy, pride, fun, and even crying are near the heart of any successful enterprise.
8. **Be interesting!** Life's too short to waste time suppressing emotions, trying to be like the others, fearing rebuffs or being fired. You will never please everyone.

So go nurture some very interesting failures and even better successes!

References

1. Office of Advocacy, U. S. Small Business Administration. *Frequently Asked Questions;* on-line at www.sba.gov: 2002.
2. U.S. Dept of Commerce, Bureau of the Census; 2000.
3. Small Business Vital Statistics. *National Business News;* May/June 1999.
4. Dun and Bradstreet Report on Entrepreneurs. In: Williams G. 2001: An Entrepreneurial Odyssey. *Entrepreneur;* April 1999.
5. National Association of Self-Employed Survey. *NASE*; 2000.
6. Williams G. 2001: An Entrepreneurial Odyssey. *Entrepreneur;* April 1999.
7. Living It Up. *National Business News;* July/August 1999.
8. Special Report: A Quick Guide for Women & Minority Entrepreneurs. *Entrepreneur;* January 1998.
9. Roper Starch Worldwide Survey of Influential Americans for Ernst & Young. In: Williams G. 2001: An Entrepreneurial Odyssey. *Entrepreneur;* April 1999.
10. Petzinger T. *The New Pioneers.* New York: Simon & Schuster; 1999.
11. Drucker P. *Innovations and Entrepreneurship.* New York: Harper & Row; 1985.
12. Kanter R. *Change Masters: Innovation for Productivity in the American Corporation.* New York: Simon & Schuster; 1985.
13. Bolles RN. *What Color is Your Parachute?* Berkeley, CA: Ten Speed Press; 2001.
14. Pollan S, Levine M. Playing to Win. *The Atlantic Monthly;* Fall 1988.
15. Kunde D. Striking Out on Their Own. *The Dallas Morning News;* Feb. 19, 1991.
16. Dodd J. Look before you leap—but do leap! *JADA:* vol. 99:4: page 422.
17. Johnson S. Who Moved My Cheese. New York: Putnam; 1999.
18. 1999 Membership Survey, The American Dietetic Association. *JADA:* 01:1.
19. Shenson H. Surefire Strategies for Making it as a Consultant. *Home Office Computing;* April 1991.
20. Peters T. Some Advice: Do. Fail. Laugh. Weep. And be Interesting. *Dallas Business Journal;* February 12, 1990.

Chapter 2

Is Self-Employment For You?

Self-employment is not a decision that should be taken lightly. It's a calculated risk that requires forethought and continuous critical thinking to evaluate the options and pitfalls as a project grows. Because it's challenging, succeeding as an entrepreneur can be one of the most satisfying accomplishments you will ever have.

What makes some individuals want to do such a thing in the first place? What drives some to do it, while others only talk about it? How do you tell if you're one of them?

There are few universal criteria that are common to all successful entrepreneurs. The personal qualities, experience, luck or financial resources necessary for one entrepreneur's success may be less important for another. Encouraging potential entrepreneurs merely to have years of experience in dietetics without regard to the type and quality of experience is not well founded. Dietitians and dietetic technicians have the basic clinical knowledge and skills upon entry into the profession. It's the other personal qualities and skills that help set people apart from their peers.

Venture capitalist, Arthur Rock, states (1), "Good ideas and good products are a dime a dozen. Good execution and good management—in a word, good people—are rare. A conventional manager isn't risk-oriented enough to succeed with a new venture, while an entrepreneur without managerial savvy is just another promoter. Good managers, on the other hand, can't lose. If their strategy doesn't work, they can develop another one. Great people make great companies, and that's the kind of company I want to be a part of."

WHAT DOES IT TAKE?

A successful entrepreneur has many areas of expertise that should be developed, which include:
- a desire and an ability to network with other people,
- a thorough working knowledge of how a business operates (often learned or observed on a former job),
- a willingness to promote yourself and the business,

- the ability to develop a quality product or service, and
- financial management skills and ability to generate capital to finance the business.

The business' strengths should be based upon the owner's unique personality, knowledge and experience. This means that you must know about yourself. You may not need specialized training beyond the dietetic education and internship.

The character of entrepreneurs is also extremely important. You need:

- high integrity,
- a fierce dedication to achievement,
- perseverance,
- willingness to take risks,
- enthusiasm or passion for what you want to do, and
- an openness to new ideas.

"Successful entrepreneurs know (or learn) how to be tough, how to accept criticism and how to make quick decisions. Personal integrity is crucial for continued growth of the business. The most successful strive for short-term excellence on every project or they do not agree to do it. They must be able to accept responsibility and stick by commitments."(2)

Business skills of successful entrepreneurs include: (1)

- must be honest with themselves—about the status of the business, its costs, personnel needs, etc.;
- know whom to listen to and when to listen, and which questions to ask;
- know when to bring in skills from the outside and what kinds of skills are needed;
- tough-minded with themselves and with their teams.

They can make hard decisions.

As a nutrition counselor, it's important to be people-oriented, empathetic, and be exceptionally good in communicating with others. Advanced counseling skills learned through additional education or training in psychotherapeutic counseling with supervision will be necessary for a long career in counseling.

As media spokespersons, public speakers, and consultants, dietitians must develop verbal communication skills and the powers to reason and organize. As you can see, formal dietetic education is just the beginning.

There is no guarantee that a new business will show an immediate profit. Individuals who start their own businesses can't be prone to discouragement or boredom. A successful entrepreneur is a realist as well as a dreamer—reaching for the stars while maintaining a firm, earthly footing. Financially, entrepreneurs learn where to cut corners to save money and where to spend their limited resources to make the best impression or serve their clients better. Entrepreneurs must learn to be brutal when it comes to cutting "bad" ideas that drain resources, but generate diversion.

Entrepreneurs must learn from others because so many new skills are unfamiliar and because most new ventures are solo projects. Many will set up informal mentor relationships with highly respected authorities who have experience and insight beyond that of the entrepreneur. At other times, they will network in dietetic practice groups and local business groups where they share ideas and problems with other entrepreneurs.

WHY CHOOSE SELF-EMPLOYMENT?

Dietitians on the verge of leaving employee status for that of self-employment find that being an employee no longer gives them what they need. It's as if they have come to the end of a certain passage. They can no longer grow in the present environment. Venturing into the unknown becomes necessary in order to continue personal and career growth.

Other reasons for becoming self-employed are to gain flexibility of time, to be your own boss, or to be home with small children. Some do it to follow patient care in a wellness setting, to create and implement programs, to do a greater variety of work, or to make more income or have greater recognition for their work.

The potential exists to make it in a big way. If entrepreneurs are successful, they can make much more money than they ever could as an employee in a traditional job because they collect both the owner's and employee's shares. However, they also pay for all the overhead and fringe benefits. There is a tremendous swelling of pride in their work and in themselves as they bring to fruition projects they originate. In society as a whole, entrepreneurs receive the approval and respect of many people who realize the enormity of the commitment and effort.

What Price Is Paid?

Many of the benefits granted the employee, for example, regular paychecks, paid sick leave, pension plans, health insurance, regular working hours, and vacation time are no longer givens when you are your own boss. It may dawn like a revelation for the new entrepreneur that if he doesn't work a day, he doesn't get paid. There are no benefits when self-employed, except what you provide for yourself.

In logical and practical terms, the possible risks of being an entrepreneur can include:

- financial and emotional insecurity (at times),
- a large time and effort commitment,
- family stress due to long hours and financial insecurity,
- no paid benefits, and
- a financial investment ($10,000-$40,000 or more initially).

Family needs, emotional support and others' schedules must be considered before becoming an entrepreneur, especially for women with children or a husband without stable work. The stress can be high when children are young, ill or very active in sports or other outside activities that require a parent to be available. Although an entrepreneur's schedule can be more flexible, once appointments and regular office hours are set, you damage your image by frequently changing appointments or closing the office during office hours. When a spouse's work is sporadic or money is tight, the stress can be high for an entrepreneur trying to make the best long-term decisions for the growing business instead of taking only jobs that produce immediate income.

Even formerly supportive spouses can become antagonistic and jealous about the time and effort an entrepreneur invests in the business. Does it help to involve the spouse in business activities? It helps some marriages because they see the work as a labor of love, sharing the workload and reducing the time needed to conduct the business. For others, it is the beginning of the end. Too many hours together may worsen tempers instead of soothe them.

Not for Everyone

As you can tell from what has been shared, entrepreneurship does intimately affect an individual. Also, the point needs to be made that you can't assume since you have good ideas, money, lots of energy, and the right credentials you should start your own business. You might also think about working as an employee in business and industry, or for a spa, caterer, cruise line, large medical clinic, or another nontraditional employment setting. As mentioned, good progressive corporations are starting to recognize the value of hiring more creative individuals who are looking for career alternatives with regular paychecks and fringe benefits.

The negative aspects of starting a business are very real but certainly not insurmountable when a person does careful research and develops well thought-out solutions. The fear of the unknown is often more paralyzing than what really happens.

MYTHS ABOUT ENTREPRENEURSHIP

MYTH: You will get rich quick! (3)

You hear about the "Miracle" franchises that make tons of money overnight or the skate boarding college dropouts who built skateboards and are now millionaires. But those are flukes, according to most entrepreneurs' experience. Most entrepreneurs find that growing a business takes time and patience. There are false starts along the way and growing pains when things catch on.

MYTH: It's all about making money.

Surveys and interviews don't support this conclusion. More entrepreneurs say they're in business for the other reasons that have been mentioned. Satisfaction comes from the thrill of the challenge and the money helps make ends meet and covers the bills. After needs and wants are met, having more money doesn't make everything exponentially better. (Tell this to struggling entrepreneurs and I'm sure they'll say, "I'd like to have that experience!")

MYTH: When you finally make it, it gets easier. (3)

After working day and night to get the business past start-up, there are all new challenges to preoccupy the owner's time and resources. As the business gets larger and more successful, there can be employee problems, increased consumer expectations, new products or services to invent and maintain, increased costs to improve the business image, more equipment to purchase, increased overhead, larger space needs, and tax commitments.

MYTH: Multi-level-marketing opportunities pay well.

Not true. According to the national association for this type of businesses, the average member of a MLM business makes less than $300 per year. It's only the first investors in the top of the pyramid of a MLM business who actually make money.

MYTH: If you build it, they will come.

Too many new entrepreneurs plan for the huge surge of patients or customers when they open their doors or throw a Grand Opening. Many meet with frustration because they never realized how much of their previous success at work was due to customers being there before they walked in the door.(4) Before starting a business, Rebecca Hart, marketing consultant (4), suggests, "I'd say you need at least 250 names in your Rolodex. They don't all have to be potential clients or referral agents, but you at least need a base of people who know you and who you can count on for information." TV book promoter, Matthew Lesko, stated in a seminar for dietitians, "I had a new MBA degree, a fancy office and new furniture, and do you know what? NO ONE CARED! I needed something to sell people wanted to buy." (5)

MAJOR REASONS WHY BUSINESSES FAIL ⸻

1. Not advertising or promoting enough. Many businesses have gone under before adequate money started coming in.(6)
2. The "product" and service are not unique enough, and there is either little demand for what you are selling, or the competition is strong so you decide to compete on price. That strategy often fails.
3. You haven't borrowed or saved enough money to run the business and pay living expenses. Or, you let your overhead get out of hand by having an expensive office, staff, and equipment before you could afford them. (6)
4. Joining forces with the wrong partner(s) has destroyed many business ventures—partnerships usually last less than 18 months.
5. You are not willing to put in the time and effort necessary to nurture the start-up process. "What separates success from failure: You have to be willing to do anything and everything to get the business off the ground." (7)
6. Starting a business is a major lifestyle decision. The business owner and her or his family must be committed to making the business succeed. (7)

RISK TAKING ISN'T RISKY LIKE IT USED TO BE⸻

Risk taking has always involved fear of the unknown. In today's dietetic market, the status quo involves fear of the unknown. Change is happening at an alarming rate. Dietitians must grow just to stay even (8).

Smart people learn how to minimize their risks. In an article, Risky Business, by Bob Winston, he points out the difference between "dumb" and "smart" risks: (9)

Dumb Risks
- When the odds are staggeringly against you.
- You've done little or no research.
- It was an emotional decision without great merit.
- You are about to change your life all at once.
- You'll make a big effort for a small return on investment.

Smart Risks
- You've researched it for months.
- The timing is right.
- You've given it your undivided attention.
- Experts support you.
- It blends well with the rest of your life.
- Your gut instinct tells you to go for it.

FIVE STEPS TO SUCCESS: (8,9)

Careful planning—but don't wait too long before acting. Which venture and when are extremely important concerns. Markets change and trends come and go. Competitors' plans can open new doors for you or destroy your plans. However, for most services, the primary competitor is apathy on the part of the patient or client, not another similar service in your region. (10)

Control the size of the risks. Consider starting slow and building your business as revenues grow. First, contact clients who already know you and like your services instead of going after all new markets. Consider working part-time for consultant positions while waiting for your entrepreneurial venture to grow. Start with services or products that are familiar to you, and try promoting them to new markets instead of inventing something totally new. Offer more than one service or product to each client you contact.

Time your risk. Learn more about the importance of the Product Life Cycle described in Chapter 3. You will be able to time the introduction of new items for more success than when you allow them to "happen" when it is convenient for your schedule.

Build a support system. To get through tough times, surround yourself with people who support you in your risk taking. Look for role models, join groups where successful people meet and get to know one another. No one expects a person who is new to business not to make any mistakes. However, there is no excuse for repeated blunders when there are so many people and resources available to help the new businessperson.

Keep cool under stress. Learn to identify the amount of change and stress you can handle comfortably. Look for signs of having too much stress, such as irritability, hyperactivity, shakiness, excessive smoking, overeating, drinking alcohol, depression and forgetfulness. If these signs appear, consider delegating some of your tasks and unnecessary busy work, take some time to relax and get away from the office.

COMMONALITIES IN PRIVATE PRACTICE

Although there is wide diversity in dietitians' businesses, the majority support themselves, especially initially, with one-to-one counseling, and more experienced practitioners begin with business consulting to established business contacts (2).

In clinical private practices, there is a shift in the type of nutrition information that is used most—from acute medical diets used in the hospitals to "chronic" or preventive nutrition with a disproportionate emphasis on weight control. Most practitioners report that at least seventy percent of their clients have weight loss as a primary or secondary diagnosis. Fat controlled heart diets, diabetic, eating disorders, sports and allergy diets are common.

Practitioners find this business is seasonal with slack times occurring usually over the holidays and in July and August. It's important to remember these times do exist. They are great times to do busy work and plan your own vacations. They should be avoided when planning group classes, mail-outs and grand openings. In the weight control business, there are two times of the year when major marketing efforts are most effective—-early fall and after the New Year.

Private practitioners' relationships with other heath professionals begin to mature to true members of the health care team. The major reason interrelationships are more cooperative is because patients are treated for chronic problems instead of acute, life-threatening ones. As an entrepreneur, more time is given to patient instruction and follow-up than is traditionally available in a hospital setting. As a result, nutrition intervention may produce impressive outcomes. Referring physicians and nurses become very supportive of effective nutrition therapists.

Money takes on new meaning to new business owners. To survive you must generate more income than expenses. It doesn't take long before new business owners learn how to call their "accounts receivable" to ask for a prompt payment, or to establish a policy where payment is due at the time of the visit. In the beginning, the fun, creative work with great future financial potential may have to take a backseat to less exciting projects that make money now and pay the bills.

Practitioners realize the beginning pace of a small business can't be kept forever. The need arises to develop projects that produce "passive" income. This is some product or service that brings in revenue without the consultant's constant input. Examples are selling products out of the office, earning book royalties, selling copyrighted teaching materials or computer programs, inventing a product, or hiring other dietitians to cover some of your client contracts. The business strategy to create passive income is responsible for some of the most financially successful businesses owned by dietitians.

As the business and its owner mature, it's common to narrow the kinds of products and services the business offers. The dead weight—fun but not profitable or profitable but no longer fun projects—are let go. The owner has learned over the years who to trust, and who has to pay up front and sign in triplicate in front of a notary. Entry-level projects that used to be loads of fun and tons of work are usually left to the newcomers. Business maturity leads entrepreneurs into working on decision-making committees, state and national dietetic offices, and Board of Directors of businesses and organizations outside of dietetics.

Q & A: COMMON CONCERNS

Q: I'm afraid I won't keep current without the input of other professionals around me like in the hospital.

A: This can be a problem. However, since your livelihood will depend upon staying up with the market you must develop some solutions. First, see if you can start an informal journal club with other dietitian business owners or at-home moms. Start subscribing to nutrition newsletters and use your computer to access databases or get up-dates online from ADA or other health services. Read the newspaper and business-related magazines regularly. Join dietetic practice groups that relate to your areas of interest. Many of their newsletters offer a wealth of information and so do their meetings. Look for self-study continuing education programs on timely topics that put you ahead of the curve for what your target markets presently know. Finally, contribute ideas for programming to your local and state dietetic program planners.

Q: I've always had difficulty getting organized, any suggestions?

A: This concern is extremely important, and it will take care of itself. You will either learn to do it yourself out of necessity, or you will have to hire someone to do it for you or teach you how, if you want to stay in business. You alone are responsible for the timeliness and quality of your output. There isn't an employer or supervisor to look over your shoulder telling you what to do and when to do it.

If you work out of your home, you will want to maintain "business hours" and avoid watching daytime TV and doing chores instead of business projects during that time. Good time management is essential. Start a notebook and list your daily "Things to do." Be sure to prioritize them—all things are not equally important. Start with the most dreaded task first and get it out of the way. Many people make lists, but end up doing only the fun, easy projects.

Q: I have wanted to start a consulting private practice for years. I have some money from the sale of our house, and I also have some income from two consultant jobs for food companies in the area. I will need a steady income to support us. How do I get started?

A: You have already started your business, since you have two consulting positions. Before you go any further, I suggest you do as my mentor, Jean Yancey, suggested, "Weed out the garden of your life." Sit down and take a good, hard look at your life and see what is draining you emotionally and all other ways. Do you take on too much responsibility at home, church or school and leave too little time for yourself? Do you have too much debt? Are there people who use you or abuse boundaries you set? Those are just a few of the weeds that must be considered and better controlled before starting your own business.

Next, go talk to your two present accounts and tell them about your plans to expand, and ask if there is additional work you could do for them. Ask if they know of other companies that might use your services.

Now, call and meet with as many other business contacts as you can to discuss what services you can offer. Many times from these discussions, new services or ideas will emerge that you never considered before. Join and become active in the ADA referral network and Dietetic Practice Groups. Use their online discussion groups and attend meetings of local industry groups. Volunteer to be on highly visible committees where you will meet potential clients, like charity golf tournaments, gala fundraisers, or solicit sponsorships for large events so you can meet company owners.

Stay visible, become current with the newest controversies and products, agree to speak for groups of potential clients, and begin to research and write articles that establish your credibility in the consulting areas you want to pursue. Good luck!

Evaluating Your Strengths and Weaknesses

It's important you look at your strengths and weaknesses objectively. You need to know what your strengths are because you will want to capitalize on them and base a lot of your business strengths on them. Knowing your weaknesses will show you where you could be vulnerable. You can seek help to supplement or retrain your weaker areas, such as public speaking, writing, marketing, computer work or whatever. The less you are able to do for yourself, the more it will cost to operate a business. The cost of delegating responsibilities and training office staff must be weighed against the value of your time in generating income.

Education

The challenges of entrepreneurship can access every brain cell and frame of reference you have. People often enter small business totally unprepared for the scope of skills that are needed. It's unreasonable to assume a new entrepreneur would know how to do everything. For that reason, entrepreneurs must accept that education will be ongoing both formally in continuing education or schooling and from life or work experience.

A dietetic technician is only limited in the clinical area of nutrition practice, where supervision by a dietitian is necessary. He or she is certainly more qualified than most of the lay counselors who work with the public in weight loss and fitness centers. By working in catering, food development or management or with "normal" nutrition, a dietetic technician can be successfully self-employed.

In a survey of successful private practitioners, Rodney Leonard, writer for Community Nutritionist, found that, "If they had to do their schooling over again, they would choose a curriculum heavily weighted toward building communication skills and acquiring a basic knowledge of business practices. They would take public speaking, journalism, marketing, public relations, bookkeeping or accounting, and economics." (2) In interviews conducted recently, entrepreneurs agreed with this list and added more advanced counseling skills.

Graduate Education or Specialty Certifications should open more varied doors in business and improve an entrepreneur's marketability. Besides nutrition, dietitians are taking advanced degrees or training in law, medicine, culinary, chiropractic, exercise physiology, communications, health promotion, food technology, business management, psychology, Functional Nutrition Therapy, Chinese medicine, and marketing, to name a few. Certification can be in diabetes, renal, pediatric, nutrition support, lactation, weight counseling, Certified Clinical Nutritionist and many others.

Practitioners do not agree on the exact role that an advanced degree will play in an entrepreneur's career. Some feel it is an absolute necessity that provides an edge in today's professional world and competitive markets. Others feel advanced degrees are perhaps only important in clinical settings, academia and government positions. Everyone agrees that a Master's or Ph.D. will not compensate for a lack of ability, skill or personality traits needed to succeed in business.

Reeducation is important when a dietitian hasn't remained current in the areas of nutrition that will be used in practice. Due to the growing nutrition awareness of the public and the sophistication of the competition, new business owners can't afford to be outdated.

When you have not practiced for some time, don't underestimate what you know. However, you should consider taking updated dietetic courses, qualifying for dietetic registration (if you aren't registered), and perhaps working in a teaching or clinical setting for a while to refresh your knowledge and improve your skills.

Experience/Expertise can be gained in a variety of ways—from working in a family-owned business, working as an employee or volunteer, or creating a business of your own. The quality of the experience and the degree of involvement are usually as important as the number of years, but adequate time and exposure are necessary.

Dietetic experience past the internship level is all but mandatory to gain composure, practical clinical knowledge, save money, build a network and to learn those things not taught in school. People presently in practice have recommended two to five years of experience in a variety of positions before starting out on your own.

There are, of course, exceptions to every guideline, and there are dietitians who have started successful businesses directly out of school. But for the majority, the added years can be beneficial in learning new ways of doing things, trying out programs in institutions where resources are more readily available, establishing good credit, and saving seed money for a new venture.

Commitment Limits

You will need to decide the amount of personal commitment you want to have to your business. There are some major questions to ask yourself and decisions that need to be made.

- Will you work at private practice full or part time?
- Will you try to keep your other job?
- Will you have a medical, commercial or home office?
- How much debt can you handle?
- Where can you get funding for the venture?
- If you have a family, how will you juggle your life?

When determining your limits, recognize that having support for your venture from your family and friends can be very helpful on your road to success. Involving other people in your decision-making may help solicit their support for your projects.

LEAVING YOUR OTHER JOB

How you leave your present job or how you handle your job while you start a new business on the side can be very important professionally. Your reputation either will precede or follow you into your new venture, so the past is never really gone. Try to leave as amicably and cordially as you can. After giving notice, use the next few weeks to let people know about your plans and generate goodwill. Hopefully, your present colleagues will become good referral agents if you have chosen to conduct a non-competing business.

If you are starting a business on the side, keep it "on the side." Don't get fired because you used the photocopier to print all of your diets or solicited patients on the floors of the hospital. Also, be aware many employers consider starting a private practice after hours as conflict of interest, and it may jeopardize your job.

Several clinic dietitians have found their employers were less than understanding when they established part-time private practices in the same community and offered services that competed with the employers' outpatient clinic services. That wasn't a smart move. Put yourself in the employer's spot—-wouldn't you make the dietitian decide which job she or he wanted more? Work in a different community or offer excellent, but noncompetitive services, such as group weight loss classes with an exercise specialist or diabetic cooking classes.

Your reputation and goodwill toward you will grow as you become known for your services. Your identity will grow separate from your employer's.

A common question dietitians ask is: "What is mine when I quit?" Generally, the rule of thumb is: Intangibles probably are yours (including the names of your contacts), tangibles (patient records, the Rolodex or palm computer provided by the employer, etc.) probably are not. If you invented or created something on your salaried time, usually it belongs to your employer unless you had another agreement. If you wrote materials that you want to use later in your business, plan to write different ones with newer information.

A former employer can't keep you from practicing your profession—-unless you signed a noncompete contract—-and even then it must be reasonable. An agreement may state that you can't solicit business from your employer's client accounts, or disclose the employer's proprietary information. You should be able to contact physicians on staff at the hospital, but on your day off, not during paid working hours.

One practitioner reported a food service company asked her to sign a contract when she first started. It stated that upon termination, or if she quit, she could not work as a dietitian for anyone for one year within a 100-mile radius of the large metropolitan area where she lived. Don't sign something like that! It's doubtful the agreement would stand up in court, but who wants the expense and bother of a court case? Talk to a good lawyer about some compromise.

SUMMARY

If you are going to succeed as an entrepreneur, you must have a burning desire to develop your idea; you must believe so firmly in the idea that everything else pales in comparison. (1) By now you can tell the commitment to become a full time entrepreneur should not be taken lightly. In the next chapters, you will learn the importance of timing, customer service and marketing to making a venture a success.

REFERENCES

1. Rock A. Strategy vs. Tactics from a Venture Capitalist. In: *Harvard Business Review on Entrepreneurship.* Boston, MA: Harvard Business School Press; 1999.
2. Leonard R. Private Practice. On Our Own. *Community Nutritionist;* 1982.
3. Chun J. To Tell the Truth. *Entrepreneur;* April 1998.
4. McCafferty D. *Are you ready to become self-employed?* CareerBuilder on MSN.com; 2000.
5. Lesko M. Speech in Washington, DC at *How to Make Money in Dietetics;* 1992.
6. Mancuso J. *How to Start, Finance and Manage Your Own Business.* New Jersey: Prentice-Hall; 1990.
7. Ciabattari J. When You Start Your Own Business. *Parade;* August, 21, 1988.
8. Helm KK. Risk taking isn't risky like it used to be. *JADA.* Chicago, IL; 89:4.
9. Weinstein B. Risky Business. *Entrepreneurial Woman;* May/June, 1990.
10. Beckwith H. *Selling the Invisible.* New York: Warner Books; 1997.

── Building a Strong ── Foundation

Words of Wisdom:

"We cannot direct the wind...but we can adjust the sails."

"Do not let what you cannot do interfere with what you can do."

John Wooden

Chapter 3

Business Strategies and Management

It's almost universally believed that customers can tell excellence when they see it; they seek the superior choice when buying as long as the price is low; and they want healthy food and quality programming on TV. However, according to marketing consultant, Harry Beckwith: (1)

- people buy what they hear about most, or what seems most familiar;
- they want to avoid making a bad choice; they seldom seek the superior choice;
- they buy from people with whom they have a relationship;
- they will pay more if the "perceived value" or image is higher than the price; and
- they aren't truthful on surveys—they say what they think surveyors want to hear and what makes them look good.

There is so much advice for new businesses on strategies for success—much of it conflicting—because "the range of options and problems is vast and most decisions are 'up for grabs.' Many new business ventures simultaneously lack coherent strategies, competitive strengths and talented employees."(2) Successful entrepreneurs encourage newcomers to create a focused, timely business strategy, execute it well, exceed customers' expectations, and keep your overhead a modest percentage of your income.

Relationships are the Key

Your marketing, talent, professional knowledge and expertise will get customers to your door, but your service business will not flourish unless you have RELATIONSHIPS with your customers.(1) This helps explain why some well-financed businesses run by highly educated people fail or make only marginal income. Customers don't return and they don't refer their friends and colleagues when your service is an "encounter" (like ordering online or buying from a vending machine) (3), instead of a relationship. As more and more businesses turn to offering services and products online with no human contact, it will be interesting to see how they try to maintain the loyalty factor with encounter services instead of relationships. Using a person's name on a letter heading or recalling their past purchases haven't proven to be very effective and aren't really relationships.

Customer service skills for front line employees and yourself are imperative in today's competitive marketplaces. For a small business with limited resources, establishing relationships is often the difference why patients are referred to you instead of the outpatient department. Additionally, it's why a food company returns to you when they need a media spokesperson, even though there are other dietitians who can speak as well or who are willing to work for less.

There are noteworthy, changing trends in some relationship services that seem to be catching on: one hour eyeglasses, buying stocks online, and Zoots cleaners with 24/7 service and online reports when clothes are ready. (3) The key may be to keep the services fast, effective, efficient, friendly and with minimal hassle.

Lifestyle Entrepreneur or Wheeler-Dealer?

When choosing strategies for your business, an important decision to make is whether you want to be a lifestyle entrepreneur, or you want to build a sustainable business (survives without the founder) that has high income potential and may eventually sell out to the highest bidder. Your goal for the business is important because the businesses are run differently and usually seek different markets. It also may be that entrepreneurs must remain "lifestyle," until they finally create the "wheeler dealer" concept that is lucrative enough to attract outside financing, crack employees and an eventual buyer.

"Lifestyle entrepreneurs are interested in generating enough cash flow to maintain a certain way of life, so they don't need to grow very large. In fact, a business that becomes too big might prevent the founder from enjoying life or remaining personally involved in all aspects of the work."(2) Their problems include: limited ability to attract good employees or financial backing, long hours, and because the owner is so closely associated with the business, selling it is difficult, and burn out or illness can threaten its stability. "With no ways to leverage their skills (except subcontracting or hiring employees), they can eat only what they kill. Factors that make it easy for entrepreneurs to launch such businesses often make it easy for competitors or employees to do what founders do."(2) These entrepreneurs pursue such ventures as one-on-one counseling, consulting to businesses for ongoing smaller projects, speaking, media opportunities, book writing, and being a personal chef or trainer.

Business owners who want to grow a venture to eventually take public, sell for a large amount, or just enjoy on a larger scale, pursue more high-dollar markets like computer programming for institutions, product manufacturing, building a retail business, weight loss for the masses, or creating a consultant firm with employees and numerous client accounts. The entrepreneur's day is spent more on management of employees, overseeing projects, negotiation, product development, financial issues, and less on carrying out the direct service or sale of the product. The most common drawbacks or stresses for these entrepreneurs are missing the day-to-day closeness with customers, employee hassles, large debt and tax issues, and uncertainties or feelings of loss when delegating.

THE BIG IDEA

At one time or another, we all have a "big" idea we know will make us a million dollars if we would just pursue it. Truth is, not many people actually try to pursue their ideas. The patent office reports that out of the 1,400 new patents issued per week, only about five percent are ever manufactured.

In his book, *The Rejects,* Nathan Aaseng explores the difficulties and negative feedback that inventors of well-known, highly successful products or services had to endure in order to make their ideas successful. (4) His examples included: Orville Redenbacher and his high priced but high quality popcorn; Frederick Smith and his idea for overnight delivery (Federal Express), and Clarence Birdseye, who drew upon his adventures in the Arctic to invent a process to freeze vegetables successfully.

The small book is inspirational because it does not highlight the "overnight" success stories. Instead, it looks at the dedication and perseverance required when you believe in your idea and it's not an instant hit. The reader sees that the thrill and satisfaction from an idea is in the intellectual challenge, creativity, camaraderie with the others involved, and the emotional highs along the way. Money is a good reward too, but for most entrepreneurs, it's the thrill of the challenge that makes them happiest.

What is it About an Idea that Makes it Unique?

It could be you and your association with it. It could be how you market it; its message. Usually, it's the fact it was first on the market, or if not first, then it was different and better. There are many ideas that hit when the timing was right; they weren't first, but the public acted like they were first. Miller Lite beer was actually the third or fourth lower calorie beer to hit the market, but when it hit, the timing was right and so was its message, "lighter and less filling," not diet.

CRAFTING STRATEGIES THAT WORK ───────────────────

Most new start-ups have to start with tried and true strategies that have worked for others because of the lack of funding and the need to gain business experience. "A new company based on hustle, like consulting or sales, can provide good income, and a dynamic and competitive market. Capital requirements are low and overhead is often lower. Surprisingly, small endeavors often hold more financial promise than large ones. Often, the founders can keep a larger share of the profits because the company grew on its own profits, instead of borrowed money. However, niche enterprises can also enter the 'land of the living dead,' because their market is too small for the business to thrive, but the entrepreneur has too much invested to walk away."(5) In this case, the venture needs to be redesigned.

> ### HOW IS AN HMO LIKE MCDONALD'S? ─────────
> By Barbara Gutek and Theresa Welsh (3)
>
> Many doctors who used to serve their patients in relationships are forced to see them in encounters:
> - Providers are considered functionally equivalent.
> - Service is standardized based on the rules of an organization.
> - All customers get the same amount of time.
> - Feedback is between the HMO and patient, not physician and patient.
> - The physician is paid the same no matter how many patients he sees.
> - The HMO measures efficiency by counting patients seen.

It's okay not to be the leader in the market—you can be a follower and still find your niche and make a decent living.(6) When you are the leader, competitors seek to dethrone you and continually point out your faults to customers. Leaders often spend more money and time trying to maintain the status of that role. At their own expense, leaders often help create new awareness in the marketplace for a new kind of product or service you can also deliver. Then you come along and capitalize on that awareness in a smaller segment of the market.

For example, the leader may be going for all households over $50K in income and you pitch to teens or to single parent families with a similar product or service.

A 1990 National Federation of Independent Businesses survey of almost 3,000 start-ups found that entrepreneurs who spent a large amount of study, reflection and planning were no more likely to survive for three years in business than people who seized opportunities as they presented themselves without much preplanning.(7) Successful entrepreneurs adopt practical approaches that are quick, inexpensive and timely.

Bhide, a venture capitalist and Harvard visiting professor, gives four helpful guidelines for aspiring founders: (5)

1. Screen out unpromising ideas as early as possible through judgment and reflection, not gathering loads of data.
2. Realistically assess your financial situation, personal preferences and goals—they will gauge your passion for the idea.
3. A niche venture can't justify too much advertising (but it must advertise); it must work within its budget and available distributors and referral agents because it can't support huge investments. In other words, you work smart—use local printers to save on shipping and network with people you know, as well as referred colleagues.
4. Integrate action and analysis. Don't wait for all the answers, and remain flexible and ready to change course.

PRODUCT LIFE CYCLE

The product life cycle concept can be applied to products, services, market trends, and even careers and professions. Just as trends come and go so does market potential. By understanding the graph (see Figure 3.1), an entrepreneurial dietitian can better anticipate the levels of consumer demand and competition, and better estimate the amount of capital needed to enter a market. The more established the competition (mature market), the more it will cost to create an identity for a new service or product.

As illustrated in Stage One of the chart, Infancy, describes the period when a new trend is just emerging, when a new idea is at the cutting edge, as was wellness in the '1970s.' A few people were talking about the idea, but it didn't have mass appeal. The dietitian who wanted to become established as an expert at this stage did so at her or his own expense. However, at this stage it often doesn't take much money to become established. True entrepreneurs love this stage. They thrive on the untapped potential of the emerging trend and creative brainstorming. They often develop close professional ties with people they meet while actively pursuing the trend at this stage. (10)

Stage Two, _Growth,_ begins when the idea becomes popular and demand grows for the best services and products from stage one. Profits rise, and the new idea starts to attract the attention of other possible providers (your competitors). Competitors copy or improve on the best ideas and add lots of marketing dollars. As the market matures, it becomes expensive to enter with a new product. Businesses experiment less at this stage. Marginal services, products, staff, and marketing efforts are let go. The venture is honed to a lean, well-functioning revenue-generating business. (10)

Saturation becomes a problem in the _Mature,_ Stage Three, as too many competitors vie for a piece of the market. Sales are at the highest level since the product or service was introduced but growth begins to decline. As James Rose, RD, stated, "During stage three, the business becomes fairly routine so many entrepreneurs lose interest. A person with good management skills is needed at this stage to keep the product or service consistent in quality and efficiently produced." (11) Marketing is especially competitive at this stage with each competitor trying to attract the same shrinking target markets. If this chart represents your career, it means that what you are doing has reached its peak of popularity and you need to be investing in several new ideas in earlier stages with future revenue potential.

Finally, Stage Four, _Decline,_ arrives. The trend and its attractiveness to its present target markets are declining. There are fewer new buyers because everyone who wanted the product or service has purchased it. Sales drop and the product, service, practitioner, profession, or trend in its original form is no longer competitive. There are three options at this

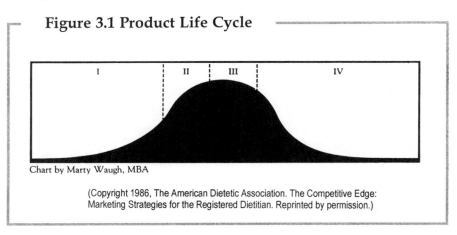

Figure 3.1 Product Life Cycle

Chart by Marty Waugh, MBA

stage. The first is to continue offering the product or service for as long as it is profitable. The second is to reformulate or repackage the concept and reintroduce it as "new and improved." The third option is a mixture. While either of those two options takes place, you can invest a percentage of your resources into a new, cutting-edge concept in stage one or early stage two. Many businesses offer several products or services, each fitting into a different stage of the life cycle.

Although many trends may take years for stage four to evolve, when something dramatic happens like a new breakthrough product or widespread negative publicity, change can happen overnight. For example, when Oprah announced she lost weight on a liquid protein diet, it gave credibility and heaven-made exposure to that industry. Other weight loss programs based on more gradual diets couldn't attract enough participants to hold class for several years. Stage four happened in a matter of weeks. However, as often happens with fads, when news hit of the women suing a diet franchise because of gallbladder problems, liquid diet programs began to fold within weeks.

BOOTSTRAPPER'S 7 SUCCESS SECRETS

by Kimberly Stansell (8)

- Think like an owner on a tight budget—not an employee.
- Avoid ideas that don't have a future—you can't afford them.
- Ignore the "free" or grant money promises on TV—your chances of getting any are very small.
- Mimic others' creative financing solutions—a good idea, enthusiasm and energy can carry you far.
- Conserve cash by exploring free government resources.
- Focus on marketing tactics that require more time than money—complete online member profiles at AOL and other email services, participate in online discussions in your business area, consider co-op advertising and bartering services for media exposure.
- Handle price objections with finesse—give comparative value and remember price isn't a problem until 25 percent of the customers complain.(9)

THE PROCESSES OF MANAGEMENT

Managers decide what is to be done and how it will be accomplished. The majority of self-employed entrepreneurs will work solo, but there will be advisors, printers, repair people, and numerous others to oversee. So, the success of their business is still based on how well they manage.

Entrepreneurs must be self-motivated and have coordination in seven critical areas, as outlined by Tom Gorman: (12)

- **Planning:** determines what is to be done—it can be strategic plans, financial plans, marketing plans and production. The business plan will cover all of these plans and should be in enough detail to steer the business.
- **Goal-Setting:** Goals should be big enough to inspire people and small enough to be achieved. There should be business, financial, marketing, and personal goals. Goals also must have the following three characteristics:

  Specific—goals must be specific, i.e. "breakeven by six months in business."

  Measurable—so you know whether or not you reached it, i.e. "contact three new accounts each week."

  Time-limited—It has a deadline and isn't open-ended, i.e. "completed by June 10, 2004."

- **Decision-maker:** A good manager is a decision-maker. Some people hate being "wrong." Actually, the business will suffer if timely decisions aren't made. Following is a process for making decisions:

  • **Define the problem.** Identify what you must solve. Gather information. Dig deep to find all the facts; talk to people, research trends and market economics, study competitors and so on.

  • **Analyze the information.** You may use the personnel policy manual, legal counsel, mathematical equations, or a computer decision-support system to help with the analysis. This step helps you understand the full ramifications of the issue.

  • **Develop options.** Options give you choices, which you need to arrive at logical, rational, legal, and practical decisions. Choose and use the best option. Now you act because you have all the information you need to make the best choice that anyone could make, given the same knowledge. Don't be paralyzed by dwelling on the need for more analysis.

  • **Monitor the outcome.** You need to know if your decision solved the problem, so you have to monitor and make another decision if the problem remains or it mutates.

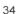

- **Delegation:** Assign tasks and responsibilities to others. This is how managers get work done through employees, and how lone rangers get more work done—by letting temporary help, subcontractors, graphic artists, and others do what they do best, while the owner gets "high level stuff" done. Others may do the work but the manager is still responsible for approving the quality of work and its completion schedule. Everyone should have clear responsibilities, and enough authority to carry them out. Everyone should only have one person to report to.
- **Support:** Employees and others who are assigned delegated work will meet with barriers or problems—some anticipated, some not. The manager can't just walk away and say, "Not my problem, you take care of it." The manager needs to be there initially to help problem-solve, establish guidelines, listen to complaints as they come in, and correct problems. Managers also need to hand out humor, encouragement, pointers, and praise.
- **Communication:** This is one of the most important skills of a manager, and one that often determines success. First, listen to what is being said. Respond in direct, precise, clear language, and then ask the person to tell you, in his own words, what you said. People like to feel needed and important; this means that others need to feel "in the loop," so share important information.
- **Controlling to Plan:** This means controlling all the elements—people, resources, time, money—to follow the plan to reach the goals that were set out in the beginning.

More on Delegation

Because entrepreneurs are so self-reliant and independent, many have trouble delegating to anyone else. They fear loss of control or loss of quality output. This may cause problems like owner burnout, frustration for anyone who has to work or live around the owner, red flags of warning for possible investors, and if the business is ready for expansion it could stifle its growth. This situation is remedied by hiring or subcontracting to very qualified people, which will take the entrepreneur some research time to find. It may take several tries, but if the person is right for the job, it should become apparent.

Strategic Thinking

Strategic thinking was originally a wartime concept, but it has come to mean the "process of reasoning that during the decision-making process is used to find the ideal route to achieving a goal or competitive advantage. People who are good at strategic thinking have developed the capacity to craft unique ideas that are practical and applicable to specific business situations and, most importantly, to bring them to fruition."(14) Robert Jonas, President of Strategy International, Inc., suggests specific tools that may be used to develop this skill: (14)

- Get training to overcome the status quo and learn strategy like in chess or manual building skills.
- Seek environmental stimulation while walking around and seeing new things, to break the monotony of mental stagnation.
- Seek generalists who more often see the whole picture, instead of "experts" who may be locked into their narrow vision of what works.
- Benchmarking has helped businesses learn from others, but not all competitors share their secrets.
- Elaboration in the forms of prototypes, models, tests, what-ifs, and risk analysis must be conducted during the discovery stage.
- Role playing to gain perspective from another's view point.
- Create an environment that accepts and fosters learning from failures.

Strategic Planning

Strategic planning is concerned with identification and actualization of long-term organizational objectives (5 or more years).(15) Short-range forecasts are revised on a quarterly basis, and medium-range plans are reviewed annually. When a venture is first planned, these stages are identified and explored. As new opportunities present themselves, the plans may be informally reviewed or revised more or less frequently.

Small business owners, especially, need to write down their plans for three important reasons: (15)

1. *Continuity and succession planning* (if the owner becomes ill, injured or dies, the mental plans go with him or her if they aren't written down).
2. *Quality of decisions improves* because the owner is forced to assess the pros and cons of ideas, which can help the best ideas come to the top.
3. *Commitment.* The plan acts as a psychological tool or contract to reaffirm the owner's implicit commitment to his or her business.

Business consultants suggest that good managers know when to micromanage a project and when to only set up checkpoints along the way. They know they will never be able to guess all the right answers before a project begins, so they develop action plans based on their best research, and then begin. They make corrective decisions along the way in order to stay on target to their goals. Entrepreneurs take risks, but they are calculated, well researched and closely managed.

DESIGNING SERVICES THAT DELIVER

Even though they are intangible, services can be subjected to the same rigorous analysis as other management operations, according to Lynn Shostack, a senior vice president at Bankers Trust, in an article in the *Harvard Business Review.(16)* She uses a blueprint concept to develop new services, to decide the steps and stages of delivery, to identify problems and potential for other market opportunities.

The development of new services is usually characterized by trial and error. However, there is no way to ensure quality or uniformity without a detailed design.(16) By adapting a work flow design, you can devise a blueprint that is non-subjective and quantifiable, one that will allow you to work out details ahead of time.(16) Simply identify all the steps of a service, adding time and costs, including any preparation time. By illustrating what you do, or plan to do, you can find possible weak points where quality may be compromised. Or, you can use the example to train a subcontractor on the finer points of a service you provide that you want duplicated.

GROWING A PRODUCT-BASED BUSINESS

The profession of dietetics can point to some very successful members when it discusses people with product-based businesses. Merilyn Cummings, MS, RD, invented The Diet to Lose & Win, a card-wallet system to control food intake, using the diabetic exchanges.

Ellyn Luros, RD, is president and founder of Computrition, Inc., a developer of foodservice operations and nutritional care software. In total, they have over fifty different products for the foodservice and nutrition markets. Computrition's products have become known as state-of-the-art in the food service arena. Sales in 2002 are expected to exceed $10 million. Ellyn says, "It takes about thirty-six months for a product to be developed, tested, refined, and packaged for the market. It takes an additional twelve to twenty-seven months for it to breakeven. Our company has over $25 million invested in its product development. But even with the high costs, having products to sell is the only way I know to make a lot of money in dietetics. Service-based businesses soon realize there are only so many hours in the day to sell. After the start-up investment, products can sell and generate revenue without your heavy input of time like with service businesses."

A FEW TERMS TO KNOW
by Mark Hendricks (13)

Balanced scorecard: As the fiasco over WorldCom proved, we expect more from a company than just financial success.

Benchmarking: Assess the best in your field and apply the lessons and strategies to help your business.

Continuous improvement: This can have powerful results—getting a little better over a long period of time.

Core competencies: These are the things you and your business are best at doing; focus on them, especially as a small business.

Customer relationship management: Your relationship to your customers is what it's all about.

Learning organizations: Knowledge is increasingly the most important asset; with so much information coming out in nutrition, keeping up takes effort.

Mass customization: Information and services meet in an effort to give customers what they want.

Mission and vision statements: Although many discount these, they're among the most popular and long-lived management tools around.

Reengineering: The 1990s were the reengineering decade, but U.S. will benefit from improving business processes for years to come.

Total quality management (TQM): Systems era of business management began in 1980 and is almost synonymous with TQM—striving toward constant and ongoing improvement through empowering employees, setting long-term objectives, using the team approach, and to "do it right the first time."

Randye Worth, RD, developed the fruit sweetened cookies you see in your grocery called R.W. Frookies and Animal Frackers. She wanted an all-natural cookie that was good for you. Two and a half years in development, and with her husband's marketing and product experience, they started with four flavors and a concept for a free standing display. She knows that with the competitive grocery market, her products must have mass appeal to be successful.(17)

In an interview, product experts, John Luther and Jim McManus of the Marketing Corporation of America in Westport, Connecticut, gave advice to people with product-based businesses: (18)

1. Don't introduce a new product unless it has proprietary competitive advantages. If it's not unique, don't spend your time and money on it. If there is no barrier to a competitor entering the market with a product that is just as good or better than yours, you'll quickly be competing on price. You could have a marketing success, but you'll have a business failure if you can't sell it at a profit.

2. Be simple and candid in your packaging and in your description to the trade. If you can't be, the product probably isn't very good.

3. Don't bet the ranch. Always hold some assets in reserve.

4. Test market by getting into the business. There is nothing theoretical about it. Just do focus groups in at least two geographic regions to get a reality check that you are on target with colors, flavors, attributes, marketing messages, and so on. The old thinking was that you test marketed a product in a representative city and if they liked it, it would sell nationwide. *That did not prove to be true.*

Two very interesting books on product development are *How to Create Your Own Fad and Make a Million Dollars* by Ken Hakuta (19) and *Toyland: The High-Stakes Game of the Toy Industry* by Sydney Stem and Ted Schoenhaus.(20) Although these two books talk about the toy industry, the manufacturing trials, competition, retail problems, and so on are often similar to those in other markets.

Your library will have many more references for you to read and consider before starting a product in any market. There are several universities in the U.S. that have departments that will analyze your product and its marketing plan for a fee of $200 or so to determine whether they feel it has a chance for success. Products can be extremely successful; and they can be very time consuming and expensive pastimes.

Your ideas for your business may change many times, as you conduct market research and talk to people. The most important point is to remain open-minded, but analytical and thorough in your quest.

BUILDING A MATURE BUSINESS

What do you do differently when your business matures? Your reputation is established, you have a stable relationship with clients, and your days are filled more with income producing projects than get-your-foot-in-the-door freebies. This is the time to establish stability and savor what you have created. Read the books, *Rich Dad Poor Dad* (21) and *The Millionaire Next Door* (22), and see that it's common folks who save the money and invest in assets that end up having financial security and fewer sleepless nights. Spending every cent that comes in is a common practice and tempting, but foolish. Even if it's for the newest technology, if you really don't need it to increase business revenue, don't get it.

The keys to prosperity are:
- Save a percentage of your income that you can afford every month—pay yourself first before you pay the bills (21).
- Invest in assets first (real estate, small apartment building, stocks, bonds, etc.) that grow in value, instead of liabilities that eat your cash flow and depreciate (fancy home, expensive car, the most expensive technology and toys) (21).

- Watch out—don't live on credit cards and leveraged assets, so your income is spent on big interest payments.
- Don't buy new assets or liabilities until you can afford them—learn to delay gratification and live within your means (21,22).

Maturing businesses also can mean a lot more of the same work the entrepreneur has been doing for years. All of a sudden, the physicians are referring, more food companies need menus analyzed, the media want more interviews, and somewhere in there your family wants to see you too. What can you do? Don't quit and walk away! This is what you worked for all these years. Try these ideas:

1. Get rid of the most time-consuming jobs that pay the least—or hire someone to cover them, as long as you still make a decent profit as manager.
2. Say "no" to volunteer or lower paying jobs that don't really need your skills, unless you love them—then do fewer.
3. Do the work and then find interesting activities to do outside of work—with your family and friends or by yourself—this changes the pace, while improving your attitude and you still reap the benefits of your years of labor. Sometimes surges in workload are just temporary and don't warrant any major changes.
4. Cut back on your workload since it's more lucrative now and refocus your career to include activities you have always wanted to do, like speaking, writing, cooking, or mentoring young entrepreneurs.
5. Create a parallel career in something you enjoy that doesn't involve nutrition, like music, art, selling real estate on the side, or managing your apartment complex.

Subcontractor or Employee?

Expansion is not to be taken lightly. It must be well planned, adequately financed, and you must be willing to accept new additional responsibilities, especially management and leadership. Your accountant, lawyer and business advisor(s) need to be consulted before any steps are taken in this direction.

Don't bring on a subcontractor to help you, if only your needs are presently being met. Don't jump prematurely. Many business advisors suggest having enough work for one-and-a-half full time dietitians before a part-time associate is added. The other option is to have a consultant work as needed to cover new projects, client accounts or office patients in order to free your time to pursue new client accounts. First, get more business, then subcontract or hire an employee—in that order.

Dietitians who own businesses that subcontract to or hire other dietitians or any employees report it can be a big challenge. You can't expect that other practitioners will have the same dedication as you do to your business. You must take the time and spend the money to interview, hire and train good people to act as subcontractors or employees. Then you work with your client accounts to accept and trust a substitute for yourself, usually by working together with the new subcontractor or employee at the accounts.

Your job changes from a virtual consultant to overseeing accounts and personnel. Unless there is sufficient profit coming in, you personally may have a resultant short term loss of income when the overhead expenses increase for local travel, added secretarial services, telephone, insurance, printed materials, bookkeeping, legal fees to write agreements, and so on.

If you split the revenue generated by the subcontractor, for example 50-50 or 60-40 percent, after you deduct the added overhead (according to two business owners), you may make less than 10 percent of the money generated by a subcontractor. When you consider your earlier loss of income and time spent managing, that could be breakeven. According to these same practitioners, unless you can bill three times the hourly wage you pay the subcontractor, it's probably better to bring people on as employees. In some industries, like public relations, media work and consulting to business and industry, fees are high enough to easily subcontract.

The IRS is very particular about who can be called contract labor and who is an employee, working under the titles "consultant" or "subcontractor." If you set the person's hours and days of work, offer training on how to do the job, pay by the hour, and the other person only works for you and does not have other clients, she meets the IRS criteria for an employee. When a person is an employee there are federal and state taxes, workman's compensation and unemployment taxes to pay. If the person has worked for you several years as an independent contractor and then the IRS rules the person has always been an employee, there may be back taxes and penalties to pay. Check with your accountant and see Chapter 14 to avoid getting into trouble.

In his book on entrepreneurship, Joseph Mancuso discusses how to choose the team members that work best with an entrepreneur.(23) The best choice is not an energetic, go-getter like the owner. That person may become frustrated and refuse to take orders, or become an in-house competitor instead of an aide. You want to choose a bright, but otherwise committed (family, small children, not a leader, etc.), person who benefits your company through good ideas, loyalty and team spirit. Dietitians have had luck with subcontractors who complement their own personality traits. If the owner loves to market or sell, the subcontractor may enjoy counseling patients in a well-run office.

A contract or letter of agreement should be signed and reviewed by your lawyer. If a subcontractor or employee is placed with a client's account, have the client agree to it in writing, and visit the client every four to six weeks. Replace the person if the client is unhappy instead of losing the account. Keep business as business.

YOU KNOW IT'S TIME TO CLOSE WHEN...

After all you have invested, you know it's time to close the business when: (24)

1. You become emotionally detached from the business and dread going to work.
2. You struggle to pay the bills month after month, taxes go unpaid and you start paying bills with credit cards.
3. There is a marked increase in customer complaints, or established customers are cutting down on business or not coming back—and you have been trying to correct things for some time.
4. You are in strong denial about how bad things are really getting—or have been for some time. You realize you haven't been listening to your banker, accountant or family when they tried to identify what was happening.

INTERVIEW WITH BECKY DORNER, RD
Owner of Becky Dorner & Assoc., Akron, OH

What kind of business do you have?

I have about 20 employees and two sub-contractors; together we cover over 130 accounts, plus temporary staffing for vacations, etc. We consult to skilled nursing facilities, assisted living, retirement villages, acute care facilities and MRDD group homes.

What did you feel when you were no longer satisfied with just growing the business larger?

Obviously, my family is most important to me. However, my business and career are a huge part of my life. I derive a great deal of my self-value and satisfaction from working. In one year, I doubled the business income by working day and night. I made

---

changes in systems, developed new policies and procedures, hired and trained a lot of staff, and increased staff benefits. And with all the hard work and success, I found I was miserable. I was not happy with how I was spending my time—it was no longer fulfilling.

What did you do to restore your enthusiasm?

I spent a lot of time soul searching and worked with a business/career coach. I discovered what I truly love to do—what I am passionate about—and started spending more of my time on that (speaking, writing, marketing, and product development). I delegated what I did not enjoy—it took years to train other people to take over those jobs, but I am much happier now! I use the talents and skills of others to do what they do best. The business is a great success and everyone wins!

Why did you buy your office space?

I bought and renovated a Cape Cod-style house in a commercial area and converted it into offices. I felt it was a good investment. I can potentially earn income down the road when I choose to sell it, rather than just throwing my money away on rent. And best of all, it is very comfortable for my staff.

Some other signs of trouble may be excessive employee turnover (often a sign of a failing business) and excessive price cuts to move inventory or attract business (reduces profits and cash flow causing an even worse downward spiral). These signs can also be a call to action to do something to correct them.

SUMMARY

The keys to a successful business are:
- Work on having a relationship or quality encounter with clients.
- Have good products or services and great customer service.
- Provide good management to keep services consistent and on your budget.
- Keep an open mind and be flexible to make changes when needed.
- Have credibility and shared loyalty with customers.
- Invest hard work and have perseverance.

REFERENCES

1. Beckwith H. *Selling the Invisible.* New York: Warner Books; 1997.
2. Bhide A. The Questions Every Entrepreneur Must Answer. In: *Harvard Business Review on Entrepreneurship.* Boston, MA: Harvard Business School Press; 1999.
3. Gutek B, Welsh T. *The Brave New Service Strategy.* New York: AMA-COM; 2000.
4. Aaseng N. *The Rejects.* Minneapolis, MN: Lerner Publications; 1989.
5. Bhide A. How Entrepreneurs Craft Strategies That Work. In: *Harvard Business Review on Entrepreneurship.* Boston, MA: Harvard Business School Press; 1999.
6. McGarvey R. #1 Why Playing Second Fiddle to an Industry Leader May be Music to Your Ears. *Entrepreneur* magazine; January 2001.
7. 1990 Survey of Business Start-ups. *National Federation of Independent Business;* 1991.
8. Stansell K. Bootstrapper's Success Secrets...7 Golden Rules for Working on a Shoestring Budget. *National Business News;* May/June 1998.
9. Beckwith H. *The Invisible Touch.* New York: Warner Books; 2000.
10. Helm KK. *Becoming an Entrepreneur in Your Own Setting.* Chicago, IL: The American Dietetic Association; 1991.
11. Rose James. *Cooper Memorial Lecture.* Presentation at ADA Annual Meeting; 1987.
12. Gorman T. *The Complete Idiot's Guide to MBA Basics.* New York: Simon & Schuster Macmillan Company; 1998.
13. Henricks M. Management. *Entrepreneur* magazine; January 2001.
14. Strategic Thinking: A Vital Skill Set for 21st Century Survival. *National Business News;* May/June 1999.
15. Sobel M. *The 12-Hour MBA Program.* New Jersey: Prentice Hall; 1993.
16. Shostack GL. Designing services that deliver. *Harvard Business Review;* January-February, 1984.
17. Dietitian and Product Development. *Courier.* Chicago, IL: The American Dietetic Assoc.; 1990.
18. Richman T. *How to Grow a Product-Based Business.* INC.; April 1990.
19. Hakuta K. *How To Create Your Own Fad and Make a Million Dollars.* New York: Avon Books; 1990.
20. Stem S, Schoenhaus T. *Toyland: The High-Stakes Game of the Toy Industry.* Contemporary Books; 1990.
21. Kiyosaki R. *Rich Dad Poor Dad.* New York: Warner Books; 1998.
22. Stanley TJ, Danko WD. *The Millionaire Next Door.* New York: Pocket Books; 1996.
23. Mancuso J. *How to Start, Finance and Manage Your Own Small Business.* New Jersey: Prentice Hall; 1978.
24. Wuorio J. Know when it's time to close up shop. *Home Office.* Downloaded on July 15, 2002 from MSN.

Chapter 4

Building Your Credibility

Not being taken seriously is a common complaint of new entrepreneurs. It's a problem if you work out of your home, or you look or sound very young. Institutions still discriminate against self-employed people. Banks, for example, categorically used to refuse credit card merchant accounts to home-based businesses, and some temporary employment agencies won't send personnel to a home office. (1) These problems are improving but for individuals who look young or inexperienced, they are very real. The longer a person stays in business and gains more credibility, the more these barriers diminish.

THREE SOURCES OF POWER

In his book, *Games People Play,* Dr. Eric Berne describes the three sources of power he feels lead to credibility: (2)

Position power is authority and respect you command because of the position you hold within an established organization. Ways to capitalize on position power are:

1. Refer to yourself as "President, Owner, Senior Partner, or something similar;"
2. Highlight former positions like "Former director of..." or "Former consultant to...;"
3. Take a part-time teaching position that will show authority "Instructor at...;"

Become active in trade and professional organizations where you work to be elected to positions of authority and visibility; and try to land a position on the media or as a columnist in a newspaper or magazine.

Cultural power arises from the values of the culture within which you work. The academic degrees you hold, the schools you attended, the people you know, the clients you've served, the way you dress—each field and each community has its own set of expected credentials.

Look the part. Successful people look and act a certain way. How you look and act are your affair but if you want the approval of others in power, it helps to look successful.

Become involved in business and business organizations so you know the unwritten way to do things. It will give you more power, more clout and probably save you money.

Personal power is the authority you command by the force of your own personality and the results you produce. The other powers may get you in the door, but only if you produce results will your credibility grow.

CREDIBILITY IS THE GOAL (3)
(Adapted and used with permission)

Credibility is a perception others can have about you. It means they believe and trust you. Having credibility with others gives you freedom to act because others trust you will do it well.

Studies of the most important qualities in scientists, managers, business and religious leaders, and salespeople always put credibility at or near the top. Most health care providers believe credibility is essential to their effectiveness.

Strong credibility can sustain a professional relationship even in severe adversity. Credibility is the basis of all lasting and fruitful human relationships. It forms the basis for open communication, teamwork and mutual respect.

Strong credibility is difficult to build, but once established, it's very resistant to erosion. However, once destroyed, credibility possibly will never be reestablished. It's curious how so many politicians have been re-elected after they have been convicted of crimes. Of course, some have been re-elected after they died!

Components of Credibility (3)

Four terms act as building blocks in helping develop credibility. Those terms are: honesty, responsiveness, consistency or reliability, and forethought. Since having credibility is so important to a career, these four terms will be described in more detail.

Honesty
The primary building block of credibility is honesty or truthfulness. People must feel you are being honest with them. Credibility will never be built if others think or even suspect you are lying. Credibility can be tarnished whether or not you knowingly tell an untruth.

Honesty generates confidence. If people think you are telling the truth, they will tend to have confidence in what you say. If people (patients, clients, peers, employers etc.) have confidence in what you say, they do not need further verification beyond your word.

Confidence means people do not second-guess you. You say it and the matter is put to rest. There is not endless debate about what you "really meant." Where confidence does not exist, your statement is the beginning of the matter not the end of it.

The perception of honesty means people believe you. Communication is clean, clear and efficient. Messages are taken at face value, not analyzed and reprocessed. People listen for your content rather than your motive.

Responsiveness

Responsiveness occurs when others believe you will come through for them. They feel you have access to the resources needed and you have the intelligence, energy and ability to make something happen.

Promises must be kept. Responsiveness is built on honesty, but it goes beyond honesty. When your weight loss proposal arrives at your client's office on Tuesday as promised, or when you call back your clients in a timely manner, your credibility is established. When you have to state honestly that the proposal was mailed on time and you don't know what delayed it, credibility tends to deteriorate.

The perception of unresponsiveness, sometimes seen as irresponsibility, is deadly to credibility. Others often perceive you as being half-hearted or only giving "lip service."

On the positive side, responsiveness generates loyalty. If others think you will "come through" for them, they will do so for you. Responsiveness is actually a form of loyalty, the best form. If people perceive you have that kind of loyalty, they will return it. This is not a loyalty born of obligation. This is a reasoned loyalty, earned loyalty, loyalty rooted in legitimate self-interest. If credibility is strong this loyalty will endure. Others will stay with you in a crisis; in other words, you have a right to ask for their loyalty when times become rough for you.

A dietitian who offers extra time or energy to a consultant account or client shows responsiveness and, of course, expects loyalty in return. If loyalty is not forthcoming, the client's credibility may be lost, and the dietitian may not choose to be responsive in the future.

Following is a good example of how responsiveness works in brief encounters: if a patient requests an appointment for a diet consultation at 7:00 am (before normal working hours), but then the patient fails to show up, it is doubtful the dietitian will agree to reschedule at the patient's convenience again. Loyalty was not returned and therefore, the patient's credibility was compromised.

Consistency or Reliability

When you are consistent and reliable, others believe they can depend on you. They believe you will not give your support one day and retract it the next day. You do not change your personality or behave erratically as far as other people are concerned.

Your credibility will suffer if you constantly change career courses or begin a new job before adequately finishing the last. It will suffer if you switch loyalties too often. Someone given a task should not have to be concerned whether you will change course and leave him or her with many hours of wasted energy.

Sometimes reliable simply means that you are available and present. Reliability adds depth to responsiveness over time. There is a quality of constancy about your working relationship. Others have access to you; they can find you. You will not scare them off with mood changes or messages that you are too busy for them.

Credibility not only means that others believe what you say. They also believe what you say today, you will say tomorrow. This quality is really stability, a decision-making process that reaches conclusions sound enough that frequent changes of mind do not happen.

Forethought

Forethought means what you say makes sense to other people. The things you say seem to be based on sound suppositions, on researched information, and logic. You show a command of the topic or situation. You seem to understand the way things really are. This aspect of credibility is often overlooked, yet its absence erodes credibility. It appears a person does not use forethought when inappropriate, quick, off-the-cuff remarks are made. Comments also may be poor due to the speaker's lack of expertise, knowledge or intelligence.

Forethought generates respect. Respect is really a sense of security. Others feel secure you know what you are doing.

Respect also means other people feel you understand enough about a situation to make intelligent statements on it. Dietitians who do not know enough about sports nutrition and the requirements of training or competition lose credibility with athletes by making statements that seem irrelevant and uninformed.

Being knowledgeable is essential to building credibility. Using your knowledge to say things that make good sense is a critical part of the perception of credibility.

(Adapted and used with permission)

Since having credibility engenders many deep emotions, it is often confused with other feelings that people have for one another.

Credibility Is Not Rapport

Many people confuse credibility with being personable, well liked or sociable. It's possible to have excellent rapport with someone and yet fail to have any credibility with him or her at all.

Credibility never covers all areas, issues and topics. You may have credibility as a clinical renal dietitian, but totally lack credibility as a wellness dietitian. If you have no wish to establish your credibility as a wellness dietitian, there is no problem.

The credibility issue arises only in those areas in which you want to build or maintain credibility. If you want to be credible as a renal dietitian, and you are not, you have a problem. Others may think you are a wonderful person, but you may still lack credibility as a renal dietitian. The rapport is no substitute.

In addition, the credibility issue arises only with those persons with whom you want to establish credibility. You may want credibility with your clients as a culinary expert, but have no wish to establish your credibility as a dietitian with your preacher. You may want to establish credibility with your preacher as a choir leader.

So, you may have rapport with someone at all times, but you can't possibly have credibility with someone in all areas, or with all people in any one area.

While rapport is useful and positive in a relationship, it's not essential to credibility. You can have very strong credibility with someone who would not spend one more minute than necessary with you.

Confusing credibility with rapport can cause anxiety and hurt feelings. For example, as a consultant, you may fail to sell yourself to a potential client who is also your friend. The client may not believe your argument that you are best qualified for the job.

Credibility Is Not Authority

Managers often confuse their organizational power or authority with credibility. He is wearing the badge and giving the orders, so he feels he has credibility with his people.

Credibility is built between one person and another. It is intrinsic to the relationship between the two people. If you have credibility with other people, they believe certain things about your character, competence, experience, and knowledge. They learn these things about you as you relate to one another. Your authority is not something they learn; it goes with your position within that organization.

You may be obeyed because you have authority. Others may show you respect because you have authority. But you will never have credibility with them simply because you have authority.

Interestingly, credibility can give you a kind of authority. If you are credible on an issue, you are perceived as "authoritative," having sound knowledge and competence in that area. This quality can cause people to follow you even when you have no formal authority at all. On the other hand, subordinates have been known to abandon ship on a manager with all the authority in the world—the manager lost credibility!

Credibility Is Not Fear

You may have power over other people, either organizational or brute power. Others may do your bidding, but you will not necessarily have a shred of credibility with them. In fact, people who use intimidation frequently damage their credibility when they intimidate.

Credibility Is Not Submissiveness

All three of the above, rapport, authority and intimidation, can bring about submissiveness even if they do not engender credibility. Because you are personable and popular, you may cause some to follow your wishes, perhaps because the person does not perceive himself to be very popular.

If you are submissive, there is an undertone of coercion. You are acting against your will. If you go in someone's direction because of his credibility, there is never coercion, or the feeling of coercion. You go because you believe in him or her.

Credibility Is Not Awe

Finally, someone may be awe struck, enraptured by you and your charisma, but you may fail to have a shred of credibility with him. If you perform some spectacular stunt or feat, you might well engender feeling of awe, but you will have no more credibility than a waterfall. You will have credibility as someone who can engender awe in others.

Credibility is always built over time, as a result of sustained contact between two people. Awe comes in a sudden flash and can leave just as suddenly. Credibility, once built, never leaves suddenly, except through some calamitous event.

Remember: Credibility always has a basis in reason and logic. It is always built over time, and brings about a feeling often different from awe.

PROXY CREDIBILITY (3)

(Adapted and used with permission)

Proxy credibility is any perception that eases or shortens the process of building credibility with you. Examples are reputation, rumor, rapport, and several other personal promotional tools.

Reputation

If you are well-regarded, well-credentialed or have a good record of performance, your reputation is enhanced, creating a favorable climate, building credibility for yourself, your company, your profession.

If someone likes you, enjoys your company, shares common interests, feels comfortable with you, the path to credibility is smoothed.

CONCLUSION

Credibility is essential for a long, sustained career in any field. It makes day-to-day dealings with people more productive and pleasant. Credibility opens doors of opportunity to you and lowers resistance to ideas you want to develop. Credibility is built day by day as you work and interrelate with other people. High achievers place attaining credibility as a top priority.

REFERENCES

1. Edwards P, Edwards S. How to Win Credibility and Respect. *Home Office Computing;* May 1991.
2. Berne E. *Games People Play.* New York: Ballentine Books; 1985.
3. Adapted from a presentation by Orlando Barone, *Credibility.* Used by permission; Copyright 1986.

ANOTHER NON-TRADITIONAL CAREER IN DIETETICS

Carol Meerschaert, RD, LDN

What was the biomedical company you started? What was its business concept?

I was the President of a biotech company, Genesis Biologics, Inc.; it was started to work on AIDS vaccines. Although I am not a research scientist, my RD skills sure came into play. I knew how to search the literature and get up to speed with scientific topics enough to follow the RFP (Request For Proposals) that NIH (National Institutes of Health) issued and let the scientists on staff do their work. We were awarded two SBIR (Small Business Innovative Research) grants that totaled over $200,000. This amount included a salary for me as company president. While we did not cure AIDS and the company had a short run, the experience was one I'll never forget. I really enjoyed discussing business with scientists at CDC, discussing consulting agreements with world renown scientists at Johns Hopkins and running a business beyond dietetics.

My RD training and my experience in running a small business applied: science, logical thinking, negotiating contracts, taxes, payroll and lots of other business skills.

In your observations, why are some dietitians more successful at being an entrepreneur than others?

You have to have courage. This includes courage to fail. Not everyone will love you and we are trained to please. To be an entrepreneur you must be willing to put yourself out there and that is scary. As a clinical RD, I was trained to wait for a doctor to order what must be done before I could do what I knew had to be done. As an entrepreneur, you must see what needs to be done and do it! You need to convince people they need you, your services, your skills and everything you have to offer and then convince them to pay you for it. That takes self-confidence and pride in your knowledge and skills. If you don't think your talk is worth $800 or your counseling is worth $100 per hour, your potential clients won't either.

Carol M. Meerschaert, RD, LDN is Your Favorite Dietitian in Falmouth, Maine. She is currently a corporate consultant, freelance writer and Executive Director of the Massachusetts Dietetic Association.

Chapter 5

Nurturing Your Creativity

Creativity remains the lifeblood of continued growth in a career. Creativity can mean a new invention or insight, or the ability to overcome obstacles by approaching them in novel ways.

Psychologists now believe we are born with creativity but allow it to atrophy, as we grow older. They believe it's our social conditioning that teaches us to squelch curiosity, fear failure and inhibit any new, nontraditional ideas. Eventually, we become so used to conforming that creative thought becomes uncomfortable. Ashley Montague once said that all man wants today is "a womb with a view." (1)

Many businesses are just beginning to recognize the importance of having new, exciting ideas. They are developing innovation committees, creative think-tanks and rewarding new ideas. Some companies have been doing it for years. The 3M Company has allowed its researchers to spend fifteen percent of their time on whatever project interests them, since the 1920s. (2) Corporations are sending their employees to training programs run by "creative consultants." Some business schools now teach creativity along with other basic courses.

As Teresa Amabile, senior associate dean for research at the Harvard Business School, found in her research, "In many companies, new ideas are met not with open minds but with time-consuming layers of evaluation." (3) She found managers in successful, creative organizations rarely offer financial rewards but instead freely and generously recognize creative work, while managers who kill creativity do so by failing to acknowledge innovative efforts or greet them with skepticism. (3)

INTELLIGENCE AND EDUCATION

As nutrition professionals with scientific training, we often discount the importance of creativity. Creative ideas may be seen as non-scientifically based. Could our entrenchment in this way of thinking be why so often we are hired to carry out a layman's nutrition ideas? Why aren't more of us at the forefront of the nutrition trends?

Nobel Laureate, Jonas Salk, inventor of the polio vaccine, once said, "When I became a scientist, I would picture myself as a virus, or a cancer cell, and try to sense what it would be like to be either."(4) He often referred to himself as both a scientist and an artist. Intelligence is by nature creative. Creativity helps develop ways to better use our intellectual capabilities.(4)

By teaching and only using today's generally accepted nutrition ideas and strategies, we are doomed to follow, instead of lead in our field. Trying to make dietitians or dietetic technicians think just the same is a grave mistake. Yet, so often we are hesitant to try new ideas ourselves or to support our peers when they try something new like nutrition in complementary medicine.

Personality

Creativity is not just a matter of intellect; it is a factor of personality. Experts describe a highly creative person as one willing to live with ambiguity. He does not need problems solved immediately and can afford waiting for the right idea. Creative people are often unconventional, curious and highly motivated, but easily bored.(4)

Creative people are often depicted as leading chaotic lives. The truth is that business executives could learn a lot about organization from artists. According to Stephanie Winston, author of The Organized Executive, "Creative people are extremely disciplined in their use of time, control their environment, and are capable of focusing their attention like a laser. They are essentially not distractible, whereas many of my business clients can be distracted by the drop of a pin."(5)

Other people sometimes perceive creative people as being "different" or so ingenious as to be a "threat" to the comfortable status quo on a job. For a self-assured supervisor, these people won't pose a threat but, instead, an opportunity to have wonderful energy and new ideas coming into the system.

Often creative people work best while alone. They can also be productive in a supportive environment where other people with greater skills in management or technical expertise refine and carry out their ideas. By complementing each other's areas of specialty, each person's capability for creativity can blossom. Work output is sometimes brilliant.

"Stuck"

The opposite of creativity is being "stuck," or habitual thinking. When a quick answer will not come for a problem, many people doggedly stick to the same problem-solving processes they have used all their lives. (6)

When people are "stuck," they often jump to conclusions before they have full understanding of the situation. On the other hand, creativity allows a good problem-solver to look on all sides before committing to a solution. (4)

MYTHS ABOUT CREATIVE GENIUS

In an article, "Strokes of Genius," psychologist Perry Buffington, PhD, explores the myths around the idea that very creative people are "different" from the rest of us. He suggests that "genius may be nothing more than certain style of thinking."(6)

Because most people do not feel they are capable of advanced thinking, they often fail to live up to their full potential. However, genius may be the result of using the creative potential of the brain, instead of being born with a "special" brain. (7)

When Albert Einstein's brain was donated to science, it was found that it did have more glial brain cells. It is thought these cells contribute to amalgamation of information from other areas of the brain. In fact, the extra brain development in Einstein may have been the result of his genius ways of working and thinking, rather than the cause of it.(8)

Myths about creative genius need to be explored in order to negate the powerful hold they have on our perceived ability to grow and be creative. Buffington identified the following five myths: (6)

Myth: A Genius Creates Masterpieces or Invents Revolutionary Theories Overnight

This is not true. Much like the average person, a genius develops ideas via incremental critical thinking and a special type of worry. For example, there is no doubt that Ludwig von Beethoven was a genius. Yet, inspection of his sketchbooks with over 5,000 pages of preliminary musical scores makes it clear he worked hard to perfect his work. (6)

Inherent in this myth is the idea that creative ideas all of a sudden appear without any previous thought. According to Buffington, "It appears that efficient problem-solvers 'creatively worry' and carry a problem around with them mentally even while doing other tasks. What appears to be a sudden solution is actually the result of days or weeks of detailed thoughts, incremental changes and critical evaluations, eventually allowing the solution to arrive."(6)

Myth: Geniuses Are Born

Although slightly true, there is evidence to suggest that a genius' abilities are due to practice. Ten years of practice seems to be the amount required.(6,7) A period of time is needed to learn the rules of the trade or field of study. Even a would-be genius must study and learn the necessary building blocks. For instance, a master chess player must develop at least 50,000 patterns with four or five pieces in each pattern. These building blocks are developed over time: ten years and 25,000 to 30,000 hours of actively studying chess. (6)

Motivation and commitment are key variables in the definition of genius. Dr. John Ketteringham, co-author of, *Breakthroughs!,* states originators of great ideas "come from all strata of society, and can be anyone from distinguished research scientists to high school drop-outs."(9)

Myth: An Individual Genius is Consistently Creative Through-out His or Her Life

This is not true. For example, Einstein rejected statistical laws of quantum mechanics as an explanation of how our universe works and as result removed himself from the forefront of new thought in this area. In later years, Einstein himself stated that this inability to see far enough into the future made him and his views a "genuine old museum piece."(8)

Until recently, dietitians have had the image of being slow to accept or apply new ideas in nutrition. This slowness often has made our programs and business ideas "also-rans," instead of on the leading edge of nutrition innovation. It's encouraging to see support for programming on herbs and alternative therapies and enthusiasm for the Nutrition in Complementary Care Dietetic Practice Group among members.

Myth: To be a Genius One Must Create Original Works

Often the creative genius lies in the ability to do a common thing "different or better." It's not necessary to create a "breakthrough" idea to be considered immensely successful in life.

A "breakthrough" is defined as a product or service that proves to be much more than a fad or trend. It can change the way people live, and can create huge new markets where none existed before, like gourmet bottled water or the microwave.(9)

Copying others' work is certainly not suggested, since it shows lack of creative thought and respect of ownership. Learning from another is the way most ideas are developed.

Myth: Genius Is Always Respected and Acknowledged

Not so. The true worth of a person's ideas may be seen after the person's death or fall from popularity. Genius in one set of circumstances may be simple mediocrity in another. In other words, the acknowledgement of creative genius is an interaction between the artistic work or scientific theory and the current needs of the audience.(8)

"The popular myth is that inventors see a need in the marketplace and try to satisfy it. In most cases, we found they were driven by their own intellectual curiosity and personal need to solve a problem."(9)

CREATIVITY TRAINING

The purpose of creativity training is to help people avoid becoming "stuck" or escape from it to find better solutions. For years experts have been trying to find out how people come up with creative ideas.

The moment of creative insight often does not come when a person tries the hardest, but when he least expects it. In most cases, creative people had been grappling with the problem consciously and subconsciously for a long time before their sudden insight. (1)

The major contributors to the development of creative thought are the commitment of adequate time, energy and free flowing thoughts. Old barriers (time, money, resources, etc.) and old ways of doing things should not be allowed to influence the flow of ideas. Reality can be dealt with later, after the full potential of the idea has come forth. Another idea to help stimulate creativity includes associating with other creative people who encourage new ideas to flow. Whenever a person is "stuck," he should alter his pace, change rooms, or go for a walk. Let his subconscious mind work with the problem while he does something else. (4)

TECHNIQUES

Faced with the job of fostering new ideas on a daily basis, business people soon develop their own style. Some common techniques follow:

Brainstorming vs. Creative Thinking

In the 1950s, Alex Osborn developed the notion of brainstorming, initially designed to increase the creativity of American scientists and engineers. The technique allows any idea to be put on the table. Criticism is not allowed; bizarre ideas are welcome; quantity is encouraged; and no critiquing takes place until a full range of ideas are generated. (6)

Recent studies have compared brainstorming groups and critical thinking groups (creative worrying practiced by most geniuses). The result supports the genius way of thinking. Two groups of undergraduates were chosen as participants. Both groups were asked to invent brand names for a deodorant and an automobile. One group was allowed to use the brainstorming technique with no instructions. The other group, critical thinkers, was offered instructions that placed more emphasis on analyzing the ideas as they were produced. The names generated were then rated on a quality scale by another group of students. As was expected, the brainstorming group generated more ideas than the other group. However, upon closer inspection, they did not create as many "great" ideas. In other words, critical evaluation, or creative worrying, increases the quality of ideas. Critical judgment is essential from the moment the idea is conceived, and is what separates average ideas from genius-type ones.(6)

HOW CAN BUSINESS FOSTER CREATIVITY?

There is no set formula for fostering creativity. The company that designs a "creative work place" has no more chance than any other company of engendering a great idea. Ketteringham states, "We found that breakthrough ideas grew in rich soil, poor soil and no soil at all."(9)

Management can help by allowing teamwork and exchange of new ideas to take place; and by not over managing a new idea. New ideas need to be given time and room to develop to the full potential in a supportive atmosphere.

At 3M they use the "lead user" approach, which means they collect information from the early users of new ideas, not from the people who follow the crowd once the idea is a hit. When 3M team members have the beginning of a good idea, they know there are probably lead users in the public who are many stages ahead on the development. Through networking and following leads to authors of articles, speakers, government researchers and amateur inventors, they track down the people who are on the leading edge of a new concept. These experts help the 3M people understand the breakthrough idea they are seeking and save untold amounts of trial and error as well as years of invested time to assess the idea's potential and whether it should be developed. (10)

Sarah and Paul Edwards, authors of *Making It On Your Own,* a book on how to start a business from home, give the following suggestions on "what to do when you don't know what to do:" (11)

1. **Don't worry.** Decide instead that you need to solve the problem and then go after it.
2. **Trust your gut.** One way to make sure you do something right is to do it wrong first, but not for long. However, intuition can often be accurate and a very dependable barometer for how you really feel about something.
3. **Focus on the desired outcome.** If you're caught up in the problem, the solutions aren't readily apparent. Look at it objectively.
4. **Think of several solutions.** Generate as many options as possible before you decide which is best.
5. **Talk with an outsider.** Talk it through with someone and look or listen for new ideas or perspectives. Seek out people you respect who listen well and don't always agree with you. This may be a good time to consider talking to mentors, peer confidants or professional advisors.
6. **Don't just stand there, do something.** Often, lack of action sets you back as much as taking the wrong action. Try out an option in a small way if you can, to see if it works.

Every business venture has problems and every businessperson has times of indecision. The successful businessperson is the one who learns to solve problems, come up with new options, or react to situations that need feedback quickly and efficiently.

REFERENCES

1. Ingber D. Inside The Creative Mind. New York: *Success;* 1985.
2. Hoffer W. Innovators At Work. New York: *Success;* 1985.
3. Amabile T. How to kill creativity. *Harvard Business Review;* September-October 1998.
4. Neimark J. Intelligence vs. Creativity. New York: *Success;* 1985.
5. Feinberg A. Artists of Organization. New York: *Success;* October 1987.
6. Buffington P. Strokes of Genius. Dallas, TX: *Sky;* February 1987.
7. Weisberg RW. *Genius and Other Myths.* New York: W.H. Freeman and Co; 1986.
8. Yulsman T. Einstein Update: The Better Brain. *Science Digest;* July 1985.
9. *For Members Only.* American Express. Interview with John Ketteringham, author of Breakthrough!; 1990.
10. von Hippel E, Thomke S, Sonnack M. Creating Breakthroughs at 3M. *Harvard Business Review;* September-October 1999.
11. Edwards P, Edwards S. *Making It on Your Own.* JP Tarcher; 1990.

Chapter 6

Ethics and Malpractice

The ethical manner in which people conduct their businesses determines to a large extent the loyalty of clients and the support of peers. Clients want to feel they are being honestly served for a fair price. Our peers expect us to conduct ourselves professionally, honestly and within the law. They expect us to give accurate information and not engage in questionable dealings.

Commonly, business or professional people who get into trouble ethically, legally or from malpractice close up shop because business becomes so poor. Occasionally, there is that rare instance where the person benefits from all of the publicity and ends up with a booming business. If the breach is bad enough, a lawsuit, or loss of license or professional membership may occur.

All too often in the past, health professionals were ridiculed or ousted from their professional groups because they tried or believed in something new and different, but completely ethical and legal. For a profession and its members to lead in their areas of expertise, exploration of new ideas is mandatory. When judging the merit or ethical nature of a new idea, peers and organizations must show some tolerance.

WHO JUDGES ETHICS?

Ethics in private practice may be "judged" by our professional and business peers, by government agencies, such as the judicial system, the Internal Revenue Service, the Public Health Department, and by business organizations, such as the Better Business Bureau and the local Chamber of Commerce. As long as no one complains, no one probably will ever be concerned about you or your business. That is one good reason to take complaints seriously and follow them to resolution. However, fear of ethical breaches should not paralyze you or make you compromise on all matters that you feel very strongly are right.

25

Professional Process

If the person is an employee or contractual consultant, an ethical matter could be simply addressed in-house. If the person is in private practice, more than likely it will be the local or state dietetic organization or state licensing board that first questions a professional ethics problem. If the matter is serious enough, the House of Delegates Ethics Committee of the American Dietetic Association will review the case in terms of considering censoring or revocation of membership.

Peers have the obligation to handle an ethical review in a professional manner and not commit slander, libel and character assassination. The accused individual has the basic right to be considered in the right until proven otherwise.

The Individual

Ultimately, of course, it is individual practitioners who must live with their own decisions. We all have varying degrees of restrictions we place on our actions, according to our value systems. We tempt our ethical boundaries every time we don't simply refuse a physician who wants a kickback, or when we give less than our best care because we run short of time, or when we discuss our fees at the local dietetic meeting (could be interpreted as price-fixing).

Honesty in Business

In an article, "Why be honest if honesty doesn't pay?" authors Bhide and Stevenson found in extensive interviews that treachery can pay. (1) There is no compelling economic reason to tell the truth or to keep one's word. In the real world, punishment for the treacherous is neither swift nor sure, even when wrongdoing has been clearly shown. Conscience, rather than calculation, explains why most businesspeople keep their word and deal fairly with one another. It is the absence of predictable financial rewards that makes honesty a moral quality to be cherished. (1)

Because of Enron, WorldCom and other corporate fraud instances, laws are being changed to help protect investors and insure the reliability of a corporation's financial books. But the line has been crossed and it will be hard to have businesses return to valuing honesty and credibility, when the financial reward is so great and the punishment so small.

WHAT THEN IS ETHICAL?

The American Dietetic Association and its credentialing agency, the Commission on Dietetic Registration have written a Code of Ethics for the Profession of Dietetics. A copy can be obtained from the ADA at 800-877-1600. The main components of the standards include the following: (2)

- That members provide professional services with objectivity and sensitivity with respect for the unique needs and values of individuals, and does not discriminate.
- That professional qualifications are presented accurately.
- That sufficient information is provided for patients to make informed decisions.
- That conflicts of interest and the appearance of conflicts are avoided.
- That competency of practice is maintained.
- That the professional does not engage in sexual harassment.
- That confidentiality of information is respected.
- That controversial material is substantiated and interpretation is based on scientific principles.
- That advertising statements and product representation are truthful and do not misrepresent the products nor mislead consumers.
- That a member practices honesty, integrity, and fairness.

Up-to-Date Knowledge

As professional dietitians and dietetic technicians, we are expected to give the best quality of work we are capable of doing. To do that, we have an obligation to remain current and up-to-date in our field of knowledge. Our knowledge is what we have to market. Therefore, every effort should be made to have our knowledge timely, unbiased, well thought out, and of such quality the competition can't compete.

Self-referrals

26

Established private practitioners normally consider it ethical to accept new patients who refer themselves. The professional relationship is between the patient and the practitioner, similar to when a patient goes to see a family guidance or stop smoking counselor—no referral is needed. Why would eating food be controlled by a medical referral? The dietitian is the trained expert in the nutrition field, and nutrition is the area of service. Nutrition practitioners do not make medical diagnoses from symptoms. They make nutrition assessments and provide nutritional care plans. Patients who need medical care are given the names of competent medical professionals or are referred to the local medical society.

Computing Diets

Computing diet limits for all patients is commonplace in private practice. Most private practitioners find that as referring physicians gain confidence in them, diet orders change from specific limits or chemical scores to just the diagnosis. It seems we have all come to realize it is premature to guess a calorie level before a diet history and assessment is made.

Confidentiality of Patient Records

Your patients' records need to be kept confidential. A patient has the right to see his own chart; therefore, care should be taken when comments not related to the patient's nutritional care are made or even repeated by you in the chart. If a patient requests that his records be sent to his physician, clinic or other dietitian, get it in writing and photocopy the materials—keep one copy and send the other. It's recommended you keep the old patient charts for as long as you are in business. If office storage space becomes a problem, box the charts that have not been used for many years, label the box, and store it in the attic.

Referrals to Other Professionals

It is considered good patient care to refer patients to other professionals you feel could help the patients with their problems. This is often done in the cases of anorexia nervosa, when suicidal statements are made, when the patient needs medical care, or when more testing is needed. If the patient has a referring physician, you should try to work through that physician to help the patient.

Referring patients to other professionals does carry some risk with it for you, especially if you only give one or two names. You may be held responsible if patients are very unhappy with the care they receive from the other professional—both of you may be sued. Therefore, give several names of specialists you highly respect, also suggest the patient seek help from the local medical society, the county health department or look in the Yellow Pages.

It is ethical to suggest to patients to seek a second opinion in matters of health and treatment. Care should be taken not to alarm the patient unnecessarily or to condemn their medical care. Consulting nutritionists state that seeing questionable medical care is not an uncommon occurrence.

Questioning Diet Orders

It's ethical, if not mandatory, for a nutritionist to question a diet order that is not clear, reasonable or correct. Part of what the patient and the public expect from a professionally trained nutritionist is that decisions are made in the best interest of the patient.

"Ordering" Laboratory Tests

According to Sue Rodwell Williams, PhD, RD, from California, some private practitioners "order" appropriate laboratory tests for their patients through arrangements made with a local physician. To do this, at least two major criteria must be met. First, the dietitian must be a clinical nutrition specialist and be recognized by the medical community as such; and second, sound protocols must be written jointly by the practitioner and a physician and filed with a nearby reputable clinical laboratory. The protocols should be periodically reviewed and updated by the dietitian and physician. Additionally, there should not be hesitancy by a practitioner to recommend to a physician that certain tests would be appropriate for nutrition assessment. Mutual respect and good working relationships are prerequisites for this kind of trust to take place. (See "Finger-Stick Blood Screening" under the "Malpractice" heading.)

Selling Supplements and Other Products

Considering the competitive nature of health care today, some practitioners increase their income and the convenience to their patients by selling products like recommended cookbooks, herb books, kitchen gadgets, and nutritional or herbal supplements. (3) Many health professionals have been doing this for years with prescriptions, eye glasses, prosthesis, braces, crutches and so on. The products are legal and selling them is ethical and legal—but care must be taken to allow the patient the option of buying the products somewhere else. The fear is that the health professional may unfairly influence the patient to buy a recommended product from the health care provider without comparing prices elsewhere and not having adequate time to determine whether the product is wanted. On the flip side, some products are hard to find and it will save patients time and money to have those products available.

Guidelines for selling products by health professionals have been published for years and can be summarized: (4)

1. Provide patients with enough information they know what they are being asked to buy and what to ask for if they go to another retailer.
2. Disclose that you are making a profit from the sale of the products.
3. Tell patients they are free to buy the products wherever they like, but stress the minimum quality standards or recommended brands.
4. If possible, offer several products with a range of prices.
5. Don't recruit patients in any manner for multi-level marketing programs or buying clubs.

WHAT IS UNETHICAL?

Other than failing to follow the previously mentioned ethical practices, it is also unethical to commit theft, fraud and other illegal acts. Many activities are open to interpretation, while others are very clearly defined by the local and federal government.

Deceptive Advertising

If an advertisement is deceptive, it's unethical, regardless of its intent. (5) Although enforcement may be a problem, the law supports this position.

Bribery or Kickback

Bribery is action on the part of a employee or consultant that permits a third party to gain unfair advantage in dealings with the employer or client account in return for being enriched (e.g. kickbacks). This is both unethical and illegal. (5) Gifts can also be a form of bribery and many companies and government agencies set stringent limits on the value of accepted items (usually under $25). (5)

As it relates to our profession, a "kickback" is a payment resulting from non-contractual favoritism, usually involving restraint of trade. For example, a referring physician or clinic wants to charge a percentage of your fee merely for the referral of a patient, and if you refuse, the referral would be made instead to a competitor. It also can occur when a consultant dietitian awards a contract for a client account to a food service company in return for receiving remuneration "under the table."

The government feels that patients should not have to pay to be referred for proper care (fees would no doubt be raised to cover the cost of kickbacks). Client accounts should be able to have fair, honest contracts without the negotiator making a profit, unless that was part of the hiring agreement.

A point of clarification should be made here concerning office sharing and paying a percentage of your income for it. If office space or services are being exchanged in return for you seeing patients, it isn't considered a kickback to pay for the space.

Conflict of Interest

The rule of thumb centers on concealment and whether all parties are aware the professional is "wearing more than one hat." (5) For example, it is very common for sponsoring organizations to ask their speakers if they work for a food or pharmaceutical company and whether its products will be mentioned in the speech. The concern is whether the audience is getting unbiased information or commercial announcements. Conflict of interest also happens when a contract is awarded to a relative or close friend when the client account is unaware of the relationship. If the client knows the relationship and agrees with the decision, it's not a conflict

Firing Employees

From legal and ethical standpoints, employees don't want to be fired "at the whim" of a supervisor or employer. They want due process where they can state their case and be judged fairly. (5) The employer must justify why the employee is being terminated. It helps to have documentation and show that attempts to work with the employee/employer have been made.

Ignorance of the Law

Ignorance of the law does not constitute a defense or justification from a legal or ethical standpoint. (5)

Informed Consent

Simply put, if someone is potentially going to be at risk for using a product (for example due to side effects to a prescription drug or possible allergic reaction to a herbal supplement), the consumer should know about it ahead of time. The information can be on a label or accompanying pamphlet. If the consumer knowingly buys the product, consent is implied. Failure to obtain informed consent is unethical and may subject the offender to damages under civil law. (5)

Moonlighting

Moonlighting is neither unethical nor illegal. There may be a problem, however, if you work on the side for a competitor or customer of your major client account or employer (may be seen as a conflict of interest).

Price Fixing

Price fixing is conspiracy by "competitors" to set prices and is both unethical and illegal. This exists when professionals discuss in writing or verbally what to charge for services. Or, when you encourage a new practitioner to call around to check the "going prices" of allied health professionals in the local area it's considered price fixing as well. The concern is that the buying public is not getting the best deal because everyone who provides a certain service is influenced to charge a certain fee—instead of allowing competition to prevail. This being said, physicians and clinics have reported that managed care and insurance agencies have been practicing price-fixing for some time. When physicians want to charge a lower or higher price than the area "going rate," they often are penalized and reimbursed at a smaller percentage.

Practicing Medicine

State medical licensing boards and medical societies are very concerned when they feel people are overstepping their professional scopes of practice into practicing medicine. The line is not always clearly defined, but it usually involves making diagnoses from the patient's symptoms and tests (X-rays, CAT scans, blood tests, etc.), and representing oneself as "curing" a patient.

Screening for glucose or cholesterol problems is now so common in grocery stores and wellness health screens that by itself without diagnosing, it's not considered practicing medicine. Laboratory results must be reported as compared to "normal" ranges. When the results are out of the norm, people should be referred back to their physicians.

Several physicians or medical societies have accused private practitioners of practicing medicine. The known instances revolved around allergy testing, passing out a medical diet based upon symptoms, and poor word choice in an advertisement. The problems were resolved but only after much trouble and embarrassment. Care must be taken not to insinuate that diagnoses are being made.

Misrepresentation of Ownership of Ideas

Ideas have value. To protect the ownership of new ideas the government created copyrights, patents and trademarks. Most ideas are evolutions or conglomerations of thoughts from many sources. "New" ideas are often better ways of stating or doing an old concept.

As we progress in business, we evaluate our ideas and keep the ones that work and discard the rest. We also evaluate ideas, programs, materials, speeches, and business techniques that we see around us and adopt what we think will work for our business.

Ethically, the important point to remember is we should respect the legal protection offered by the copyright, patent or trademark. Also, there may be a unique business concept closely associated with a competitor in your market. If you copy the idea, don't be surprised if the person feels you have infringed upon her or his business. Although you haven't broken any laws, you may be generating unnecessary bad will for your business.

Given the opportunity, many people are happy to give a copyright release or negotiate some equitable agreement. All too often it seems the very people who become upset when their own work is used without permission, don't give a second thought about photocopying someone else's chart, teaching materials or book chapter.

Certainly, not all ethical and legal issues have been discussed, just some of the major reasons for concern of private practitioners. For answers to other questions, call the appropriate legal or business advisor or the American Dietetic Association.

MALPRACTICE

Nutritional malpractice occurs when a dietitian fails to meet the accepted standard of care and the action results in harm to the patient. Although there have been cases where dietitians have been sued for malpractice, the possibility of more cases in the future is very real. As dietitians become more visible professionally, as they take the initiative to prescribe diets, as malnutrition is diagnosed in institutions more often, and as more attorneys use "blind pleading" in suits for their clients, where more professionals other than just physicians are implicated, the risk of a suit is more likely. (6)

Life and business are not risk free. However, having a basic understanding of the legal system as it applies to malpractice may help to minimize the risk, and its accompanying expense and embarrassment.

Legal Principles

In their article, "Malpractice Law and the Dietitian," (7) Elizabeth and Daniel Reidy state, "Each person is required by law to exercise a certain standard of care in order to avoid causing injury to the person or property of others. If a person fails to meet that standard and that failure causes harm to another's person or property, then the person is liable for the damage. This is the basic law of negligence. Dietitians—like physicians, lawyers, accountants, and other professionals—must exercise the skill and knowledge normally possessed by members in good standing of their profession."(7)

There is no theoretical minimum harm a patient has to prove. Simply demonstrating that negligence of proper care on the part of the dietitian caused discomfort or delayed the recovery process constitutes the basis for a lawsuit. However, if the patient does not prove the dietitian's care caused some injury to him, there can't be a finding of liability against the dietitian. (7)

Possible Liability Situations

Whenever dietitians practice their profession, whether or not they are paid for it, they are potentially risking liability and must meet the professional standards of practice. Other instances where liability may be tested are in situations where food from a kitchen gives food poisoning, where a nursing home patient dies and/or is diagnosed with malnutrition, and where there are miscalculations on diet instructions, such as protein or potassium on a renal diet. (6) Dietitians violating accepted management principles run the risk of being charged with administrative malpractice.

Protecting Yourself from Malpractice

Along with giving good care, a dietitian should stay current with new advances or practices in the field of nutrition. In a court of law, documentation of proper care and communication about the patient's poor eating habits to the proper channels is extremely important. Records should show the proper information was given to the patient, his progress was adequately followed, or if he did not return or follow it, it should be so stated, and the referring physician was advised of the patient's progress in writing.

Finger-Stick Blood Screening

According to an announcement in the May 1990 ADA Courier, "Members covered by ADA-sponsored liability insurance are protected against malpractice suits when performing finger-stick blood screening, a procedure many dietetic professionals include in their practice as a client service. This simple screening technique can identify possible health problems related to blood sugar and cholesterol. When questionable results are obtained, the client is referred to his or her physician for further laboratory analysis. Diet modifications are made only after the client's condition has been assessed. Malpractice insurance coverage for eligible members is effective, provided the RD practitioner has received training on the finger-stick blood screening techniques."(8)

WHAT IS LIBEL AND HOW IS IT DIFFERENT?

Legally, libel is any statement or representation published without just cause or excuse, or by pictures, effigies or other signs tending to expose another person, corporation, or product to public hatred, contempt or ridicule.(6) Calling someone a "quack" or "incompetent" could cause defamation. However, you should not be discouraged from stating the facts as you know them, backed up with scientific evidence. Such subjects as the danger of a severe low calorie diet regime and the nutritional inadequacy of some foods are important to the public, and it's the responsibility of our profession to warn the public.

Don Reuben, an attorney for Reuben and Proctor in Chicago, Illinois, has stated that in cases where a dietitian makes a public statement about an issue, "A dietitian's key defense against a public person (corporation) or government official who sues for libel is that the suing party must prove the dietitian knew it was libelous at the time of the statement. A dietitian is an expert and professionally trained authority who has the right to express nutrition facts as she sees them under fair comment protection."(6)

Victor Herbert, who is both a physician and a lawyer, has stated, "If a private individual or company sues you for speaking the truth as you see it, without malice, countersue on the grounds of malicious harassment and abuse of process. Ask the court to order the plaintiff to pay your legal fees, as suggested by Federal Judge A. Sofaer in NNFA (National Nutritional Foods Association) vs. Whelan and Stare (78 Civ. 6276 [ADS], U.S. District Court, Southern District of New York) (1980)."(6)

Betty Wedman, RD, who was threatened with a libel suit by a food company for a statement she made, has stated, "From personal experience let me emphasize the need for daily, detailed logs of conversations that could be used in a court of law, if litigation were pursued. Keep records and be widely read; check out your facts with reference books and other professionals, and you need not be intimidated by the food industry, drug manufacturers, physicians, or patients."(6)

Malpractice insurance coverage will usually cover your court costs and up to a maximum amount for a settlement for nutrition-related libel suits. Check with your insurance agent or policy concerning all items covered.

SUMMARY

The dietitian's main concern should always be the welfare of his or her patient. Excessive measures need not be taken to practice differently just out of fear of liability. By offering quality, humanistic care, good management practices, and taking the steps to document their services, practitioners should be able to conduct business with a minimum fear of risk.

REFERENCES

1. Bhide A, Stevenson H. Why be honest if honesty doesn't pay? *Harvard Business Review;* September/October, 1990.
2. Code of Ethics for the Profession of Dietetics 1999. The American Dietetic Association. *J Am Diet Assoc.* 1999:99:109-113.
3. Practice Points. Ethical considerations in dietetic practice. *J Am Diet Assoc.* 2000;100:454.
4. Guidelines for Selling Supplements to Patients. *American Nutraceutical Association;* 1997.
5. Sobel M. *The 12-Hour MBA Program.* Paramus, NJ: Prentice Hall; 1993.
6. Baird P, Jacobs B. Malpractice your Day in Court. *Food Management Magazine;* February 1981.
7. Reidy E, Reidy D. Malpractice Law and the Dietitian. *J Am Diet Assoc;* 1975:10:75.
8. News Notes. *Courier.* The American Dietetic Association; May 1990.
9. King K. *Starting a Private Practice,* Study Kit # 3. The American Dietetic Association; 1982.

ORGANIZATIONS AND RESOURCES

Academy of Ethical Studies
117 W. Harrison Building, 6th floor
Suite I-104
Chicago, IL 60605
800-423-3844

Ethics Resource Center
600 New Hampshire Ave., N.W.
Suite 400
Washington, DC 20037
202-333-3419

Chapter 7

Creating a Good Business Image

Every new business and its owner will eventually develop an image in the mind of the public. The important thing is for the image to be a good one. Having a positive, successful image is what many large corporations, politicians and movie stars spend untold amounts of money to achieve. They know their image will usually decide success—whether their products sell, they get a vote or remain a star.(1)

Consultant nutritionists report that as their professional images grow to look successful, their businesses attract new clientele with a minimum of effort. Good images make patients, physicians and business people want to use their services. Everyone likes to feel their nutritionist (also physician and dentist) is the best, the most sought after, the most qualified and successful.

"Until you've bought from a business and tested it, all you have to go on is image. Image is where many small businesses fall down, however. Started on too tight a budget or operated too casually, a home or small business can look like an amateur effort." (2) Image also extends to packaging, for example if you sell cookbooks out of your office, do you put them in a used grocery bag or a paper bag printed with fruits on the outside? Many wholesalers carry these bags for a reasonable cost.

YOUR OWN STYLE

When creating an image, the first thing that comes to mind is physical appearance. But it's most important who we are, what we stand for, our "message," tactfulness, stability, credibility, and appearance of success.

Successful entrepreneurs have a variety of professional approaches. Some are very conservative in dress and manner, and traditional in instructing patients or consulting to business accounts. Others have flashy appearances and seek out unconventional nutrition information. As long as the person's practice is ethical and meets the clients' needs, it's not necessary for everyone's approach to be the same.

Creativity and uniqueness in the development of a business will help create an image that is distinctive from its competition. One image is only better than another, if the practitioner feels more comfortable with it, or if it's more successful in reaching people and producing more income. It doesn't matter if the practitioner's peers like it.

WHO WE ARE AND WHAT WE STAND FOR

Choose battles carefully. Others' opinions of us are greatly influenced by what we choose to defend, our honesty and how we fight our battles. It's important that we have opinions and that they are well thought out and researched. Do not appear to be a person who lacks loyalty and changes opinions to please whoever is ahead. Defend your arguments with facts and fairly listen to other points of view. Also, be willing to accept a majority vote or new evidence that substantiates another point of view. Become known for your honesty, integrity and fairness.

APPEARANCE AND FIRST IMPRESSIONS

Because of stiff competition and the fast-paced nature of this society, a person seldom has the opportunity to make up for a poor first impression. A well-qualified dietitian may never get the chance to show what she knows because she did not "first get her foot in the door."

Having a good appearance increases the chances that a consultant's creative ideas will be heard. A counselor's effectiveness on the job is also influenced by appearance. Part of whether a patient or his family responds to counseling is dependent upon their first impression of the counselor, and whether credibility and a relationship have been established.

Although it may seem vain and foolish to put too much emphasis on outward appearance, it is equally foolhardy to put too little value on it. A story about an East Coast student illustrates the importance the public places on overall appearance and clothing. A student was dressed in two different ways on two different days and then went to ask people for money in a New York City subway. He used the same words both days, "I've lost my wallet; can I borrow 30 cents to get home?" The first day, the student had a day's growth of beard and was dressed slovenly in old clothes. The second day he was clean-shaven and dressed in a three-piece suit. The difference in the amount of money he collected was astounding—about $19 the first day and over $300 the second day! The public responded to how he took care of himself, his dress, the status or power it implied, and whether the fellow was telling a lie (begging) or not (really lost his wallet).

To show examples of how dress and appearance influence feelings about someone, think how you would feel when:

1. A very close relative of yours is in the hospital and while you are visiting, a young medical person comes into the room. The fellow is wearing a white jacket with a stethoscope around his neck. He is also wearing a colored paisley tie. Do you wonder whether he is really the physician in charge, a student or a nurse? Do you question his seriousness?

2. You are down to the two final candidates to be the head dietitian for a corporate wellness fundraising campaign. You must hire the best one for the job. Both women speak equally well and have similar grooming. One candidate has worn floral shirtwaist dresses to both interviews and the other wore a linen suit the first interview and a black suit at the second interview. Do you feel a tendency to hire the candidate who dresses more like a corporate executive?

A dietitian should strive to be a good example of the nutrition and health professions and "practice what she preaches." That means he or she should have near normal weight, eat well and have a healthy appearance. Carolyn Worthington, a registered dietitian who specializes in recruiting dietitians, states that, "Nothing diminishes a candidate's job prospects more than being very overweight. The overweight dietitian destroys her or his credibility with clients and medical staffs." Just as a cardiologist who smokes or a preacher who swears loses credibility in the eyes of some of his clients, extreme obesity and poor health habits can create a credibility problem for a dietitian.

Other aspects of a good physical image and appearance are posture, direct eye contact while speaking, a firm handshake, and body language that is confident and positive, not filled with nervous movement. Speaking in a clear, bold manner and making sure the statements are well thought out also contribute to good image.

TACTFULNESS AND MANNER

Along with physical appearance, people notice and respond to a professional's tactfulness and manner. The old adage holds true, "He was right, but he lost the argument because of the way he handled it." People in business find they are not only selling a commodity or service, but also themselves to the client, their families and professional peers.

Business people have the task of finding the happy medium between being aggressive and knowing when to be passive and pull back. They must learn when to make a point and when to let another person's point-of-view dictate. Novices tend to experience greater swings and react in one extreme manner or the other. Experience and self-confidence help develop a more self-assured, moderate attitude and approach. This transition is difficult for most. Until the last thirty years, women have never been encouraged to be assertive. Consultant nutritionists have definitely experienced this confusion, coming from meeker hospital roles into trying to distinguish themselves as businesspersons. Time and experience in the field prove to be the best teachers.

The "Rule of 250," developed by a sales trainer, briefly states that every person we meet has a sphere of influence with other people, such as employer, family, neighbors, and so on, that may affect as many as 250 other people. That means a tactless comment or a bad encounter or a very positive experience can have influence on a potentially large number of people. A businessperson's image in the eyes of the public is greatly affected by the small day-to-day dealings and the manner in which they are handled.

Some suggestions that could improve tactfulness with your patients, clients, referring physicians, leasing agents, professional counselors, etc., include:

1. Be very cautious about what is said when you feel you have been attacked. Becoming defensive and "striking back" is not the best response. Instead, try to relax and state something like, "I am sorry you feel that way" or "I don't feel that was necessary to say."

2. Be brief and direct in your word choices and speak in a slow, non-emotional tone. Conduct your business directly with the individuals involved and do not leave long messages with spouses or secretaries. Second-hand messages have a way of being misinterpreted.

3. When people ask, "Are you worth that much money?" consultants can answer by saying, "I certainly am; let me explain what I can do for you."

4. If a physician states that he or she only charges $65 for a visit, why do you charge $85, a good answer is, "That is true, but the difference may be in how long we spend with the patient. I spend one hour with a patient for that fee."

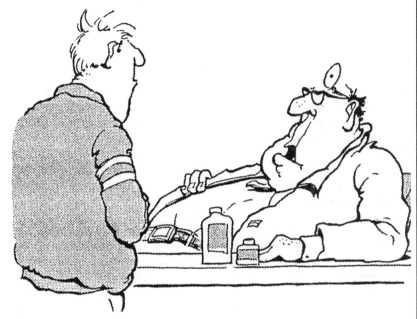

HERMAN

" Are you eating properly and getting plenty of exercise ?"

5. If a patient is not responding to the counseling and probably has no intention of doing so, it's not out of line to suggest that, "We evidently do not respond well to each other, and I feel perhaps another counselor could help you more. Would you like me to refer you to someone else?"

6. If a professional advisor (lawyer, accountant, etc.) has not performed your work well, talk directly with the individual and state, "I am not happy with what I see of your work. Are you interested in my business and, if so, what can you do to take care of this situation?" or "Your work is not the quality I expected and I am disappointed. Some of it is not what we discussed. I would like you to reevaluate the charges on the bill you sent me."

STABILITY AND CREDIBILITY

In his book, *Winning Images,* Robert Shook states, "People need to know that their relationships with you are durable. Everyone realizes that flash-in-the-pan types cannot be counted on, and such an image scares people away."(1)

A service type of business, such as nutrition counseling, is intangible; therefore, its need to look stable and credible is even greater. Most beginning practitioners will not be in a financial position to afford an expensive office in the best location, so other means to look stable and prosperous must be found.

Using high-quality business cards and brochures, as well as handout materials, gives the appearance of professionalism and can engender a sense of trust in others. Offering personalized instruction and development of high-quality programs gives a business and its owner credibility. Completing projects by the deadline and within the projected budget builds a good reputation. Doing something when you say you will sounds simple, but it is a rare individual or company that actually follows this principle.

Keeping appointments and arriving on time are important and appreciated. Clients and patients also expect to come and meet with a consultant nutritionist at or near the appointment time. Physicians who are notoriously late in seeing their patients are finding patients will not accept this discourtesy, as they used to.

Second chances are seldom given today to professionals who don't perform as promised. Many people whose talents border on genius achieve only mediocre results from their careers, because they lack the necessary follow-through and persistence to perform well. In business, less-gifted people continually outperform highly educated and gifted persons because they provide consistently good service. (1)

To enjoy a long and rewarding career, an entrepreneur should provide outstanding work and good, timely information. The clients should feel they receive full value of the services rendered.

SUCCESS BREEDS SUCCESS

People like to deal with successful people because being successful must mean they are good at what they do. When given a choice, people want to deal with the best. To create an image of success, do outstanding work and become successful. The performance and reputation of a professional will attract the public and bring in business referrals as time passes.

When starting a new business, there are some lessons that can be incorporated to reduce the amount of time needed to appear as a winner.

First, appear busy to the clients. Patients question how good a professional is if they can make an appointment at any time on any day they call. It's not misrepresentation to state several available appointment times during the week instead of saying, "Any time you want Tuesday or Wednesday—I'm open." One practitioner found that as she traveled on business and became less available in the office, demand for her services increased because her professional image was becoming more successful.

One practitioner in California, after being in business for three years, had an actual eight-month waiting period for non-emergency patients to get an appointment. Patients must have felt privileged to see such a successful nutritionist. Why else would they have agreed to wait so long? The practitioner now has two associates, and the three of them see several hundred patients per week.

When working in a medical complex or clinic area, it's not suggested that a professional regularly take extended breaks in the public areas. Prospective clients and referring physicians take notice of others who appear not to be busy.

Framed diplomas, degrees or awards displayed on office walls are also a graphic way to show success and accomplishment. Desk sets and trophies have adorned businessmen's offices for years, so there is no reason for plastic food models and free calorie charts to be the only highlights of a nutritionist's office!

The image of success is undoubtedly the most significant reason many people are able to demand such high prices for their work. The artist, for example, who establishes the reputation of being distinctive and expensive, may soon get more for his work than many unknown artists, who have as much or more talent. The secret is in his ability to build a winning image, not in his talent to paint on canvas. (1)

CONCLUSION

When entrepreneurs become successful in business, they usually find that other people who could not be bothered before now seek advice and agree with them on the issues. Referrals of new clients and jobs are received with minimum effort, as compared to that needed to start the business. Fees go up to improve the profit margin. More importantly, job satisfaction increases because more options open in the nutritionist's life.

REFERENCES

1. Shook R. *Winning Images.* New York: Macmillan Publishers; 1977.
2. Edwards P, Edwards S. *Working From Home, 5th edition.* New York: Penguin Putnam; 1999.

Chapter 8

Counseling Expertise

Paulette Lambert, RD updated by Kathy King, RD

EXCITEMENT IN THE COUNSELING AREA

Since the last edition of this book was written, a lot of changes have taken place in the counseling arena. The ADA coined Medical Nutrition Therapy (MNT) to better identify dietitians' services in health care. Reimbursement for MNT services for counseling Medicare patients with diabetes and renal disease passed Congress and is now a reality. In the mid 1990's, several Dietetic Practice Groups created subgroups specializing in improving practitioners' counseling skills: Nutrition Therapists subgroup of the Nutrition Entrepreneurs and Disordered Eating Networking Group within Sports and Cardiovascular Nutritionists (SCAN).(1)

Nutrition Therapists

Counseling in the outpatient setting has continued to evolve into the long term relationship-based psychotherapeutic style of counseling identified in this chapter 18 years ago in the first edition. Counselors in private practice found that what they had been taught about counseling in the medical model of therapy (short term intervention with loads of information for the patient) often didn't change behaviors nor produce the outcomes patients needed to be healthier. Change is difficult and more information won't necessarily make it happen—there are other barriers and variables with which to work. Nutrition counselors needed more therapy options, and more training and supervision by other more qualified counselors.

A definition offered by the Nutrition Therapists' subgroup states, "Nutrition Therapists integrate theories and techniques of counseling psychology into nutrition practice to facilitate changes in clients' beliefs and choices related to food, health and weight. Ideally, they have training and education in counseling, psychology and practice in a multidisciplinary framework."(2)

Our success as nutrition therapists depends on our ability to help clients learn and apply new information and skills. Dietitians who become counselors need to realize their counseling expertise determines the quality of their output. When counselors have problems getting their businesses established, it may be for several reasons. One major reason may be their lack of counseling skill.

Developing high quality counseling skills is a time-consuming, complex task. It often means changing old familiar, but unsuccessful, counseling habits. Do not expect to achieve perfect skills within a few weeks or months. It takes time to practice the new techniques learned through course work, seminars, self-study, and supervision. Every new client walks in the door with an interesting, challenging mix of expectations, preconceived ideas and food preferences. What works for one client won't necessarily apply to another. A counselor must work with many strategies.

The day-to-day job of counseling clients can be extremely stressful and draining. You need the ability to "turn off" your business when you're not working, to better protect yourself from being emotionally drained and burned out.

This chapter and others intend to share some basic insights and ideas for producing successful counseling sessions. Advanced counseling skills are beyond the scope of this book. Please refer to the resources at the back of this chapter for more in-depth information.

Successful practitioners have their own style of patient counseling. The amount of information, number of sessions, and emphasis on wellness, non-diet, behavior modification or psychology is a counselor's decision and varies with each patient.

Nutrition Education, or Psychotherapeutic Counseling?

For too long dietitians used nutrition education as counseling. Experience has shown us handing out lists of foods, calculating diets and explaining the physiology of the disease will not necessarily create compliance or motivate clients to change their behaviors. We know what's best for them, they just need to do it! This approach works when the client makes the effort to read, learn and apply the content. (3) Dietitians couldn't take much credit for change, except for teaching the content. What then is the difference between nutrition education and more advanced counseling skills? (See Table 8.1.)

Advanced counseling skills include: (1)
- relationship building skills: empathy, warmth and genuineness;
- helping skills: attending, helping a client explore, active listening;

- ability to gain collaboration and empower the client;
- sensitivity to multicultural and other client-specific uniqueness;
- ability to sustain a long-term counseling relationship; and
- ability to assess and teach developmental skills.

Goals of Counseling (1)

- Increase clients' self-awareness, decrease denial of problems that affect the person's nutrition or weight, and give encouragement these problems can be resolved.
- Help client become aware of inner strengths in order to function independently and challenge old beliefs.
- Help client feel responsible for his own feelings, thoughts, behaviors, and relationships instead of holding onto the "victim" role.
- Help client take more risks like being more flexible or tolerating more incongruities.
- Help client trust more and give new behaviors and thoughts a chance.
- Help client become more conscious of alternative choices when responding to stress, and not always turn to food.
- Help client achieve self-acceptance.

Table 8.1

Nutrition Education vs. Client-Centered Counseling (4,5)

Content-Based Education	Psychotherapeutic Counseling
1. Short-term	Open-ended (based upon client's needs)
2. Content-based (learning assumed)	Relationship-oriented; counselor is trainer
3. Improve knowledge & skills	Resolution of issues & barriers
4. Work on behaviors	Work on thoughts, feeling & behaviors
5. Address cognitive deficits	Address motivation, denial & resistance
6. Success measured objectively (e.g. knowledge, behavior change)	Success measured subjectively (e.g. happiness, mood shift, relationships)

QUALIFICATIONS OF A COUNSELOR

Not everyone has the personality and patience to be a good counselor. The personal attributes usually associated with a successful counselor include: empathy, optimism, good communication skills, sensitivity, patience, creativity, teaching ability, and enthusiasm.

Clinical judgment is imperative to good nutrition counseling. The American Diabetes Association's position paper on consultation emphasizes a minimum of three years experience in clinical, administration and education. Without this practical experience, it is difficult for a nutrition therapist to be proficient at counseling or to have developed sound clinical judgment. A consultant must be aware of common drugs and their side effects, know how to do simple assessment tests, and be aware of the laboratory chemical values as they relate to health and nutrition.

Relationship-building skills are necessary for effective counseling. Before counselors can develop plans for a client's behavior change, the counselor must understand the client's needs.(3) The development of a "helping relationship" that projects empathy, understanding and trust needs to precede any development of plans and strategies.

The nutrition therapist encourages clients to talk about themselves and their feelings. A client needs to feel safe in reporting failures so adjustments can be made to the care plan.

Being a good nutrition counselor involves possessing interpersonal skills that promote positive outcomes in counseling. A successful counselor is one who genuinely cares about and is committed to patients.

Although a counselor wants to be warm, caring, empathetic, and so on, it is important the counselor remain professional. Exercise caution. There is a point in counseling where becoming very close and familiar with patients may jeopardize your ability to act as a counselor to them.

Several other traits are helpful. A positive attitude keeps the client and you interested in continuing to work together. One needs to be positive and even-tempered to deal with counseling on a day-to-day basis. Being assertive in a caring way and not being afraid of dealing with issues that inhibit progress is important. Nutrition counseling is not passive, but a very active procedure.

Behavioral therapy skills are important to counselors. Along with the ability to dispense information, a practitioner needs to be able to promote behavior changes. Behavioral therapy skills include being able to define a problem, design strategies to treat a problem, and to evaluate and make necessary changes. Behavioral therapy uses various techniques, such as behavior modification, stimulus control, and cognitive restructuring, to assist in helping the client change his behavior.

For example, if your client admits having many failed attempts at weight control, find one eating behavior that is causing the biggest problem and work with the client to come up with a solution. Start with one incremental step. For many clients it may be merely reducing fat intake at dinner or avoiding the morning donut.

An understanding of psychology is important to a counselor. By understanding clients' motivations or barriers to different choices, a good counselor can then facilitate the clients finding ways to satisfy their needs in non-self-defeating or food-oriented ways. An appreciation for psychology also helps in perspective—the counselor is part of the solution, not part of the problem. As an example, if the counselor fails to comprehend a patient's frustration with changing his diet and lectures him, any possibility of helping the client may be lost. The counselor must know about cognitive restructuring—how to help a client confront irrational thoughts and choose new ways of thinking.

Teaching skills help ensure the patient learns the new information. The content must be geared to the client's level of understanding. A patient is often "turned off" by language and nutrition information that is either over his head or too elementary, and thus, unchallenging and uninteresting. Presentations should be organized, since random discussions are hard to recall. A good teacher knows how to help patients reach their goals by using a variety of teaching methods and only the information the patient "needs" to know. As a patient's needs change, a good teacher should be flexible enough to adjust the patient's care plan to handle new problems. If a patient doesn't respond to one type of approach, try another.

The ability to sell is a vital skill often overlooked. Selling is based on meeting the client's needs and convincing him of the importance of nutrition intervention. For example, a client may not realize why the physician wants him to lose weight in order to decrease his blood sugar. The counselor needs to convey benefits to the client.

In nutrition counseling you sell the client, his family, the physicians, and all others involved in the value of counseling. You sell the program and the changes the client needs to make in order to be successful. If you look at the many fad diets that materialize each year, you soon realize the power of the ability to sell.

When counseling is totally dominated by client requests and tangential topics, little psychological or behavior change will take place. A session totally dominated by the counselor, who provides only advice without listening to the client's concerns, can be equally unproductive. The ideal is a mix of client and counselor interaction.

Two very good books on the subject of counseling are *Nutrition Therapy: Advanced Counseling Skills* (1) with 36 contributing authors and Linda Snetselaar's *Nutrition Counseling Skills* (6); please refer to these resources for more in-depth discussion.

Client expectations of what the counselor will be like can greatly influence how receptive he or she is to counseling. If a client expects the counselor to be domineering and antagonistic, or friendly and helpful, the client may treat the counselor as if he were actually playing that role.(6) Through experience, counselors learn to perceive what the client is expecting from them. Qualified counselors then try to correct or validate clients' preconceived beliefs.

Clients also come to nutrition counseling sessions with feelings about themselves that may act as barriers to behavior change. A young, obese woman may say she wants to lose weight, but may be so fearful of attention from men, she keeps her weight stable. A man may come for nutrition instruction for hypertension, but he may want his wife to feel responsible for what he eats. A counselor learns to perceive a client's needs and level of motivation. The client is then motivated to change and take responsibility for his own constructive behavior.

Wellness Approach

A counselor may choose to incorporate emphasis on the "wellness" approach in nutrition consultations. This approach believes that nutrition information should not be separate from other life-style decisions. Counseling sessions could include evaluation and discussion of the client's fitness and exercise program or referral to a fitness specialist.

The counselor may identify a client's inability to handle stress or a dependence on alcohol, drugs or smoking. The client is then encouraged to consider a change in behavior and perhaps a referral to another program or specialist. To be qualified to discuss these other topics, a nutrition counselor must be familiar with health risk factors and their effect on health. A nutrition therapist might take course work or seminars on wellness, health education and exercise physiology.

Non-Diet Approach

The non-diet approach to weight issues is growing in popularity with health professionals, especially with the rise and fall of each new fad diet. This philosophy basically centers on size acceptance, and relearning eating habits and exercise. The past years of "diet" foods and miracle diets have not reduced the overall weight of the population. Emphasis on being super thin and fit has not worked for the majority, so what's left?

The non-diet approach involves learning to eat a variety of healthy foods in modest amounts and moving your body to have fun (e.g. riding bicycles with the kids, taking a tai chi class, meeting the ladies for a dawn tennis match, and so on). And, in addition, loving yourself and feeling good about yourself, no matter your weight.

VARIOUS APPROACHES ALL "SELL"

Experienced nutrition counselors bring a wealth of practical knowledge. Counseling sessions are usually a mixture of what has worked in the past, along with a few ideas the counselor has learned from someone else. Here are examples of different approaches:

Many practitioners do not give a diet plan at the first counseling session. They feel the initial session should be used to establish a relationship, collect data, teach patients how to measure foods for computer analysis, make assessments, and determine habits and needs.

A later session is used for more instruction after the assessments are completed. Another practitioner sees sports patients initially for thirty minutes to instruct the clients on filling out the computer food intake record, then begins counseling at the next session.

Some practitioners offer instruction in "packages." A consultation for diabetes or heart disease is sold in a group of three or more visits to assure understanding and compliance. A weight loss program may be eight to twelve weeks of individual or group sessions.

Other practitioners provide written nutrition instructions at the first visit, of approximately one hour or two hours, and schedule follow-up visits every one to two weeks, while setting no limitations on the duration of therapy.

Practitioners may incorporate a variety of activities in their programs: computer nutrient analysis, menu planning, grocery shopping, skinfold analysis or impedance body analysis, individualized fitness program and workout, and long-term follow-up. Sometimes the nutrition consultant handles all of these functions, and other times it's in association with a fitness specialist.

Practitioners sometimes choose to send their patients lifestyle or food questionnaires in advance, or ask they arrive 30-minutes early so that session time is not spent filling out the forms. Others want to fill out the questionnaire with the patient in order to interpret insinuations and body language.

Other practitioners who work with obesity spend time on psychological issues related to food and lifestyle choices and do not use scales or other measurements at all. They work with the non-diet approach and relearning eating and exercise habits. Effort is made to improve the person's self-esteem and feeling of self worth.

THE SESSIONS

Before beginning with a new patient, a counselor should prepare for the role of diagnostician by reviewing all available data on the patient.(6) If the patient's chart is accessible, it should be reviewed. However, in private practice and outpatient clinics, it is usually necessary to start your own chart and put in chemical scores, intake analysis, anthropometric results, interview sheet, progress notes, etc. as you have them.

The Introduction

The patients' first exposure to you and your office begin to form their opinion of your ability to help them. Trust and respect for the counselor are important motivators to patients. Small, fairly simple actions on your part can help engender good feelings. Try to start counseling sessions on time. Make the office warm and inviting. Greet the patient and his family. Offer a beverage to drink. Begin with exploring small talk about the patient; share some of yourself. Find out about the patient and his needs. It sounds so elementary, but many counselors and medical professionals are so consumed with their counseling or the patients' diseases they forget that it's the person they are working with.(6)

The Interview and Assessment

The session begins with an explanation of the counseling relationship, describing enough so the client knows precisely what will take place.(6) If the client has other expectations, this is the time to have them known. You act as a diagnostician and evaluate the client's nutrition status and relate food intake data to behavioral indicators. (6)

Assessments can be made of many categories of information:
- Biochemical studies
- Anthropometric studies
- Vital and health statistics
- Socioeconomic data
- Additional medical information

A client's behavior must be assessed: (1,6)
- General health practices
- Attitudes, beliefs and information
- Physical activities
- Educational achievements and language skills
- Economic considerations
- Environmental considerations
- Social considerations

Motivation must be assessed since it is essential for compliance. Clients are motivated by their own needs, more than by the counselors' desires.(6) Therefore, in order to assist the somewhat motivated clients, you need to determine their stage of change and what you can do to help the client progress through the stages by determining what is important to them. Clients also become motivated when they see results. To that end it is important for the counselor to initially encourage more intermediate, easily reached goals.

Nutritional care or treatment plan can be developed once assessments are made and problems are identified. In the treatment phase the counselor assumes the role of both expert and mutual problem solver. (3,6) Most novice counselors tend to follow one extreme or the other—expert or empathizer. The counselor who knows everything and makes all of the decisions may overwhelm patients. On the other hand, as mentioned earlier, counselors may become ineffective if they become too friendly or liberal with clients and their diet limitations. Clients often seek assistance in setting limits for themselves. A good balance of the two roles is optimal.

In the treatment phase, problems, behaviors, inconsistencies, and wrong beliefs are matched with possible solutions or rational alternatives. Desired changes or goals are ranked, and the client determines which small achievable goal he will work on first.

When assuming the training role, the nutrition counselor facilitates change, and the client practices new choices and behaviors until they are achieved. At each visit, the client shares the successes, challenges and problems since the last visit. Solutions are discussed that are acceptable to the patient—considering what is known about him now. The patient has time to react, ponder, argue, and provide input. For many reasons, if the counselor determines it's necessary, a patient may be referred to another health professional.

Good counselors attempt to keep instructions as simple as possible. People remember more of the information they hear in the beginning of instruction, so discuss top priority items first. Most patients who come to see nutrition counselors have already decided to give the counselor "a chance" to help. The important determinants are whether the patient and his family understand and respect what the counselor says, and whether the changes are reasonable, given the patient and his lifestyle.

Factors associated with compliance:
- Belief that following a diet is necessary for good health
- Supportive family members
- High level of concern over consequences of noncompliance

- Eagerness to reject the sick role
- Feeling comfortable about ability to cope with the diet

Factors associated with noncompliance:

31

- Living alone
- Lack of symptoms or pain
- Failure to communicate purpose of diet treatment adequately
- Multiple restrictions
- Poverty or unemployment
- Depression

When teaching nutrition information, a counselor produces her best results when she uses a variety of tools and methods. We remember 10 percent of what we read, 20 percent of what we hear, 30 percent of what we see, 50 percent of what we see and hear, and 80 percent of what we ourselves say. To increase compliance, combine visual aids, verbal instructions, written instructions, and learner feedback.

To improve adherence and understanding, it is important the patient receive only the instruction materials and handouts that apply to his lifestyle changes or eating pattern—not every free booklet on low fat foods or diabetes. If the patient or his family expresses an interest for more recipes or other material, additional materials can be offered.

To conclude a session, it's suggested the client summarize the agreed upon goal for the next visit and most important points to remember from that day's session. Except in very rare cases, patients need follow-up visits in order to make permanent changes in their behavior. Clients like to know they can contact you in between visits by phone or email.

Evaluation/Follow-Up

The counselor uses the follow-up sessions as a time to reinforce the positive behaviors and provide immediate feedback on any completed projects, behavior records or questions. In evaluating clients, counselors again become diagnosticians.(6) If no solution to the problem has been reached, counseling reverts to the assessment or treatment phase.

Ending Care

When it is time to conclude therapy, the practitioner and client should come to a mutual agreement that the client is ready to stop, or that any possible benefits from counseling have been achieved. Monitoring the patient with appointments (emails or phone calls) every three to six months helps identify and solve problems that tend to appear when living in the real world.

While the goal of the counseling is to provide clients with long-term, self-management goals and skills, many clients may need to remain in treatment longer to maintain the change in eating habits. By being available by phone and appointments after structured care has ended, a counselor can help a patient better handle relapses and new problems. Also, clients that were unmotivated earlier may feel comfortable about re-entry into counseling at a later date.

Self-evaluation

Since a practitioner's success as a counselor depends to a large extent on the patients' outcomes, a counselor needs to evaluate whether his patients succeeded. It's the patients' responsibility, not the counselor's, to make changes in their lives. The counselor's responsibility is to make the patient aware of the food and lifestyle habits necessary for good health, to help the patient identify and alter barriers, and to facilitate changes in motivated patients. A counselor can build on experience to improve present skills.

Documentation

Records should be kept on each patient and his progress. The information is not only important and useful to the consultant, it may prove essential in a dispute or malpractice suit. In courts of law the statement is often made that if the service wasn't documented, it didn't happen—where is the proof?

Whether a practitioner uses the SOAP method of recording or just states the pertinent facts is not important. The most important point is for objective changes, such as improved chemical scores or anthropometric values, to be documented along with behavior and belief changes.

COUNSELING ONLINE

As explored by Linda McDonald, MS, RD, in *Going Global with Nutrition Counseling* (7), "Counseling and educating by e-mail is a developing communication method that links professional expertise with consumer needs in a convenient, informal format." Clients like having timely feedback, and not taking off work to go to appointments. Counselors like the convenience of answering e-mails (or email--both spellings are correct) in their free time when they have more time to ponder client questions. They also enjoy generating income while wearing their sweats.

Courts of law have found that e-mail communication is a unique medium for conflict resolution. Some divorced spouses who haven't been able to get along in person are court ordered to use e-mail since it makes handling problems more objective and less emotional.(8) Clients sometimes open up more in e-mails than in person—it's less threatening and personal to say something to a screen than to another person.

Communicating with your patients is one thing, but other dietitians are also giving nutrition information and advice from their websites. Some dietitians charge for their services and others offer free nutrition assessment, diet analysis or diet plans, which are actually paid for by selling advertising to companies who want exposure to the people coming to the site or they sell products.(7) See Chapters 21-23 for more discussion on the creation of such sites and legal pros and cons.

CONCLUSION

Creating realistic expectations of what your clients can do and guiding them through the changes are of the utmost importance. Change is difficult to achieve. The belief held by some clients and many third party payers that lasting changes in food behavior require only a few therapy sessions is an illusion. Change has a complex nature. Nutrition counselors and clients should not feel as if they failed when a perfect, smoothly functioning set of skills are not achieved in a few weeks. The goal of nutrition counseling occurs when the client integrates healthy nutrition guidelines for a lifetime.

REFERENCES

1. Helm KK, Klawitter B. *Nutrition Therapy: Advanced Counseling Skills.* Lake Dallas, TX: Helm Publishing; 1995.
2. Nutrition Therapist Subunit. *Ventures;* Summer 1998.
3. Snetselaar L, Schatt H, Iasiello-Vailor L, Smith K. Model Workshop on Nutrition Counseling for Dietitians. *J Am Diet Assoc.* 1981; 79:678.
4. Roth J. *Comparison of Nutrition Education and Psychotherapeutic Counseling;* 1993.
5. Shortridge R. The Perceptor. A manual of training behavior for professionals, Dairy Council of California; 1980.
6. Snetselaar L. *Nutrition Counseling Skills.* MD: Aspen Publishers; 1997.
7. McDonald L. Going Global with Nutrition Counseling. *Today's Dietitian;* 1999.
8. Personal interview with Suzanne Levisay, LSW, professional counselor with years of court experience in Denton, Texas; 2002.

RESOURCES

Nutrition Counseling Skills, 2nd edition, by Linda Snetselaar. Aspen Publishers: Gaithersburg, MD; 1997.
Nutrition Therapy: Advanced Counseling Skills, 2nd edition by Kathy King and Bridget Klawitter, editors. Helm Publishing, Lake Dallas, TX; 2003.
Eating Disorders: Nutrition Therapy in the Recovery Process by Dan and Kim Reiff.
Moving Away From Diets:New Ways to Heal Eating Problems and Exercise Resistance. by Karin Kratina, Nancy King and Dayle Hayes. Helm Publishing, Lake Dallas, TX; 1998.
Winning the War Within: Nutrition Therapy for Anorexia & Bulimia Nervosa. by Eileen Stellefson Meyer. Helm Publishing, Lake Dallas, TX; 1998.

—— Managing Your —— Business

Words of Wisdom:

"Unless you try to do something beyond what you have already mastered, you will never grow."
Ronald E. Osborn

"To dream anything that you want to dream. That is the beauty of the human mind. To do anything that you want to do. That is the strength of the human will. To trust yourself to test your limits. That is the courage to succeed."
Bernard Edmonds

Chapter 9

Business Plan

Successful dietetic business ventures are started in many different ways and under a variety of circumstances. Some business opportunities are handed to the nutritionist by a physician or client, others are outgrowths of jobs, and still others start without contacts or encouragement from anyone. Many businesses are painstakingly researched for years and others are created over lunch on a napkin.

DEVELOPING THE VENTURE ON PAPER

Business consultants agree that a potential business owner should put his plans in writing while doing research on the feasibility of his future venture. The tool used to do that is called a business plan. Its purpose is to share information, find problems, organize the business, and raise capital. This business tool has more written about it and more resources to help you create it than any other in business.(2) There are online web sites, software templates (online and at office supply stores) and business consultants ready and willing to help you produce your plan.(3) Some available resources are listed at the end of this chapter.

Unfortunately, it's not rare for a future entrepreneur to be so sold on an idea for a new business that he is totally blind to obvious reasons why the idea has a poor chance at success. Some examples are locating the business too close to the strongest competition——a nationally know hospital with a free clinic——or wanting to become a nutrition consultant to only Greek restaurants in Omaha. Although these ideas have a chance of working, it may take too long before you generate adequate income.

An experienced businessperson or professional advisor can look over the executive summary and business plan and find over-looked problems. Having your ideas clearly stated will help reduce the amount of time needed by paid advisors to assess your business needs. Many banks and all potential venture capital investors will request this information when considering a loan or investment. Business people take the time to prepare these documents because they are useful, provide insight, and give the appearance of having one's act together.

EXECUTIVE SUMMARY

If you had to rank all of the components of the business plan, the executive summary will float to the top. Why? The executive summary captures in less than one typed page (and one minute of reading) the general excitement, potential success, and resources required for a new product line extension or new business venture. The proposed scope of a new business—what you will sell, to whom, where, how, when—can all be stated briefly in the executive summary. It introduces the concept to the decision maker. It must stimulate them to read on, to analyze, and to buy into the idea. Without that stimulation, without that decision maker beginning to grasp the concept and share its excitement, the chances are remote there will be full consideration of the business plan.(4) If the plan is being used to attract financial backing, the executive summary should briefly spell out how much money is needed.(5) (See Figure 9.1.)

Although it's at the beginning of a Business Plan, the executive summary should be written after all the facts are in. The executive summary should: (6)

- Describe in detail the business and its goals.
- Identify the business ownership and the legal structure.
- Discuss skills and experience you (and any partners) bring to the business.
- Identify advantages you and your business have over your competitors.
- Identify your financial needs to create the venture.

Jim Rose, RD, former food service director and entrepreneur stated in Hospital Food and Nutrition Focus, "Write your executive summary in present tense, active voice. Avoid the 'shall's' and 'will's." Use verbs that show action and presume existence of the project. Make sentences short. Make paragraphs short. Use some bold or highlighted text—sparingly. But don't be too dramatic, trite or obviously overblown either. Include all the essential information. The executive summary must be possible to read in less than one minute. The first fifteen seconds of reading are critical; during that period the decision maker determines whether to 'put it aside,' trash it, or continue reading."(4)

When writing the executive summary, think of it as a promotional description of your venture. Avoid unnecessary details and concentrate on the strong, salable points.

BUSINESS PLAN

The business plan starts with a title page, followed by the table of contents and then the executive summary. By the time the rest of the plan is researched and written, you should have enough information to evaluate whether your business concept is viable, and you can estimate how much the venture will cost. Your plan can help you organize your venture and set priorities for better time and resource management. The

Figure 9.1 Example of Executive Summary (4)

The lines in our hospital cafeteria are getting longer, especially at lunch. Why? Our reputation for good food has spread. The local business community is routinely dining here—-paying premium prices, providing us with excellent profits. However, seating is at a premium, serving areas are congested, and customers are turning away.

Creating a deli operation in the vending area (now rarely used except during off-hours) that is contiguous to the cafeteria opens up opportunities for take-out services, tapping into new target markets and improving returns on profits.

A 50-seat deli operation faces no real competition within six city blocks. Only five percent of the potential population is now dining with us but the percentage is growing—-due to office building expansions with no food service operations included. Deli sales are growing in this region by twelve percent per year.

A capital investment of ___ provides a net return on investment of ___ on annual operations. Breakeven is at month _____. Operating breakeven is at ___ in annual sales. All gross revenues are based on an aggregate ____ cost of goods sold.

Renovation of the vending area requires $____. The current vending activities are incorporated into the deli operations scheme, offering expanded selections during off-hours.

Adequate labor pools exist, with recruitment simplified by our current food service recruitment programming. Management talent is already on staff.

marketing plan (Chapter 10) will be needed to fill out the business plan and to make an accurate assessment of what will "sell."

Business consultants will charge from $1,500 to $15,000 or more to research and fill out a business plan, but you can do it yourself. An accountant can be very helpful with much of the information. Typically, a plan will be five to thirty pages long, but consultants report they have seen ones with hundreds of pages when the project necessitated it. The larger size in no way improves the plan's acceptance; it may turn many readers away completely. The important point is to cover the subjects well with pertinent information. The plan should be assessed annually and updated and changed as needed.

A banker or venture capitalist uses a plan to evaluate whether he wants to invest in your business. In truth, the chance of venture capitalists being interested in a new service business is almost non-existent; they look for faster growth markets and entrepreneurs with extensive business experience.(7)

In his book *How to Start, Finance and Manage Your Own Small Business,* Joseph Mancuso, goes into great detail about what a plan should include and highlight.(8) He also shares results of his research on what items "sell" a venture capitalist or banker on a plan.

How a Business Plan Is Read

Although a business plan needs to be complete and thorough, the average investor only spends five minutes looking it over. Therefore the plan's layout and highlighted information are extremely important. In his research Mancuso found that there are typical steps in those five minutes of reading. (1,4,7,8)

Step 1. Determine the characteristics of the project, industry and company. Is this a growing market of interest to the public? Is competition doing well? Is anyone making much money in this field? Could this company or project do well?

Step 2. Determine the caliber of the people in the deal. Turn to the back of the plan and scan the resumes. This step, most venture capitalists claim, is the single most important aspect of the business plan. The employees' names, or founders, board of directors, current investors, and professional advisors' names are scanned in hopes of finding a familiar name. The reputation and quality of the business team or entrepreneur will sell a plan better than any other single item.

Step 3. Determine the terms of the deal. What is being offered in return for the money? How much is needed, and how will it be used?

Step 4. Read the latest balance sheet. Is the company making a profit or just scraping by? Are the income projections reasonable considering the balance sheet? Do the managers plan to pay themselves salaries that are reasonable?

Step 5. Determine what is different about this deal. This difference is the eventual pivotal issue for whether an investor chooses to back a business venture. Is there an unusual feature in the service or product? Nutrition is "hot" but are your programs designed to take advantage of it; are they exciting? Does the company have a patent or a significant lead over competition? Does the company's strength match the skills needed to succeed in this industry? Does the inexperienced owner recognize his limitations and have good advisors? Or is there an imbalance? Good ideas or products that are better than others will attract capital.

Step 6. Give the plan a once-over lightly. After the above analysis, the final minute is usually spent thumbing through the business plan. A casual look at product literature, graphs, unusual exhibits, published articles, and letters of agreement support the argument for unusual enclosures. Although additional items seldom make a difference to the outcome, they can extend the readership.

If the plan is rejected, it's customarily returned to you. When trying to interest a banker in your venture, it is not out of line to ask why it was rejected. If the banker wants to work with you, he or she may suggest ways to improve the plan, or offer a smaller loan, or ask for more collateral to secure the loan.

When an investor looks at business plans. Mancuso found that four elements determine which one is the chosen first: (8)

- the company, department, or persons submitting the plan,
- its geographic location,
- length of business plan—shorter ones are read first—and,
- quality of cover—interesting but not necessarily expensive.

William Sahlman, chairman of the board for the Harvard Business School Publishing Corporation, asks, "What's wrong with most business plans? Most waste too much ink on numbers and devote too little to the information that really matters (the people, opportunity, the big picture and risks or rewards). Financial projections for a new company—especially detailed, month-by-month projections—are an act of imagination. Don't misunderstand me: business plans should include some numbers (for a nutrition therapist it could be projected referrals and follow-up visits). The business model should also address the breakeven issue: At what level of sales does the business begin to make a profit? When does cash flow turn positive?"(1)

Writing a Business Plan

A business plan is a personal document. Yet there are some common ideas that should be considered when writing a plan. The different segments of the plan can be written in narrative form, as an outline, or in numbered, highlighted points. The easier it is to read and grasp the unique features, the better.

The order of the business plan is not as important as what information is included and how the information is highlighted. Adding too much detail can be a mistake. All of the following points of explanation do not have to be included; choose those that fit your needs.

SIX-STEP OUTLINE FOR BUSINESS PLAN

Introduction Title page, Table of Contents and Executive Summary.

Company Profile What is your company's mission? What is your company going to sell—products and services? Describe any unique features of your company. What are the business' short term and long-range goals? What objectives will be used to reach those goals? List the anticipated stages of growth and development. Identify any proprietary information or trade advantages your company may have (patents, copyrights, trademarks, established brands, etc.)

Market Analysis This section describes the market environment your business wants to enter. It shows whether you have carefully assessed its opportunities (new trends or ventures that could help your business) and threats (new negative trends or strong competitors who could stifle your business). You discuss why you are unique within the market as compared to the competition.

Marketing Plan   This part should detail your business position, brand development plans, sales, pricing and product strategies, promotion plans, referral agents, and potential strategic alliances. (See Chapter 10 for more details.)

What is the business position? How will the brand be developed? Who will sell the services and how? How will the business be advertised? What budgeted amount will be spent for promotion?

Who are the end users of your services? Describe them demographically. How will they be reached? Who are intermediate referral agents (physicians, clinics, corporations, hospitals, etc.)? How will they be reached?

Is business seasonal? Are there any proposed government regulations expected to affect your business (new regulations that do not include the RD or DTR, coverage for MNT, etc)?

Financial Plan You will need to offer financial reports. (You may need some help to produce projections on a company without any financial history. Ask your banker which reports he needs.)

If you are already in business or purchasing an ongoing practice, show present and past balance sheets, tax returns and profit and loss statements.

If just starting out, list projected start-up costs. Present pro forma balance sheets giving the effect of the proposed financing. What is your repayment plan? Give yearly projections of revenues and earnings for two to five years (don't waste too much time on this, as everyone knows it's being fabricated). Be positive about your potential but be honest as possible when projecting future business revenues. Bankers and others have seen hundreds of plans and often discount ones with obvious padding.

Appendixes   Your resumes can go here along with any published articles defending your market projections, your unique product brochures, product samples, newspaper articles about your business, letters of agreement and so on.

This business plan should be considered a working tool, one that is just as valuable for internal audit as external promotion or fund raising. A well-thought-out executive summary outlining your expectations for your business venture and a plan to carry out those concepts are invaluable in translating your ideas into a successful business.

REFERENCES

1. Sahlman WA. How to Write a Great Business Plan. In: *Harvard Business Review on Entrepreneurship*. Boston, MA: Harvard Business School Publishing; 1999.
2. Johnson D. Business Planning Made Easy. Home Office Computing; November 1999.
3. Haskin D. Business Essentials. *Home Office Computing;* November 1999.
4. Rose JC. Business Plan. *Hospital Food and Nutrition Focus.* 1989;4:10.
5. Business Plan. The Small Business Encyclopedia, Vol.1. Irvine, CA: *Entrepreneur Magazine Group;* 1996.
6. *The Facts About...Starting a Small Business.* Washington, DC: Small Business Administration; 2001.
7. Bhide A. Bootstrap Finance: The Art of Start-ups. In: *Harvard Business Review on Entrepreneurship*. Boston, MA: Harvard Business School Publishing; 1999.
8. Mancuso, Joseph. *How to Start, Finance and Manage Your Own Small Business*, Prentice- Hall, New Jersey; 1978.

RESOURCES (BUSINESS AND FINANCIAL PLANNERS) (3)

BizPlan Builder Interactive	$90	www.jian.com
Business Plan Pro 3.0	$90	www.palo-alto.com
Cash Plan Pro	$80	www.palo-alto.com
Plan Write Expert Edition		

Chapter 10

Marketing

Kathy King Helm, R.D. and Marianne Franz, MBA, R.D.

In the last twenty years, the need for marketing became obvious to practitioners in the dietetic profession. We now know that having educational credentials, good products or services and licensure will not make clients flock to our doors. It takes more. Clients must need or want what we have to sell.

By 2005, it is estimated that eight in ten Americans will work giving service instead of selling products. Dietitians will be counseling, consulting, working in long term care, marketing for grocery chains, disseminating information and so on.(1) Even if your business sells a product, like a handheld computer for patient assessment, customers come to you because the product is good, for the ease of purchasing, customer service follow-up and product support.

Too much of our past marketing strategies were based on the product model.(1) According to Harry Beckwith, marketing expert with 30 years of experience, the service marketing model is based on newer information: (1,2)

- **In our increasingly busy and over-communicated society, nothing works more powerfully in marketing than simplicity.** Market one focus with one positioning statement about your business. Don't confuse customers by being the jack-of-all-trades. You may offer more services, but market the most significant one.
- **When choosing a service business** (for example, when a physician refers the client for counseling on a low fat cardiac diet), customers generally do one of three things: 1) nothing at all, 2) do it themselves (go on the Internet or call the American Heart Association), or 3) use your services. Seldom do they go to a competitor.
- **It's all about relationships,** people will buy from people they like and with whom they have relationships. It's very hard to compare services.
- **The fastest, cheapest and best way to market your services is to do it yourself or through your employees.**

- **People want to avoid making a bad choice; they seldom seek a superior choice.** That's why they will go to someone they "know" who did a good counseling job for a neighbor instead of trying someone new, and why "building a better mousetrap" doesn't always guarantee business success.
- **People tend to buy what they hear most about or what seems most familiar.** That's why you should take the time and spend the money to advertise your presence in your marketplace--create your "brand." Name brands are sold in 13 out of 14 sales. People don't have the time to look around and over time they learn to trust a brand's reputation for good service, which is important since they can't see the quality of a service before it's purchased.
- **Don't assume that behaviors will follow attitudes.** Just because people think they should eat healthy or stop smoking, doesn't mean they will. Remember that next time when you think about starting a "healthy" fast food restaurant.
- **Research and data have a remarkable ability to fool people.** Focus groups don't tell more about market dynamics than a good critical thinker can. Look for people to give you advice who think for themselves and draw from a wide perspective.
- **Even if you have an "inferior" product (experts agree Microsoft DOS was inferior to Apple) from a technical or critical standpoint, you can still make money if your product solves customers' problems.** It just becomes more important to get the other elements in the marketing mix right.(3)

How will people know what you sell? Eventually, they will know it by word of mouth. However, in today's competitive markets with limited budgets and shortened timelines, most businesspeople find that organized, aggressive marketing is essential.

Marketing's goal is consumer satisfaction. Too often in the past, we only offered what we felt our target markets should have. That has changed. Good tasting food--gourmet or gluttonous--and information on nutrition are "big business" now, attracting many people into the fields that were once ours by default.

MARKETING IS NOT NEW

Marketing is not a new philosophy. Basic ideology stems from the mid-1600s, when a Tokyo merchant named Mitsui opened what might be called the first department store. His intent was to serve his customers by offering a selection of products that were designed to meet their needs and backed by a money-back guarantee.(4)

In the mid-19th century Cyrus McCormick invented more than just a mechanical harvester. Mr. McCormick invented basic tools of marketing; namely, market research, customer service and installment credit. He also introduced the idea that marketing should be a central function of doing business.(4)

Marketing spread rapidly among firms that produced tangible products, such as industrial and consumer goods. Marketing intangible services caught on much more slowly. The American health sector tried hard to resist the encroachment of marketing philosophy. Marketing activities, such as sales and advertising were not viewed favorably in an industry traditionally grounded in helping and caring. Because medical care is a God-given right, health marketing seemed to be an oxymoron or at least "commercial" and nonprofessional. Yet, when the costs of health care began to spiral upward, and the number of patients began to decline, a few innovative hospitals hired marketing professionals. Competitive change was launched. Today, billions of budget dollars are dedicated to consumer health care marketing activities.

MARKETING DEFINED

To encapsulate the many formal definitions that have evolved to describe the function of marketing, it simply means: Those activities necessary for the delivery of services or products from the producer to the customer, to satisfy the customer and to meet the business' objectives.(5) These activities include:
- Product or service development
- Market research
- Advertising
- Public relations (product publicity)
- Sales promotion
- Customer service
- Sales

The above definition requires two visions: 1) assessing and reacting to trends in the marketplace and 2) the higher purpose of your business or "mission" that should keep you focused and on track.

Trends

First, the marketing function involves an ongoing process of anticipating problems and opportunities through regularly analyzing the trends in the marketplace. Trends can be local, national or global. Examples of "big" national trends include:
- Continuing changes will come to health care: cutting costs, merging tasks
- Population growing older with a huge baby boom group about to hit

- Obesity is the number one malnutrition problem
- Large number (44 million) of Americans are uninsured for health problems
- Big interest by some in culinary skills, Whole Foods Markets, and good food while the majority of Americans are seeking "ready-to-serve homemade" carry-out
- Too much junk mail-30% of all mail is thrown away before opening
- E-commerce will catch on more and change the way we live, market and communicate

Strategic Assumptions

In response to trends, you then develop strategic assumptions on what you expect the market to do. Strategic assumption statements should be concise and easily understood. They help you by excluding activities and investments that, although they seem attractive, would deplete the company's resources if you followed them.(6)

These assumptions could be as simple as, "The population base in my Phoenix area will continue to grow older faster than the U.S. population," or "As long as this region is in a deep recession, wellness is not a high priority for most corporations, except as a health care cost-cutting tool." By deciding what the strategic assumptions are for your business area, you can better anticipate what will sell and how to sell it.

You base your short and long term marketing decisions on your assumptions, and alter them as your assumptions change. Continuing with the examples, during the recession, you know in the short term you should immediately change the marketing focus for your corporate weight loss program. Your pitch should change from highlighting the satisfied participants and pounds lost, to how much less would be spent on health care during the year following the program. Long term, if you live in Phoenix, you may decide that over the next three years your major services or products will be changed to satisfy the needs of people over sixty years old.

Mission

A second vision associated with marketing is your business mission. A mission statement tells the "higher purpose" why your business exists. It could be "To provide high quality catered healthy gourmet entrees and low fat desserts to the city of Midland," or "My mission is to become a consumer-educator in nutrition through the broadcast and newspaper media with special emphasis on disease prevention and vegetarian eating." The mission statement sets your course. It helps you decide what your goals should be in order to keep your allocation of resources focused. You may have many different business or career opportunities that present themselves during the course of the day or year. Underlying your decisions on which ones to take should be your ultimate dedication to your mission.

MARKETING DEFINITIONS (6,7)

ADVERTISING
Advertising is a paid form of non-personal communication about an organization and/or its products that is transmitted to a target audience through a mass medium.

BRAND
A brand is a name, term, symbol, design, or combination of these that identifies a seller's products and differentiates them from competitors' products.

MARKETING
Marketing is those activities necessary for the delivery of services or products from the producer to the customer in order to satisfy the customer and to meet the business' objectives.(5)

MARKET NICHE
A niche is narrow segment of the potential larger target market that your product or service can satisfy best without as much competition. Marketing dollars are often invested more wisely when pursuing the correct niche.

MARKETING MIX
The marketing mix consists of four major variables: product, price, place or distribution and promotion.

MARKETING PLAN
The plan is the written document or blueprint for implementing and controlling an organization's marketing activities.

MISSION STATEMENT
This statement declares what business you are in and its "higher purpose." It sets your course, improves focus and helps you decide what your goals should be.

PRODUCT or SERVICE
Anything offered in the marketplace to be exchanged for something of value, i.e. money, commitment to change, etc.

PUBLIC RELATIONS
Marketing activities designed to create a positive image for you or your business in which to do business, earn recognition and gain acceptance.

PUBLICITY
Publicity is free media coverage of some newsworthy story or event. Look for a news "hook" that will interest the media and its audiences.

SOCIAL MARKETING

Social marketing influences attitudes, beliefs, or lifestyle choices for the benefit of a person or the public. Media campaigns for stop smoking, pro-literacy, low cholesterol diets and anti-abortion are all examples of social marketing.

STRATEGIC ASSUMPTIONS

These are statements about trends in the external environment that will affect the future and may present opportunities or threats to your business.

SWOT ANALYSIS

An analysis used to assess your internal or personal Strengths (S) or Weaknesses (W), and the external Opportunities (O) or Threats (T) in the marketplace that may affect your plans.

TARGET MARKET

Primary customer group targeted for the marketing campaign. The group members usually have similar needs, wants or desires.

MARKETING MIX ————————————————————————————

The four P's of marketing are the variables you have to work with to influence the buyer to purchase your product or service. The standard marketing mix concept was developed by professor Jerome McCarthy in the early 1960s.(8)

1. **Product.** This refers to the product or services the business sells.
2. **Price.** The money customers must pay for it.
3. **Place.** Location or where the customer will purchase the product.
4. **Promotion.** The marketing or advertising used to attract customers.

By altering the above variables, a business can attract different target or niche markets. For example, by choosing a place or location in a very wealthy area of town, the practitioner has committed to produce a more comprehensive, high-end product, at a higher price to cover increased costs with more expensive looking packaging and stylish, tasteful promotion.

According to marketing expert and author, Philip Kotler, "the four P's are from a seller's point of view. The four C's are from the customers' viewpoint. Marketers sell products, but customers buy customer value. Customers are interested in more than the price; they want to know the costs of obtaining and using the product. Customers want convenience when seeking to buy; and finally, customers want two-way communication not promotion."(8)

MARKETING STRATEGIES

Entrepreneurs soon learn that it's easier to sell something else to a satisfied customer than it is to find another customer. Some marketing experts estimate that businesses spend five times more to attract new customers than they do to keep old ones.(1) In fact, the most successful service businesses become that way because of repeat customers.(1,2,8) The strategy is to "grow" a customer; the key is to move the customer through a series of stages that strengthen the relationship between the customer and business: (8)

- First-time customers have no history or commitment to your company-keep them satisfied.
- Repeat customers not only buy again, but they may spend more.
- The one-on-one client relationship is next with personalized care and attention.
- The best customers become advocates and tout your business to others.
- In some industries the customer is so close the relationship becomes a partnership, like when an independent caterer becomes the exclusive provider of catered meals in a banquet facility.
- The highest view of the customer is the part owner, where the customer actually becomes part of the enterprise through an investment or bartered agreement.

If a patient is referred to you for a lower calorie diabetic diet, what else could you sell that person? What about a group weight loss class with an exercise component, or grocery store tour, nutritional supplements, or low fat cooking classes, or cookbooks discounted ten percent from bookstore prices? By having a line of products or services, you can satisfy your patients' needs better and generate more revenue. This is called **Concentrated Marketing**-identifying one target market but selling multiple products or services to that market.

If you have a catering business and someone comes to you wanting food for a special event, what else could you offer that person? What about flowers, table decorations, musicians, linens, theme parties, or photography? You may only do the catering and managing everything else could be subcontracted to others.

Another strategy, **Differentiated Marketing,** repackages a proven or new product to fit the needs of new target markets. This could be as simple as adapting a group weight loss program to fit the needs of patients in cardiac rehabilitation. You could offer a "senior meal" selection in your cafeteria at a lower price to attract a new target market.

Keep good records on your clients or patients. Try to identify who are your best buying customers and keep in touch with them through a newsletter or year-end thank you note. The goal is to develop ongoing relationships that don't end when a consultation session or catered event is over. Every client has a sphere of influence that could mean increased business for you.

The third marketing strategy is *Undifferentiated Marketing,* which involves introducing only a single version of the product in the hope it will appeal to everyone. The original Coke was a good example of this strategy, but so is a nutrition presentation on healthy eating or one on disease prevention through nutrition.

An OB/GYN physician in Lewisville, Texas, sends a year-end and signed letter to each of his patients thanking them for their business and discussing what new benefits he offers. His office also sends very attractive thank you cards for patient referrals and reminders for yearly pap smears. He keeps two large scrapbooks of baby pictures and thank you notes from happy parents on the lobby coffee table that help establish his credibility with expectant mothers. After delivery of a baby, he brings new mothers a baby picture frame and a newborn t-shirt that says, "Hand Delivered by Dr. Franklin." He happens to be popular with the nurses, not because he is easy to work with but because he has empathy for his patients and gives good medical care. He is an example of the kind of health care specialist who will succeed in the future-- patient-oriented and skilled in marketing as well as his specialty.

Market research and your own creativity and ingenuity can help you find niches in the marketplace where your products or services with the right mix can flourish without heavy competition--at least initially.(10) You will make better marketing decisions if you use the product life cycle model described in Chapter 3. Choosing the right point on the curve to enter the market is an art as well as a science. See Chapter 20 on Promotion ideas.

SOCIAL MARKETING

Social marketing focuses on changing personal or social behavior for the benefit of the public. It is used to accomplish three objectives: (11,12)

- Disseminate new data and information to individuals like why to reduce their intake of high trans fatty acids or high aspartame-containing foods.
- Offset the negative effects of a practice or promotional effort by

another group or organization like warning the public about the megadoses of individual mineral supplements.

- Motivate people to move from intention to action like motivating clients to take control of their weight.

For a program to succeed it must have the following conditions: (9)
- Adequate resources
- Strong support from agency administrators and community leaders
- Marketing skills and savvy
- Clear authority to make the necessary marketing decisions and implement them in a timely fashion

SELLING YOURSELF

While credibility and visibility are necessary to successful marketing, they aren't the total package. You must also know specifically what message you want to communicate. What benefits does your business provide? Key words can form your message. For example, "I'm a registered dietitian who has counseled over 6,000 patients in the past 30 years. My business provides the public with easy to understand, state of the art nutrition presentations and personal consultations."

In addition to credibility, visibility and a message, you need to create an image. Image determines how people view you, how much they value you and whether they are attracted to you. Social and psychological research has found that the more similar you are to your audience in terms of attitude, values, interests and background, the more attractive you will be to them.(12)

Your image is the first impression potential customers receive about you. It must convey your expertise, professionalism, responsiveness and reliability, as well as creating warm, positive expectations.

A recent survey on marketing techniques by small-business owners found that informal speaking was the most effective means of promotion. You can talk to colleagues, the media, local business and professional groups and work as a volunteer.

Following are six marketing rules that can help you get your message across in any kind of informal speech: (12)

1. **Appearance.** Use your attire and posture to project confidence, competence and status. Strive for a look that emphasizes quality and conservatism in both dress and gestures. You don't have to have an extensive wardrobe, but do have several "President of the Company" suits to wear when power and prestige are called for. In

other circumstances, like when working with sports teams, wear appropriate sport clothing. Work on looking and acting successful.

2. **Nonverbal behavior.** Make direct eye contact. Combined with smiling and nodding, eye contact helps create an image of social attraction, power and credibility.

3. **Verbal behavior.** Use simple, direct language without jargon; speak clearly and concisely. If you need a speech coach to get rid of poor grammar, slang, a bad accent, or whatever, hire one!

4. **Involvement.** Listen actively and carefully; tailor your message to your audience--whether one person or a thousand.

5. **Illustration.** Your words should paint pictures in the minds of your audience. They will remember better what you have to say. Support important points with examples (and references if necessary).

6. **Control.** Stay in control of your image, your message, and your audience's response by deciding ahead of time exactly what you're going to say and how you're going to say it.

What *Not* To Do in a New Business (13)

Mistake #1: Don't have a plan how you are going to create and market your business. You have a good education, successful job history, and decent relationships with clients and colleagues, and you want to be a consultant to sports teams; what else is there to know?

Mistake #2: Jump in full-time without a golden handshake from your job. You need to test the waters to see if there is business potential out there for you before you quit. Try working your venture on the side to work out the bugs while you stay employed. If there is an opportunity to get severance pay for reduction-in-force, consider taking it.

Mistake #3: Believe empty promises of future work. Get it in writing, and if you can, start the work while keeping some other stable income coming in. It's easy to underestimate what it will take to survive as an entrepreneur. Don't count on others handing you a business.

Mistake #4: Don't call people you don't already know. You must network and let everyone know who you are and what your business does. You have to make phone calls and join organizations to become known.

Mistake #5: Waste a lot of money on dead-end marketing and buyers who aren't serious. A small business can't afford to waste money or time on non-productive marketing. Drop things that don't work. Ask direct questions like: Do you have the authority to sign an agreement? What is your timeline on this project? When will you buy?

Mistake #6: Underestimate what it will take to start the business and cover living expenses. Don't live off credit cards except in an emergency. Don't live beyond your means. Cut back until the money comes in on a regular basis.

Mistake #7: Poor time management can cause poor output. Business life can be feast or famine. If several jobs come in at once with similar deadlines, hire an assistant to help relieve some of the pressure and assure adequate time to maintain quality.

MARKETING AN INTANGIBLE SERVICE

In most cases, dietitians deliver intangible services, instead of tangible products. Service marketing has some unique concerns. First, the service provider is selling something the potential customer can't see, feel or evaluate before he buys it. He can hold an attractive brochure, or see quality in the business card and other surrogates that represent the service. Secondly, the production, delivery and customer evaluation of the service occur at the same moment in time. If the customer does not like the quality of the service, it can make things very awkward. The buyer places a high degree of confidence in the abilities of the service provider. In return, the provider must be sensitive to the needs of the buyer and adapt the service as it is happening, to fit those needs.

Because services usually are one-on-one, customers will seldom tell you what they think-if they are unhappy, they just don't return. So, don't assume everything was okay if no concerns were mentioned. During the delivery of your service, ask questions, actively listen, and backtrack if you have to in order to assure understanding, smile and show approval.

It's your job to create a high-perceived value about the benefits of your services through advertising and other forms of promotion.(14)

Use a distinctive looking "brand" on all of your promotion materials--that is, use your logo and business name on your business cards, brochure, letterhead, advertisements and so on. This makes you appear more successful and organized. Plus a brand creates the benefit of instant recognition. When a customer thinks of a culinary RD, he thinks of Anne Piatek or Chef Kyle. When he wants a sports nutritionist, he thinks of Jacqueline Berning. Or, for continuing education self-study courses, I want him to think of Helm Publishing.

MARKETING AN INVENTION

When you want to sell an invention there are several things you must do. First, manufacturers are contacted by thousands of people each year who have "good" ideas for new products. So don't be discouraged if they want you to sign a form stating the manufacturer doesn't owe you anything if they thought of it first. Also, most large manufacturers have their own Research and Development departments that come up with new ideas, and they often discourage bosses from buying an idea that could be developed in-house.

If you can't patent your product (in other words it doesn't have any new ingredients or process or outcome), then often its value isn't as great because other companies can copy it legally and exactly, if it becomes popular. Also, if you have an unrefined product that still needs work, or one that is only for a small select population, such as for patients with high uric acid levels, or one that has never proven itself on the market, it's usually not worth as much to the manufacturer.

Today, because of the cost of introducing a new product on the market, many companies would rather buy out a small profitable company with products that are selling than start an unknown product. Today, according to *Advertising Age*, it costs $10-20 million to test market, advertise and then introduce a new product nationwide into grocery stores.

Charlie McCann, a former new products manager for Coca-Cola of New York, once told me that the only way a small, under-financed company can make a lot of money on a new idea is as the granola inventors did. Come out with a product that sells like wildfire and then sellout to General Mills or Kellogg before everyone else jumps on the bandwagon and puts you out of business. There are numerous exceptions to that rule, most notably, Ben and Jerry's Ice Cream, Stephen Job's Apple Computers, Celestial Seasoning's teas and American Beverage Company's Soho.

Along with product samples, a "package" to interest a manufacturer could include a proposal with a market analysis and the product positioning. It could have a label sample, package design, and trademarked slogan and logo. The positioning entails determining whom the product is designed to sell to, and why they would buy it.

When you have developed a product you are proud of, it's time to contact a patent and contract lawyer to get feedback on how to protect your specific product. You also must determine what you want from an agreement with a manufacturer. A businessperson with experience in this area is also very valuable, especially in determining whom to contact and how.

If you have any contacts with someone who could open doors for you or introduce you to the right people, use them. In some instances you may choose to use someone as an agent who knows the industry and offer him a finder's fee if he brings a buyer to you. From my own experience, don't expect someone else to come in and do all the work unless you can pay them well or they get part ownership in the product.

Several Options For Selling A Product

A manufacturer may show more than a casual interest in your product and want to offer a 90-day contract to look it over. You will have to decide if you want to take it off the market for that period and allow a company to get to know the product inside out. It may be your best chance to make a sale (and to make some money because you will charge for the contract), or it could be a mistake. If several companies want it, others might not be interested if the first one rejects it.

One option is an outright sale of your product to the company that will manufacture it and take it to market. Some companies have a policy of always owning everything they manufacture---it's cleaner that way---no inventors get in the way. You could sell outright for one lump sum or sell for an up-front sum and a percentage of future sales.

Or, to make the agreement work, you may accept only a percentage of sales, but that's risky unless you really trust the company will produce as promised. The more risk you take, the more assurances you must have the manufacturer will not sit on the product, reduce the quality of the product below the expectations of the target market, price it above what the market will pay, package it poorly, or not promote it.

Another option is a license-use agreement where you retain ownership of the product but sell the manufacturer the exclusive or nonexclusive right to produce the product for a specific period of time and/or location. This offers the advantage that you still ultimately own the product, but if you chose the wrong partner again, the product may not be worth much when it's returned. When you still own the product and a customer is hurt by it, whether from the original formulation or how it was manufactured, you could have liability risk.

Dietitians have become partners with programmers, venture capitalists, small manufacturers, marketing specialists, and others in order to get their products to market. Call your advisors and lawyer, and involve them in securing a contract that will protect you and your product.

There are no guidelines on how much you can sell a product for or how much percentage to negotiate for. It all depends on how much a buyer is willing to pay and how bad you want to work with that buyer. The value is influenced by the uniqueness of the product, the size of the potential market, the markup and profit potential, the strength of the competition, and whether the product is already a proven success with packaging, trade name, patents, and copyrights established. The more you have done on the product, the greater the value.

THE MARKETING PLAN

For many projects, the marketing plan serves as the sales tool. Along with a business plan, a marketing plan is essential when you start a business.

Once you have identified one or more "big ideas" in Chapter 3, work through the following eight steps and evaluate the market potential for your concept(s). The trick is to adopt an objective approach and to thoroughly analyze as you go.(14)

Step One: Identify the Product Line and Target Market There are three basic parts to this step: identify the major product, narrow possibilities, and identify other opportunities.

- **Identify the major product and target market:** What is the "big idea?" What are the services or products you could sell? Who will buy it? Too many people wrongly believe they have universal products or services that everyone needs. They are surprised when only a few want them. The target market is the market segment that you intend to satisfy with your product or service. Therefore, it should fit their needs best, and be packaged and promoted to attract that group. Traditionally, markets were subdivided by geographic area. Today, customers are more likely to be differentiated by sex, age, income, educational level, profession, and other measurable personal characteristics. The newest market segmentation schemes are based on particular lifestyles that predict customer purchase decisions.(15)

  Profitable survival requires an edge derived from some combination of a creative idea and a superior capacity for execution. Entrepreneurs can't rely on just inventing new services or anticipating a trend. They must also execute well, especially if their concept can be easily copied.(6)

Successful ventures don't always proceed in the direction they started, a significant proportion develop entirely new markets and products. If prospects that were expected to place orders don't, the entrepreneur must rework the concept while looking for new opportunities to exploit.(6)

- **Narrow the possibilities:** Ask yourself questions that will define areas of concentration. Think in terms of three- to five-years period. The purpose of this section is to make your target market as specific as possible. Who do you like working with the most? What client settings do you enjoy the most? Who will buy your product the most? Describe the characteristics of your target market.
- **Identify other opportunities:** During your evaluation phase you may have thought of secondary target markets that could use your service. Identify them, but concentrate on your primary market.

Step Two: Conduct Market Research Here you will begin to find out if your assumptions about your "big idea" and its target market will work. Without knowing it, you probably have started your market research already. Have you started talking to people about the possibility of your venture? Have you started attending seminars or reading about ventures similar to the one you want to start? If so, you have started to test the waters.

- **General Situational Analysis:** What are the general characteristics of the market where you want to sell your product or service? What are the trends? Is the marketplace expanding? Shrinking? Is technology coming in rapidly? Are your current skills capable to meet the needs? What does your target market spend its money on? Primary market research is the research you conduct yourself. Secondary research involves statistics and information collected by someone else, such as business, trade, government, university and professional groups. Use both sources to be assured that you have thoroughly researched the concept.

Talk discretely to potential customers and trusted referral agents or business associates about your plans. Ask open-ended questions and get them to give you feedback on the concepts.

Mailed surveys today must compete with mounds of junk mail and solicitations. Don't mail surveys! Call people, you may find that a few minutes on the phone with someone could give you all the information you need in a fraction of the time and effort. Write out questions and have them ready when you call.(2)

- **SWOT (Strengths, Weaknesses, Opportunities, and Threats) Analysis:** The strengths and weaknesses are internal characteristics. In other words, what do you (or your employees) do well that could make this project a success? What are your weaknesses that must be delegated, retrained or compensated for to make this project work? Opportunities and threats are in your external environment or marketplace. The opening of a new fitness center or research unit could offer you an opportunity to use your new product or service. Things that could threaten the success of your project are like an oversupply of outpatient dietitians, changing government regulations, or a war overseas that frightens customers and creates a recession here.
- **Analysis of the competition:** Go deeper in your analysis. Identify your competition, its locations, its products or services, and any advantages or disadvantages it may have. The purpose is to find niches or weaknesses that the competition has in order for you to position your services or products as "different or better." When entering the marketplace, it's important to determine if you are a leader or a follower. A leader sets the pace and usually has the largest market share, such as Quaker Oats in the oat cereal market. A follower like Total oatmeal marketed itself as being different and better in the one area in which Quaker Oats was weak: fortification. Without an advantage over its competition, a product or service must either compete on price or spend lots of money on advertising to make a niche for itself.

Step Three: Setting Goals and Objectives. Define what you want to achieve, given the mission you have chosen. Make goals as succinct and measurable as possible. Identify short term goals that can be accomplished in several months to a year and long term goals that will take three to five years. Reevaluation of the marketplace through trends and strategic assumptions is a continuous process that will help keep the business goals on target. Think about the driving force of your project or career---the ultimate goals that will make you feel you succeeded professionally. Write down specific profit and marketing objectives that will help you reach your goals. Also, write down bailout signals that if they occur, would mean it's time to change direction or abandon the project.

Step Four: Determine Major Strategies. Now is the place to determine your marketing mix, or the 4or 5 P's of marketing for your product or service: Product, Price, Place and Promotion (some people add

Packaging as a fifth option). What you decide can determine the success of your venture. You know your product or service you want to sell, but take a few minutes to describe its "positioning" in the marketplace. Your business Position message should: (2)
- have only one focus;
- set you apart from competitors; and
- its goal is to have customers think of your business first.

What is its market "niche?" What benefits will the consumer get? How is it unique? What are your pricing strategies (see Chapter 16.) Place refers to the location or distribution system where the customer buys your product or service. Is it convenient? If it's a product for the grocery shelf, where will it be sold? The key is to make your products or services as available and convenient as possible. What means of promotion do plan to use (see Chapter 20)? Specifically explain your promotion plans.

Step Five: Develop Action Plans and Assign Responsibilities. Take the strategies in Step Four and break them down into specific activities and add a timetable with dates, list of resources required, budget allocation, deadlines, etc. Assign responsibilities if there is someone other than you also working on the project, such as a printer, graphic artist, publicist, and so on. Don't assume anything. Stay on top of the project.

Step Six: Establish a Financial Reporting System. Which resources will it take to complete your project and market it? What return on investment do you expect? How much do you have to sell to breakeven? Is the return worth the effort and investment? Look at the project over a three to five-year span, not just start-up costs.

Step Seven: Measure and Evaluate Results. If your research and estimates are favorable, what criteria will you use along the way to show you are on the right track to your goals?

Step Eight: Enlist Support. If you have a client account, supervisor or family who will be affected by this plan, how do you intend to approach them? What points can you offer that will sell the concept? Will this plan need to be formally packaged and presented, and if so, to whom and when?

When you produce this tangible report of your best research on the feasibility and costs involved in promoting your product or service, you, better than anyone, will have a feel for whether the project should go forward.

USING THE MARKETING CAPABILITIES OF ADA

The American Dietetic Association has an extremely capable staff of professionals at headquarters, along with volunteers, that produce a terrific number of marketing opportunities for members with services or products to sell, or for you to gain exposure. For a few chosen members there are the Ambassador and state-sponsored Media Representative programs. You can be on the national resource list of experts who are called at times by the media, the nationwide referral network, and sometimes ADA leaders might call on you to offer your expertise.

If you have an idea for a study kit, audiotape program, book, or other publication, you can submit a proposal to ADA's Publication Department for consideration by the Publication Committee. If you have a research study or project that is unique, consider writing an article for the ADA Journal. Your idea could be a major presentation or a poster display at ADA's Annual Meeting. If you belong to a dietetic practice group, you could present the idea at a meeting or write about it in a newsletter. There is the Product Market Place for members to exhibit their products and services on the first day of the annual convention and there are commercial booths available in the exhibit area. There are many similar opportunities at the state level for leadership and marketing opportunities.

CHANGE IS NORMAL

The marketplace is always changing, and what sells today, may only sell half as well next year. Be watchful of business trends, changes in the public buying habits, stories that make the news, and the economy, as well as feedback from your clients. Ask each client how he or she heard about your service or product and then use that market research in the future.

REFERENCES

1. Beckwith H. *Selling the Invisible*. New York: Warner Books; 1997.
2. Beckwith H. *The Invisible Touch*. New York: Warner Books; 2000.
3. Gorman T. *The Complete Idiot's Guide to MBA Basics*. New York: Simon & Schuster MacMillan Company; 1998.
4. Kotler P. *Marketing Management, Analysis, Planning and Control,* 5th edition. Englewood Cliffs, NJ: Prentice Hall; 1984.
5. Sobel M. *The 12-Hour MBA Program*. Paramus, NJ: Prentice Hall; 1993.
6. Bhide A. How Entrepreneurs Craft Strategies That Work. In: *Harvard Business Review on Entrepreneurship*. Boston, MA: Harvard Business School Press; 1999.
7. Goodale J. Presentation May 2002: *Marketing for Small Business*. Corinth, TX: Dark Horse Productions.
8. Kotler P. Kotler on Marketing: *How to Create, Win and Dominate Markets*. New York: Simon & Schuster; 1999.
9. Helm KK. *Becoming an Entrepreneur in Your Own Setting,* Study Kit. Chicago, IL: American Dietetic Association; 1991.
10. Kotler P, Zaltman G. Social Marketing: An approach to Planned Social Change. *Journal of Marketing;* 35:5; 1971.
11. Population Information Program. Social Marketing Does it Work? *Population Reports,* Series J, no.21; 1980.
12. Ward M. *Marketing Strategies: A Resource for Registered Dietitians*. New York; 1984.
13. Hudson D. How NOT to Run a Business. *Home-Office Computing;* July 1991.
14. Helm KK. *The Competitive Edge*. Chicago, IL: American Dietetic Association; 1986.
15. Bagozzi R. *Principles of Marketing Management*. Chicago, IL: Science Res. Assoc.; 1986.

RESOURCES Marketing Plan Software

Business Insight 5.0	$795	www.brs-inc.com
Marketing Builder Interactive	$75	www.jian.com
Marketing Plan Pro	$90	

Chapter 11

Legal Forms of Business Ownership

When starting your business, there are three business structures from which to choose. You can go into business as a sole proprietor, partnership or corporation (C or S corporation or a LLC Limited Liability Corporation). By far the most common form is sole proprietorship, even among legal firms.

The type of structure is often vital to the success of a business:
- it can affect your ability to attract financial backing;
- it can greatly increase the cost and paperwork of doing business;
- it affects what you pay in taxes, and
- it determines the extent your personal belongings are at risk, if the business gets into trouble (or if a spouse loses a lawsuit in a community property state).

The structure also affects the amount of control you have running the business and the amount of bookkeeping you must do. Also, the more partners or investors you have, the more bookkeeping is required.(1,2)

No business form is best for all purposes. A sole proprietorship offers freedom, but if a person needs money, it may be useful to find a partner with capital. At the same time, disagreement between partners on something so simple as how to spend the profit has undermined many ventures. A corporation may require too much money and bookkeeping to make it feasible for a very small operation.

To organize your business in the most advantageous way, talk with a good small business lawyer at the outset. Because tax laws are in a state of flux, consult with an accountant or CPA. You will feel more comfortable with business, if you become familiar with the different types of ownership. (See Figure 11.1 Forms of Business.)

To be recognized for tax purposes, whatever form you choose must be a genuine business--in other words, started and pursued in good faith to make a "profit." This makes it different from a hobby or philanthropic work. It's the Internal Revenue Service, not local or state laws, that decides your federal tax and business status.(1) Your work will be classed as a business if it produces a profit in two out of five consecutive years.

FEDERAL IDENTIFICATION NUMBER ———————————

Each employer must be registered with the Internal Revenue Service on Form SS-4 to comply with Federal Income Tax, Social Security and Unemployment Insurance regulations. This form requests a Federal Identification number that should be used when filing your taxes, and when you're paid by a client, instead of your Social Security number. Your local IRS office can give or mail you the form or your accountant will have it.

FEDERAL AND STATE REGULATIONS ———————————

Employee Considerations

If you have any employees, including officers of a corporation but not the sole proprietor or partners, you must make periodic payments, and/or file quarterly reports about payroll taxes and other mandatory deductions.(3) You may contact these government agencies for information, assistance and forms.

Social Security Administration	(800) 772-1213 www.ssa.gov
Federal Withholding (IRS)	(800) 829-1040 www.irs.ustreas.gov
Workers' Compensation	(Contact your state unemployment office)

PERMITS, LICENSES, and DBA TRADE NAME FORMS ———

In most localities, a person can do a business under his own name without registering it with anyone. In other locations, certain types of businesses need a permit, a small business license, or various other documents that someone at the State Taxation Department, City Hall and the County Court House can advise you about. Some states tax professional services like counseling, or require they add sales tax to their bills, so a sales tax license is necessary.

dba

If you want to use a trade name or fictitious business name other than your own, as a sole proprietor or partnership, you will need to check county files to see if the name is available. If it is, then register it at the county clerk's office or some similar place as a "fictitious" or Trade or dba (Doing Business As) name. This form lets people know that "Seattle Nutrition Consultants" is Jane Patterson's business. This form is necessary to obtain bank accounts in the business name or to bill clients in your county. Some states also have a registration fee for small businesses of $10-20.

Figure 11.1   Forms of Business

WHAT FORM OF BUSINESS ORGANIZATION? (1,3,4,5,6)

SOLE PROPRIETORSHIP

Advantages
1. Low start-up costs
2. Greatest freedom from regulation
3. Owner in direct control
4. Minimal working capital required
5. Tax advantage to owner
6. All profits to owner

Disadvantages
1. Unlimited liability
2. Lack of continuity if owner dies
3. Difficult to raise capital

PARTNERSHIP

Advantages
1. Ease of formation
2. Low start-up costs
3. Additional source of capital
4. Broader management base
5. Possible tax advantage
6. Limited outside regulation

Disadvantages
1. Unlimited liability
2. Lack of continuity
3. Divided authority
4. Difficulty in raising additional capital
5. Hard to find suitable partners

CORPORATION (C or FULL)

Advantages
1. Limited liability
2. Continuous existence
3. Ownership is transferable
4. Easier to raise capital
5. Legal entity
6. Possible tax advantages

Disadvantages
1. Closely regulated
2. Most expensive (fees, taxes, book keeping)
3. Charter restrictions
4. Extensive recordkeeping
5. Double taxation

CORPORATION (Small or S)

Advantages
1. Limited liability
2. Profit taxed once
3. Ownership is transferable
4. Legal entity
5. Limited outside regulation
6. Only salary subject to 15.3% self-employment tax

Disadvantages
1. State fees-initial and yearly
2. Some added bookkeeping and business records
3. One class of stock; 75 max. investors
4. Money borrowed can't lower taxes of owner

LIMITED LIABILITY CORPORATION (LLC or LLP)

Advantages
1. Limited liability
2. Legal entity separate from owners
3. Profit taxed once
4. Money borrowed can reduce taxes of owners

Disadvantages
1. Legal limits not tested in court
2. Salary and profits subject to social security and Medicare taxes (15.3%)
3. Stock easier to sell than membership in LLC

SOLE PROPRIETORSHIPS

If you plan a small, low risk private practice or you don't own many assets a sole proprietorship may be your best bet. It means a one-owner (or two spouses) operation. This is the business form chosen most often by new business owners and private practitioners.(4) The owner is responsible for all debts of the business and he or she reaps all its profits. Other than for initial questions and occasional problems, a lawyer is seldom needed. It's the least involved of the business structures under the least government control.(4) It's interesting to note that in 1995 of the nation's 501,000 attorneys, 281,000 filed taxes as sole proprietorships and another 134,000 filed as partnerships.(5) Nine out of ten attorney businesses are not organized as corporations.(5)

Starting a Sole Proprietorship

Anyone can start a proprietorship by simply stating that you are "open for business." Fill out a Form SS-4 to receive a Federal I.D. number, if you have employees. To conduct business in your area, you may need a local license, permit or Trade Name form filed. Otherwise, very little is required of you.(1) You should keep business records and bank accounts separate from personal records for tax purposes.

Taxes

At the end of the year, your tax advisor can help you fill out and file the appropriate forms that briefly list your income and expenses (schedule C), and arrive at a net profit or loss. The IRS will look closely at your deductions, and whether it appears you are actively pursuing your business or just trying to write off your purchases and travel.

As a sole owner, your profits are only taxed once as your personal income. The business profit is not taxed separately. A business loss can be deducted from any other income for that year. You will pay self-employment social security and Medicare taxes (15.3% on net income). If you have employees, you also will pay payroll taxes, worker's compensation, unemployment tax, fringe benefits, and so on.(1) A proprietor may invest in an IRA (Individual Retirement Account), KEOGH (HR-10 Pension Benefit Plan), ROTH IRA, or SEP (Simplified Employee Pension) to help reduce taxable income. Changes in tax laws happen yearly, so check with your accountant before filing taxes and regularly read business news.

Advantages

Most practitioners choose the sole proprietorship route in business because it's less expensive, less cumbersome, they like to have as much control as possible and have the option of making all the decisions. There are no partners or stockholders trying to lobby you, usurp your power or change the quality of service. If you do not like the way the secretarial service answers the phone or how your lawyer works with you--you make a change. This way of doing business can be very efficient and fast with only one person making the final decisions.

A sole proprietorship can offer a business owner the opportunity to have the freedom to act out dreams or wishes with only the obvious limitations of time, effort and money. At least no person is in the position of changing your company name or the way you counsel patients unless you allow him to do it.

Lawsuits can be minimized by being very careful and clear about all business agreements and by having them in writing. Also, by carrying malpractice and other liability insurance, litigation expenses and losses can be kept to a minimum. However, if you plan to have a business that publishes controversial exposés, manufactures a food or beverage, pursues large contracts, or in other ways handles large sums of money (or you personally own many assets) for peace of mind, the corporate structure that limits your liability may be more in order.

Disadvantages

The most obvious disadvantage to a sole proprietorship is the unlimited liability the owner must assume. An owner is personally liable for all the business' debts, its obligations and suits against it. People who have won a suit against you may claim your house, car, savings and other possessions. Additionally, your business assets are potentially at risk if you have personal debts that are unpaid. Malpractice insurance will cover you in a lawsuit against your professional nutrition practice, but not for your business ventures, financial responsibilities, judgments in community property states and unpaid bills.

Another disadvantage that many sole proprietors, especially women, experience is lack of credit. Credit can be difficult to attract both personally from lack of assets and for the business due to lack of track record and business experience. Limited credit makes it hard when an owner needs extra money to expand into a new office, publish a booklet, or cover the cash flow when a big creditor does not pay on time.(1)

A sole proprietorship's success is very dependent upon the abilities, energy and output of the owner. Most of us are not good at all business functions, so we must be willing to delegate. Also, if the owner gets sick or has personal problems that affect his work, the business usually suffers. Should the owner pass away, the enthusiasm and knowledge of how to conduct the enterprise usually goes with him unless continuation plans were developed to lead the family and employees through this time until the business is sold or it functions on its own with new management. If a sole proprietorship is sold, the new owner may take over the assets and contacts, but all the business bank accounts, licenses, federal taxpayer identification number, and state sales tax number have to be reestablished in the new owner's name.(6)

All fringe benefits are at the owner's expense, but at this time half the amount paid to social security and an escalating percentage of the cost of your health insurance are deductible.

PARTNERSHIPS

Two or more people may begin business as partners. The advantage of this type of arrangement is that one partner may complement the talents or resources of another. Another alternative to a partnership could be for one person to hire the other as a consultant or employee.

Increased financial investment, a broader base of expertise, or influential personal contacts is the ingredient needed. A partner may be a well-known person who will attract business. Legally, a partnership is a group of persons having a common business interest, each doing something to make the business succeed.(2) However, because of internal problems, our mobile society, and changing priorities, the average partnership only lasts eighteen months. (4)

Partners must get along well. They should be clearly able to do better as a team than they could separately. Partnerships take special understanding and a definite amount of patience. The biggest hurdles to work out are differences in value systems and expectations, lack of delineated of roles (partners step into each other's territory), and unequal contributions of start-up money (the major contributor may expect final say on all decisions).(2)

Successful partners often attribute their working relationships to the fact they first had talked about exactly how the business would run and what would be done "in case this happens" before the partnership was formed. Also, they had to accept that in many instances, the "good of the business" had to prevail over their own opinions.

A partnership agreement should always be put in writing with the aid of your lawyer. The agreement should describe the proposed business in detail and state the business name. It should tell: (1,2,4,5)
- What each partner's initial investment will be either in money or in other valuable consideration;
- The percentage ownership of each partner and how profits and losses will be divided;
- How much time each partner will give to the business;

- Who can sign the checks or if two signatures are required;
- Who can sign contracts, incur liabilities and sell assets;
- What each partner's functions, duties and powers are;
- How the business will be managed;
- What happens if a partner wants to get out;
- How a new partner can be admitted;
- Who will arbitrate if partners disagree;
- How the partnership can be dissolved;
- How the value of any partner's interest will be computed;
- What happens when a partner dies, divorces, goes bankrupt, becomes unable to function; and
- The size and nature of "key person life insurance policies" to be carried.

Financially, a partnership may be able to get bank loans more easily than a sole owner. Often this is true because the assets of two people instead of one are used to secure the loan.

The partnership must file a year-end tax return, but it doesn't pay taxes. The return is for information only, identifying each partner and showing her or his income and deductions from the partnership. The profit or loss is divided among the owners using pre-agreed upon percentages. Each partner must attach a copy of the partnership's tax return to his personal one and pay any due tax on the year's income.

Partnership Pitfalls (1,2,4,5)

1. To be recognized as a partner for tax purposes, a person must actually contribute money, time, reputation, or something else of value. A joint venture merely to share an office or expenses is not a partnership to the IRS.
2. Conversely, people may sometimes be liable as partners as determined by the IRS or courts because they functioned as partners.
3. Bookkeeping for a partnership can become complicated if the partners own different percentages or draw unequally for expenses.
4. Partnership income is passed through to each partner each year on paper even when the partnership decides to retain the profit for future expansion. Taxes may be owed on money that is never actually received.
5. A partnership is only as stable as its weakest member. Usually, it dissolves if a partner dies or withdraws, becomes insane or incompetent or goes bankrupt.
6. The riskiest drawback is that every partner can be held liable for

what the other partners do. This means that one partner binds the others when she or he signs a contract or check. If one partner causes an accident, all can be sued. If one partner is dishonest, all may be prosecuted.

Partnership Buy-Sell Agreement (2)

In case a partner wants to leave the business, a pre-agreed upon Buy-Sell Agreement could help make the dissolution easier. Negotiate this agreement when the partnership is formed. The agreement should include the following points:
- A formula to determine the value of the business at the time of a sellout, taking into account initial contributions by each partner, assets, debts, and goodwill generated since the business start up.
- Terms governing the sale--for example, monthly payments over a 5-year period at ten percent interest.
- Provisions in the event of death of a partner to protect the survivors against the estate of the deceased. In many states families can demand that the business assets be liquidated in order to get their inheritance. To cope with the added expense of one less person running the business, partners should consider carrying life insurance on each other.
- An agreement should be made up front before it ever becomes necessary to determine how deadlocked negotiations can be resolved--probably through arbitration.

Limited Partnerships

If a limited partnership is formed, the "limited partners" have no personal liability for business debts or the acts of their partners. To have a limited partnership, there must be at least one "general" partner who is legally responsible for all business indebtedness and the acts of all general partners. A primary drawback to using a limited partnership, depending upon how you look at it, is the requirement that limited partners can't play an active role in the management of the business or the partnership affairs. Limited partnerships are used most often when the partners want to have some of the advantages of a corporation (limited liability) but pay income taxes as a partnership.(1)

CORPORATIONS

A corporation is a legal form of business granted by states. A corporation can be created from a new business or an already existing one (a sole proprietorship or partnership). The corporate structure (C, S, and LLC forms) is the second most common business form in America.

Incorporated businesses generate over eighty-eight percent of total U.S. profits.(7)

A corporation is a legal entity separate from its owners with its own property, debts and responsibilities. Even though shareholders may own the corporate stock, they do not owe on the bills, unless they helped secure loans with personal assets or with personal loans. As a shareholder, your personal property is not at risk for your business debts.(1)

State laws govern corporations and they differ on the specifics, but generally a corporation is formed by filing articles of incorporation, along with paying a fee to the Secretary of State of any state in the United States. Each state's records are checked to make sure that no one else is using your proposed business name, and the incorporation forms are checked for completeness. If all is well, you will automatically be sent a charter.

The new corporation then issues shares of its total issue of stock.(4) In a closely held corporation, only the owner's family and friends own shares. No shares are sold to others, so control of the business is maintained. Selling shares is one way to generate capital to run the business but because it dilutes control and can complicate business as you grow, many advisors recommend trying to borrow the money first. People who buy your stock take a chance that the corporation will be successful, and they don't have to be paid back if it's a failure.

The corporation name must include one of the three following words: "Inc.," "Corp." or "Ltd." It's required so that others will know they are doing business with a corporation.(1)

It's important that a business owner seek legal advice when planning to incorporate. It's possible to incorporate your business yourself. However, if you are sued or audited and the appropriate records and have not been filed or filled out, it could be far more costly to remedy. Fees charged by lawyers to incorporate a business can vary from $800 to $3500; check around to find the best fee for service. For a smaller fee, there are legal firms on the Internet that will file the forms for you. However, they may offer limited business advice that may be too general in nature for your needs, but it's an option. The more you know about corporations, the more you can do for yourself; seek out information.

Corporate Advantages

Some advantages of a closely held C or "full" corporation: (1,3)
- Owners risk only the money they put into their corporation. It can go broke, and the owners can stay solvent.

- The corporation generally has greater borrowing power than other business structures. More frequently however, banks have been asking for loans to be secured by shareholders' personal assets as well.
- A shareholder can transfer his part ownership to someone else instantly by selling it, giving or bequeathing his stock certificates.
- Corporate executives can deduct many expenses from their gross income that probably can't be deducted as a sole proprietor, for example the full cost of health insurance can be deducted and only half the deduction for social security is taken out of the executive's pay. The corporation pays the other half.
- If an executive or any employee lives on company premises "for the convenience of the corporation", he need not pay anything for it, as well as for company-supplied food, vehicle, and so on.
- Fringe benefits can be better in terms of pension plans, profit sharing and stock purchase plans.

Corporate Disadvantages (1,3)

- Incorporation is more costly--both to begin and maintain (fees, bookkeeping, records, holding mandatory meetings, and electing directors).
- Corporate income is taxed twice--first on its profits, and then share-holders pay tax on the distributed dividends.
- Owners can't write off corporate losses on their personal income tax, nor deduct personal loans or expansion money given to the corpo-ration when it's short of cash.
- Many banks and businesses will not accept a corporate signature on a loan without a personal guarantee by one or more of the exec-utives.
- An executive's salary must be "reasonable" in the IRS's eyes or it may be disallowed as a business expense.
- Shareholders may sue a director if his incompetence or misdeeds cause the corporation to lose money.
- Some states tax corporations more heavily than individuals.
- If corporate stock is offered to the public, the corporations must conform to the complicated rules of the Securities and Exchange Commission (SEC).
- Business structure is more difficult to change if your business needs change.

S Corporation Election

If a corporation has fewer than seventy-five shareholders and meets other specifications, an "S Corporation," offered by the federal government for small businesses, should be considered unless you live in California and other states that do not recognize Subchapter S Corporations. It offers the same limitation on liability as a "full" corporation, but like the sole proprietorship and partnership, the business itself pays no income tax. All profits or losses become part of the individual's personal income tax responsibility. Benefits are also slightly different from a full corporation, so talk to your attorney and accountant about the pros and cons for you. Many private practitioners have been advised to choose this business form. For more information, contact the IRS and request IRS publication 589.

Limited Liability Corporation (LLC) or Limited Liability Partnership (LLP)

The Limited Liability Company (LLC) or Limited Liability Partnership (LLP) for professional organizations is rapidly becoming a very popular business form in those states that offer the option. An LLC files "articles of organization" with the state and is governed by an operating agreement that's comparable to a partnership agreement.(5) Some states will allow only one person to form an LLC and others require at least two persons. This form of business structure is similar to a limited partnership or S corporation in that earnings or deductions are passed on to shareholders in proportion to their ownership.(5,6) LLCs limit your personal liabilities for business debt or losses. It's a fairly new structure and it has not been proven in court whether it protects as well as a corporation. You can buy books on how to form your own LLC or go on line and have a legal firm file it for you. Again, the drawback here is too little individualized advice.

Final Words on Corporations

Dietitians, as members of the health care professions are being advised to think seriously about some form of incorporation for their businesses because of the interest in suing health care professionals. If a practitioner chooses this route, it's important to emphasize that all business and contracts should be done in the corporate name. This will establish that it's the corporation doing the work. Also, try to secure loans with only corporate assets.

CONCLUSION

It's not necessary to become overly concerned about areas of business that are completely unfamiliar to you. There are many resources and advisors to offer help. You will know more with every discussion and decision you make. Rest assured also, once a decision has been made on the business structure, it can be changed, if it needs to be with some additional effort and money. Nothing is forever "cast in stone."

REFERENCES

1. Lowry A. *How To Become Financially Successful by Owning Your Own Business.* New York: Simon and Schuster; 1981.
2. Shyne D. In Business: From Friendship to Partnership. *Working Woman;* August 1983: 48-49.
3. 2000 Dallas/Ft. Worth Small Business Resource Guide. SBA; 2000.
4. Curtin R. *Running Your Own Show.* New York: New American Library; 1985.
5. Edwards P, Edwards S. *Working From Home.* New York: Penguin Putnam; 1999.
6. Eckert WK, Sartorius AG, Warda M. *How to Form Your Own Corporation,* 3rd ed. Naperville, IL: Sphinx Publishing; 2001.

Chapter 12

Protecting Your Ideas and Interests

Business owners want to know how to keep others from taking their ideas and how to protect their property from lawsuits. The best means of protection are copyrights, patents, trademarks and insurance, but there are many other options, including written agreements, personal discretion and incorporation.

With time and experience, the ability to "read" an individual or situation and evaluate the risk involved will come easily. Through contacts and networking over the years and your own savvy, the development of ideas will become relatively non-fearful.

PUBLIC DOMAIN

A distinction needs to be made about what kinds of ideas can be protected legally or claimed for ownership. Any new and original literary, graphic, audio, mechanical, video, process series, or ingredient may be protected as belonging to an individual or company. All "common knowledge" and non-unique items are in the "public domain." They can't be the sole property of any one person or business. Examples of common items are the words "food", "juice", and "nutritionist", the Food Guide Pyramid, other government materials and program ideas, and the common medical diets (although unique manuals can be copyrighted that use this information). Everyone can use all items in the "public domain."

HAVE IT IN WRITING

To avoid confusion and lawsuits, the best advice is not to assume anything about even a simple agreement; discuss it thoroughly and have it in writing and signed by the parties involved. Initially, use lawyers to look over all agreements and later use their services, especially on all risky, important and costly agreements. No one should start a job "on good faith" unless you are willing not to collect for the services.

PERSONAL DISCRETION

Many good creative ideas become public property because the originator of the idea talked about it indiscreetly. Exceptionally different and quality ideas are of great value personally, also financially, and should be treated as such. Obviously, in the development of your ideas, consultants or professional advisors may need to be involved, but there is better recourse if any of these individuals take an idea. Business people will tell you the best way to avoid being fearful in business is to work with only ethical, honest people who come highly recommended or ones you have checked out through references.

If an original idea must be discussed with a company or individual you don't know, have a trusted acquaintance present who could witness the conversation, or ask to tape record the session, or ask that a Nondisclosure Agreement be signed (see Figure 12.1). If handled tactfully, no one will be embarrassed or threatened by the precautions. You usually do not need written protection to speak with advisors like bankers, Small Business Administration (SCORE, ACE) and other professional small business advisors.

TRADE SECRETS AND INTELLECTUAL PROPERTY

Trade secrets and intellectual property are ideas and materials that make the business unique. A trade secret may be protected by not telling anyone about it, which may hinder its usefulness, or by having nondisclosure agreements. Intellectual property may be protected through copyrights, trademarks or patents.

Copyrights

Copyrights are issued by the U.S. Copyright Office for intellectual property: books and pamphlets for new diet programs with original elements that have not been used before and for other artistic, musical, dramatic, audiovisual, choreographic, or literary creations. Ownership of copyright exists when the work is completed in any tangible form regardless of the date of registration.(1) The copyright notice should appear on all published works distributed to the public. The use of the copyright notice is the responsibility of the copyright owner and does not require permission from the Copyright Office.

The copyright law grants copyright owners certain exclusive rights to their works, including the rights of reproduction and of public performance. Only copyright owners have the right to make or authorize copies of educational materials, slides, articles, or videotapes and to show their videos publicly.(2) An owner may grant

Figure 12.1 Sample Nondisclosure Agreement

NONDISCLOSURE AGREEMENT

_____ agrees to maintain the confidentiality of all proprietary information and trade secrets concerning Diet Chefs, Inc., or Diet Chefs, Inc.'s products, services and printed information of which he or she becomes aware. This obligation of confidentiality shall survive the termination of this Agreement.

Agreed and Accepted: Diet Chef, Inc.

_____   _____

_____   _____
Date   Date

---

permission to others for limited use of one or more of these exclusive rights. Some owners will charge a fee, while others will allow free use.

The copyright term is effective for the life of the author and fifty years after the author's death. Works created for hire, and certain anonymous and pseudonymous works can be copyrighted for seventy-five years from publication or 100 years from creation, whichever is shorter.

The notice should be on copies of the work in an obvious location to give reasonable notice of the claim of copyright. The required copyright generally consists of three elements.

- The first is the © symbol, the word "Copyright", or "Copr."
- the second is the year of publication, and
- the third is the name of the copyright owner.

An example of a typical copyright is "Copyright 2003 Nutrition Daily."

In books, pamphlets and other publications, a printed reminder is usually added that states, "This material may not be copied or reproduced in any manner without the written permission of the copyright owner." Lawyers who specialize in copyright law suggest that newly published material with the copyright notice be sent to someone out of state by certified mail. The postage receipt will show when the copyright was first used. In case of a copyright dispute, the documented date may prove to be significant.

Copyright forms and information may be obtained by writing: Register of Copyrights, Copyright Office, Library of Congress, Washington 20559 or a local federally authorized library, or calling (202) 707-3000 (for information) or (202) 707-9100 (order forms) (http://lcweb.loc.gov/copyright/). The copyright application filing fee is $20 plus several copies of the completed work. The registration process will take about 16 weeks and copyright registration is effective the date that all the necessary items (application, fee, and samples) are received in the Copyright Office. The form is simple enough for most persons to fill out. It's highly recommended that you register your copyright within three months of going public with the copyrighted material. (See Figure 12.2 Sample Copyright Application.)

As the copyright owner, you, not the government, are responsible for protecting the use of the copyrighted material. If the copyright is abused, you or your lawyer can send a "cease and desist" order to the infringing person or organization to ask that use be stopped. Going to court is costly, but it can be used as a last resort. If you sue someone for unauthorized infringement and you win, you may be awarded statutory damages and attorney's fees or an additional $50,000 over actual damages and profit .(3)

As an example of how a copyright infringement can be handled, one nutritionist found out that one of her contract OB-GYN clinics was photocopying her copyrighted prenatal brochure and handing it out to all new patients. She made an appointment to discuss the situation with the clinic director. She stated that her contract agreement did not allow uncontrolled use of her copyrighted materials. The clinic agreed to purchase the brochures at a bulk rate of $1 each with 500 brochures being the minimum order.

Other ways to discourage misuse of your copyrighted material include the use of:
- odd size paper that does not easily fit on a photocopier,
- blue or brown ink that does not photocopy well, and
- the new paper and inks that do not reproduce at all on a photocopier.

Formerly employed dietitians are usually in a quandary about ownership of materials and programs they developed while employed. Lawyers agree that if you were paid as an employee when you developed the copyrighted materials for your employer, and if you do not have another prearranged agreement, the employer owns them. A former employer, however, can't keep you from practicing your profession or using your expertise, so you can create different materials on the same subject. If want to develop unique materials to use at work, and you want to own the copyright, do the work on your own time and

Figure 12.2 Application for Registration of a Copyright

FORM TX
For a Literary Work
UNITED STATES COPYRIGHT OFFICE

REGISTRATION NUMBER

_____

TX _____ TXU _____
EFFECTIVE DATE OF REGISTRATION

_____

Month _____ Day _____ Year _____

DO NOT WRITE ABOVE THIS LINE. IF YOU NEED MORE SPACE, USE A SEPARATE CONTINUATION SHEET.

1 TITLE OF THIS WORK ▼

_____

PREVIOUS OR ALTERNATIVE TITLES ▼

_____

PUBLICATION AS A CONTRIBUTION If this work was published as a contribution to a periodical, serial, or collection, give information about the collective work in which the contribution appeared.   **Title of Collective Work ▼**

If published in a periodical or serial give: Volume ▼ _____ Number ▼ _____ Issue Date ▼ _____ On Pages ▼ _____

2 **a** NAME OF AUTHOR ▼

DATES OF BIRTH AND DEATH
Year Born ▼   Year Died ▼

Was this contribution to the work a "work made for hire"?
☐ Yes
☐ No

AUTHOR'S NATIONALITY OR DOMICILE
Name of Country
OR { Citizen of ▶ _____
Domiciled in ▶ _____

WAS THIS AUTHOR'S CONTRIBUTION TO THE WORK
Anonymous?   ☐ Yes ☐ No
Pseudonymous? ☐ Yes ☐ No
If the answer to either of these questions is "Yes," see detailed instructions.

NATURE OF AUTHORSHIP Briefly describe nature of material created by this author in which copyright is claimed. ▼

NOTE

Under the law, the "author" of a "work made for hire" is generally the employer, not the employee (see instructions). For any part of this work that was "made for hire" check "Yes" in the space provided, give the employer (or other person for whom the work was prepared) as "Author" of that part, and leave the space for dates of birth and death blank.

b NAME OF AUTHOR ▼

DATES OF BIRTH AND DEATH
Year Born ▼   Year Died ▼

Was this contribution to the work a "work made for hire"?
☐ Yes
☐ No

AUTHOR'S NATIONALITY OR DOMICILE
Name of Country
OR { Citizen of ▶ _____
Domiciled in ▶ _____

WAS THIS AUTHOR'S CONTRIBUTION TO THE WORK
Anonymous?   ☐ Yes ☐ No
Pseudonymous? ☐ Yes ☐ No
If the answer to either of these questions is "Yes," see detailed instructions.

NATURE OF AUTHORSHIP Briefly describe nature of material created by this author in which copyright is claimed. ▼

c NAME OF AUTHOR ▼

DATES OF BIRTH AND DEATH
Year Born ▼   Year Died ▼

Was this contribution to the work a "work made for hire"?
☐ Yes
☐ No

AUTHOR'S NATIONALITY OR DOMICILE
Name of Country
OR { Citizen of ▶ _____
Domiciled in ▶ _____

WAS THIS AUTHOR'S CONTRIBUTION TO THE WORK
Anonymous?   ☐ Yes ☐ No
Pseudonymous? ☐ Yes ☐ No
If the answer to either of these questions is "Yes," see detailed instructions.

NATURE OF AUTHORSHIP Briefly describe nature of material created by this author in which copyright is claimed. ▼

3 **a** YEAR IN WHICH CREATION OF THIS WORK WAS COMPLETED   This information must be given ◄ Year in all cases.

b DATE AND NATION OF FIRST PUBLICATION OF THIS PARTICULAR WORK
Complete this information Month ▶ _____ Day ▶ _____ Year ▶ _____
ONLY if this work has been published.   ◄ Nation

4 COPYRIGHT CLAIMANT(S) Name and address must be given even if the claimant is the same as the author given in space 2. ▼

APPLICATION RECEIVED

ONE DEPOSIT RECEIVED

TWO DEPOSITS RECEIVED

REMITTANCE NUMBER AND DATE

DO NOT WRITE HERE OFFICE USE ONLY

See instructions before completing this space.

TRANSFER If the claimant(s) named here in space 4 is (are) different from the author(s) named in space 2, give a brief statement of how the claimant(s) obtained ownership of the copyright. ▼

MORE ON BACK ▶ • Complete all applicable spaces (numbers 5-11) on the reverse side of this page
  • See detailed instructions   • Sign the form at line 10.

DO NOT WRITE HERE
Page 1 of _____ pages

at your own expense. This assumes you have not signed an agreement giving your employer rights to all your ideas while employed (common in Research & Development).

If you want to use reprints or copies of other persons' copyrighted material, articles, newspaper stories, and so on, you should request permission first. (See Copyright Release Form in Figure 12.3.)

COMMON QUESTIONS: USING COPYRIGHTED MATERIAL

I recently purchased several videotapes on exercise at the store. Can I show them during my group weight loss class at the hospital?
No. The exemption allowing teachers to show videotapes in the classroom applies only to nonprofit educational institutions, such as K-12, colleges and universities (section 110) (1).

When I give lectures, I show slides of charts and cartoons from books and the newspaper. Is this legal?
No, although it is often done, it is not legal without permission from the copyright owner. Photographs in books and magazines are protected by copyrights, just like the written material (section 102) (2).

My public library has books on nutrition. May I photocopy from them?
Yes, but only small portions may be copied. The library photocopying exception to the copyright law allows an individual to make a single copy of one article from a magazine or one chapter from a book owned by a public library , provided the copy is made only for the personal use of the individual (section 108) (2).

I live in a small town and I am sure no one will know whether I have the permission of the copyright owner to photocopy her educational materials in a book from Aspen Publishers. Aspen can't give me permission---I've already called. Why should I write for permission?
By using the material without permission, you are stealing or trespassing on the owner's rights. Infringement of copyright can result either in a civil lawsuit brought by the copyright owner and/or criminal lawsuit brought by the U.S. government, which carries heavy fines and possible prison sentence (2). Do you really want to risk getting caught when it's so easy to write? You can find publishers' addresses at the library and The American Dietetic Association will help you contact any dietitian.

Figure 12.3

SAMPLE REQUEST TO REPRINT COPYRIGHTED MATERIAL

Date

Dear

    I am preparing an educational exercise and nutrition booklet for the patients at the Medical Treatment Center, Garland, Texas. May I please have your permission to include the following:

Table 4-2 Fun Ways to Add Exercise to Your Day In: Johnson P. Exercise for the Weak at Heart. New York: Brown & Co.; 2003.

    Unless you indicate otherwise, I will use the following credit line:

Use by permission. Copyright 2003 Brown & Co.

    I would greatly appreciate your consent to this request. For your convenience, a release statement is found below. Please sign and return this letter to me. A second copy has been included for your files.

Permission is hereby granted for the use requested above.

_____   _____

Name   Date

Sincerely,

Jan Jones, R.D.
101 Harland Street
Garland, TX 75075

What if I write and I never hear back, or the owner wants me to pay $100 for the rights?

Do not use the copyrighted work unless you have written permission (keep the letters on file) and you pay whatever fee is charged. There may also be other restrictions, such as the number of copies, or size of the group or whatever.

I have a chart I want to use in my handouts for a seminar I teach. There isn't any author's name on it, and I tried contacting the person who gave it to me-she doesn't know who the original author is either. What can I do?

Document your efforts to find ownership of the chart and file it for future reference. You will have it in case the owner ever appears and you need to show you tried to find him or her. After the fact, ask the person for proof of his or her ownership and if you still want to use the chart, ask permission. If he or she gives permission, add the copyright information to the sheet. Pay any agreed upon fee.

Trademarks

The U.S. Patent and Trademark Office issues trademarks to provide national recognition of a name, logo or phrase that symbolizes certain products or services. Examples of common product trademarks include: Coca Cola ®, Kleenex ® and Crayola ®. When a trademark stands for a service offered by a business instead of a product, it is referred to as a "service mark." Examples of common service marks include: the logo of The American Dietetic Association, McDonald's name and Prudential's rock.

A trade or commercial name is a business name used to identify a partnership, company or other organization-it's not eligible to become a trademark. Incorporation of the business will protect the company name from use by others in the original state and where the business legally expands its markets. There is no provision in the trademark law for the registration of trade names used merely to identify a business. However, you can control your name if it's written or spelled in an unusual manner or it's in artwork created to stand for your company.(4) For example, Entrepreneur Business Group is a company name and it's product Entrepreneur Magazine is trademarked.

Before filing an application, a search of trademarks should be made in the Search Room of the Trademark Examining Operation located in the Crystal Plaza Building No.2, 2011 Jefferson Davis Highway, Arlington, Virginia. Any trademark that is too similar to one already filed will not be accepted for registration. The search can be conducted by any individual. Trademark lawyers have contacts with companies who can do the research for a fee. You can also call the Chamber of Commerce in

Arlington, Virginia, and get the names of several trademark search companies that will research a trademark for around $50-100. Applications and more information can be obtained from the Patent and Trademark Office, Arlington, VA 22202 or call (800) 786-9199 or (703) 308-9000 (Hotline) or (703) 308-4357 or go online (www.uspto.gov). (5)

To establish rights to a trademark, you file a trademark application with three copies of the mark as it's actually used in commerce along with the $245 fee for each class of goods. The term of the trademark registration is twenty years from the date of issue, and it may be renewed at the end of each twenty-year term as long as the mark is still used in commerce. (2) In order for a trademark to maintain its protection, it must be used.(6)

Once a registration is issued, you may give notice of registration by using the ® circle symbol, or the phrase "Registered Trademark." Although registration symbols may not be used prior to registration, it's recommended that trademark owners use a ™ or "SM" (for service mark) to indicate claim of ownership until the application for a federally registered mark is finally approved. (5,6,7)

Trademark rights are protected under common law; in other words, the mark belongs to the first user as soon as it's used in commerce, whether or not it's ever registered. However, registering a trademark does have its advantages: it shows official claim of ownership and exclusive right to use the mark on the goods mentioned in the registration. There is no time limitation on when an application for registering a trademark can be filed.

The owner of the trademark, not the government, is responsible for protecting the mark from being used by others. If you are going to go to the trouble and expense of trademarking a name, make it distinctive, as well as meaningful. Words in the public domain like "juice" and "food" are too common to be given a trademark. If the words are too common, either the trademark will not be granted or you will be in court all the time trying to keep other people from using the words. It's not worth it.

Business owners claim that trademarks are often more effective than patents because trademarks hold up in court, are less expensive to obtain, are transferable, and they last for the lifetime of the company. (6)

Patents

Patents are issued to inventors to help protect inventions from being used without the inventor's permission. To be patented, an invention must have a useful purpose for existing and it must have some new, never before patented element that makes it unique. A new patent can be issued on a new process, machine, composition of matter, or any new and useful improvements on an old patent.

A patent is effective for seventeen years. Thereafter the invention is considered to be in the "public domain" and anyone can use it. Because of this fact, some inventors decide not to patent a product that can't be easily duplicated so that they own it exclusively. The owners of Coca Cola chose not to patent their product many years ago so the formula (which was only recently disclosed) would remain a company trade secret. The President of A&W Root Beer once explained that their product didn't have any proprietary protection (patent) in the market-except for its image and reputation-and the fact people loved the root beer served in the frosty mugs.

Patent claims and/or designs must be researched either at the Patent Office or at one of the federally designated libraries across the United States. A search will tell you what claims have already been issued on similar patents. You may have to alter your product's claims after you conduct a search. A search by a lawyer will range from $500-$3500 or more depending upon the complexity of the item researched. There are inventors groups in your Yellow Pages and through other sources like the Internet that will do searches for you for about $500+, but you should thoroughly check out any firm first before using it. Trying to do a patent search on your own often proves to be a waste of time.

What does it take to patent the new product you've dreamed up? "Persistence and perseverance," says patent attorney Ken Schaefer.(4) The patenting process can be costly and lengthy, too. Filing cost ranges from $355 to $710, and the lawyer's time may add another $1,000 to $5,000 or more. If there are designs and intricate circuitry, you may need an engineer for the drawings. An attorney's legal fees for a court dispute can mount to the tens of thousands of dollars. (6) Once you get a "notice of allowance," which means your patent has been approved you have to pay an "issue fee" of up to $620. The entire process takes at least twenty months. Even with all that time and money involved, the Patent and Trademark Office issues about 1,400 patents every week, but they esti-mate only 5% of all patents are ever developed for market. More infor-mation and an application can be obtained from the Patent and Trademark Office, Washington, D.C. 20231 or forms can be downloaded directly from www.uspto.gov/web/forms/.

INSURANCE

Insurance was originally devised as a means of spreading the risk of having bad luck through a group instead of being shouldered by one individual. It has always been common to insure material possessions, but when starting a private practice, insurance to pay salary in case of disability and malpractice insurance are recommended. The costs of malpractice and office insurance premiums are deductible as business expenses.

Malpractice insurance is available to cover the high cost of legal representation and the high incidence of threatened and actual lawsuits against not only physicians but all persons who come in contact with the patient.

Disability insurance pays income when the insured person becomes ill or disabled and is not able to work up to capacity. It's suggested for sole supported, self-employed people because they aren't eligible for worker's compensation, unemployment benefits, or sick time, except through programs set up by their own company. Social Security disability insurance requires six months of no income before payments can begin. No income for an extended period could mean loss of the business as well as personal property. It's sometimes difficult to qualify for disability insurance if you have a business based out of your home, so if you work or consult somewhere else, highlight that location for disability insurance purposes.

Office insurance should include fire, theft and liability coverage. This coverage is common and can usually be obtained from a practitioner's existing home insurance company. Office coverage is necessary because many medical buildings' insurance policies don't cover tenants' furnishings, possessions, loss of business, or visitors' accidents. When working out of your home, it's still necessary to carry extra insurance for times when clients visit and to cover your computer and other office equipment.

Auto insurance on business-owned vehicles is common and necessary. In case of an accident involving the business car, the liability coverage should be especially good because the public believes that a business has more assets and the possibility of a lawsuit after an accident may be greater. The cost of the coverage is comparable to personal auto insurance, unless younger members of the family or persons with poor driving records are allowed to drive the car.

INCORPORATION

Many persons choose to incorporate their businesses to reduce the risk of losing their personal property for business dealings. A corporation is a complete, legal entity separate from its shareholders with its own assets. If all business is conducted in the corporate name and under its umbrella, the corporation's assets alone are at jeopardy for the business's failures and lawsuits (see Chapter 11 for more information).

HOW MUCH RISK IS THERE?

Starting a business venture is not a risk-free endeavor. In fact, it requires an individual to constantly be confronted with numerous important decisions, to initiate new untried ideas, to counsel patients on medical-related nutrition programs, and risk financial loss.

The best ways to protect oneself are:
- to be ethical,
- to ask advice of people who are successful in business,
- to make well thought out decisions,
- to document all important agreements and client visits in writing, and
- to learn from experience.

Most people who have been in business for some time suggest that a person take reasonable precautionary measures and then go on with business and living.

BUSINESS QUESTIONS

Q: I have a consulting business where I contract with several medical clinics to offer patient consults. Our agreements are in writing. A year ago I subcontracted with a local dietitian to cover a clinic and we had a written agreement with a noncompete clause. For the past year, she continued to cover the account and I received a percentage of her income. Now the clinic wants her to work there as an employee without my involvement. The clinic and dietitian have asked me to walk away without any compensation. Do I have any rights here? Should I just walk away?

A: Of course you have rights! You need to show your written agreements to a good small business lawyer and ask what your options are. Depending upon what your noncompete clause says, most people would agree the dietitian (or the clinic) should compensate you for giving up the clinic account to the other dietitian. If your agreements are valid and binding, I would allow your lawyer to negotiate an agreement in a meeting with the clinic business manager or director and the other dietitian. If your agreements are vague or not easily defended in court, you may have to walk away because the cost of legal action and the negative energy to you may not be worth it.

Q: A year and a half ago I subcontracted with a dietitian to cover my private practice several days each week while I pursued my master degree. We had a verbal agreement, and she was paid for each patient instruction. There was never any question that she was an independent contractor who was responsible for her own taxes and benefits. At the end of the year, I gave her a 1099 Miscellaneous Income form to file with her income taxes. Two months ago, we had a falling out over a billing issue and I let her go. To my surprise, she went and filed for unemployment benefits as an employee who was fired. The case is pending, but I may lose. What can I do?

A: Whoa! Don't you wish the agreement had been in writing? You, of course, need to see a lawyer with employer/employee rights experience. The fact that you gave the dietitian a Form 1099 will help, but there are other criteria the IRS uses to determine if a person is an independent contractor or employee--no matter what you two had agreed (see Chapter 14). The main guidelines involve whether you gave her special training or she came in with the required knowledge; whether you determined when she would work and where or she made her own schedule; and whether she only worked for you or she marketed herself and her business to other accounts. Your lawyer will advise you about the criteria your state unemployment office uses.

As you can tell, there are many gray areas. You may be surprised to hear your lawyer say to not admit guilt but settle instead of fighting. Unfortunately, many cases are solved that way because the cost of legal action may be more than the cost of the settlement. Try to stay calm and rational, you both knew what you had agreed, but you need to keep an open mind at this point and determine how to minimize your loss--both in legal fees and potential settlement. Good Luck!

(These answers should not be construed as legal advice. They are presented to describe potential business situations that practitioners may be confronted with in normal business dealings.)

REFERENCES

1. Dukelow RH. The Library Copyright Guide. *Quilting;* August 1991.
2. Sitarz D. *The Desktop Publisher's Legal Handbook.* Chicago, IL: NOVA Publishing; 1990.
3. Helm K. *Becoming an Entrepreneur in Your Own Setting,* Study Kit #3. Chicago, IL: The American Dietetic Association; 1991.
4. Have you built a better mousetrap? *Family Circle;* August 15, 1989.
5. Edwards P, Edwards S. *Working From Home.* New York: Penguin Putnam; 1999.
6. *The Small Business Encyclopedia: Vol. II.* Irvine, CA: Entrepreneur Magazine Group; 1996.
7. Sobel M. *The 12-Hour MBA Program.* Paramus, NJ: Prentice Hall; 1993.

Chapter 13

Choosing Your Business Advisors

Olga Satterwhite, RD and updated by Kathy King, RD

Now that your business venture is developed on paper, you need to evaluate who will make up your team of mentors and professional advisors. You could go it alone. However, to give yourself a better shot at success, create an informal network of advisors you can turn to when you need them. You may be surprised to discover how many people are willing to help you--if you seek them out.

Business authors Sarah and Paul Edwards tell of a sales trainer who needed more information to develop her business, and she noticed a course available at UCLA. She didn't have time to take the course, so she hired the instructor to give her a series of private instructions. The instructor became an important mentor and introduced her to many business prospects.(1)

A team of advisors could include a lawyer, accountant, banker, insurance agent, business consultant, and a marketing, advertising, investment counselor or public relations consultant. You will benefit from each profession's expertise and learn different perspectives on the same issues. These advisors will evaluate your business, its liability, marketability, and legalities.

In their column "Working Smarter" in Home Office Computing magazine, the Edwards' give a few steps to attract benefactors (1):

1. Go to the source. Go to the best. Go to the people who are clearly authorities. If they can't help you, they may know people who are even better for you to know.
2. Ask specific questions. Many mentors and advisors will want to help, but only if it appears that you have done your homework first.
3. Be willing to pay. Most people take it as a compliment when you ask for their help. But if what you need requires more than a short phone conversation or taking them to lunch, offer to pay for their expertise. Certainly, asking lawyers and accountants for advice on your business will cost you

when they work on your business. A private consultation with an expert shouldn't cost more than $50 to $150 per hour. With the right expert, it will pay for itself many times.

4. Accept and try their advice. Of course, evaluate whether it fits your needs, but if it fits, put in enough effort to see if the idea works. Or, be willing to explain why you didn't try it.

5. Express appreciation. Most people like being appreciated, that's one of the reasons they help each other. A phone call, note or thoughtful gift can go a long way in building a relationship. Also, let your benefactors know they can call on you if they need to.

6. Pass on good advice. Establish yourself as a resource for others, someone others can turn to. You'll be amazed at the doors it will open for you.

LOCATING PROFESSIONAL ADVISORS

When seeking good professional guidance, obtain several different names of highly recommended specialists. Ask for referrals from your friends, other small business owners and the Small Business Administration.(2) Look for names of recommended professional consultants or free advisors from SCORE (Service Corps of Retired Executives) who have experience setting up and working with small businesses.

Be specific in what you are looking for. Remember too that you interview the consultant. They work for you, so don't be intimidated and feel you must hire or work with the first person you interview. Consider the following questions as guidelines when discussing a paid business consultant's services and her or his suitability for your practice:

1. What is the consultant's experience in your area of business--a divorce lawyer or large corporate banker or accountant will not fit your needs?

2. What specific services does the consultant propose for your practice?

3. Approximately how much will you be charged? If it will be on an hourly basis, obtain an estimate of how many hours the consultant feels your practice will take.

4. Will phone calls be charged? Although fees are important, be aware that bargain rates sometimes get you bargain services.

5. Does the professional advisor have the time to give you? Will you get both adequate advice and reasonable turn-around times on contracted work?

The better you know your needs, or the more work you can do for yourself, the less you have to pay someone else. Before you commit yourself to a specific consultant, ask yourself:

- Was I comfortable?
- Did the advisor seem interested in me and my practice?

Keep records of all correspondence with a contract consultant. Follow up any telephone conversations with a letter reiterating any points you feel uneasy about or that you feel were important to highlight. Keep a copy of the letter for yourself. Don't assume anything about an agreement---always ask! Change to another consultant and transfer your records if you are unhappy with the work you receive. As a rule, don't hire family and professional friends to do your work because it is so hard to fire them when the job isn't done right or on time.

Learn how to use each consultant's expertise to your best advantage. Talking with other business owners and professionals will help supplement the research and reading you must do before going into private practice.

ATTORNEY

Look for an attorney you can trust with reasonable fees. Trust means you believe the attorney can do the job, is competent, and cares about helping you.(3) Finding the right person can be a real challenge.

The legal fee quoted to you may be misleading. Often, the lawyer with the lowest hourly rate is not always the lowest total bill, especially if the attorney is not familiar with the legal problems of your type of business. An attorney may spend a lot of time at your expense learning what to do. Legal services are the last of the "cottage industries," meaning that each item is custom made-usually from preformed documents on software.(3) There is a great deal of discretion involved as an attorney does his or her job, so take the time to find a good one who takes your business seriously and has the time to work for you.

On matters such as suing or counter-suing, obtain a second (independent) decision before pursuing it. Make sure that you agree with the language and possible consequences of any legal action before you let your lawyer take action in your name. You have to live with the results. Once you consider all sides, the costs and probable outcome, you may decide to walk away.

Good legal advice at the beginning of your practice can prevent problems in years to come. A lawyer will help you understand regulations and licenses. He or she can write or look over all your contracts or letters of agreement. Most importantly, a lawyer will help you develop the appropriate structure for your practice--sole proprietorship, partnership, LLC, full or S corporation. A lawyer can help you copyright materials, trademark your business logo, or patent a product. Attorney fees range from $100 per hour in smaller communities up to $300 per hour or more for specialized work. They usually charge for phone calls.

ACCOUNTANT

Accountants are divided into two groups: those who are Certified Public Accountants (CPAs) and those who are not certified. States award certification and verify the recipient has completed a two-year apprenticeship under a CPA. The person must pass a series of difficult tests in the areas of auditing, accounting, theory, and business law. CPAs are accountants with an assured high level of skill; however, other accountants may be highly qualified, but not certified. In most states, a bookkeeper is not required to meet any standards to use the title, but he or she may be knowledgeable and perfectly matched for your business. The main thing you need is someone with practical small business experience and that person is hard to find!

As you look for an accountant or bookkeeper, ask other business people whom they use. Your best source of information is a satisfied customer.

Your accountant should help structure your practice to your best tax advantage. He or she will be valuable in helping choose a book-keeping or record system that will fit your needs. If the system is set up correctly and simply, you should be able to do the bookkeeping yourself, aided by year-end income tax assistance. An accountant can prepare financial reports that help determine business strategies, or marketing and tax analysis, or help obtain financial backing. Some accountants also give advice on how a business should be operated, called management services.

The hourly fee for an accountant or CPA usually ranges from $75 to $175 per hour or more. A bookkeeper may charge $30 to $60 per hour. Always ask for an estimate of time and fees before the work begins. Inform your financial advisor of any time limitations you have and request the work be completed by that date. Beware of "bargains," such as new people on staff that just arrived from a large corporate position, or a new graduate for "special" rates. They may take twice as long, and a supervisor may charge full price to look over their work. Even more critical, the person may not have any small business experience, and an accountant should be a valu-able business resource.

BANKER

Get to know your area banks and the services they offer. Even if you don't intend to borrow working capital from a bank, your business accounts will make you a welcome customer. Get to know a bank officer. A friendly banker is more important than which bank you use. Discuss your plans for your practice with him or her. An experienced banker can give you a wealth of valuable business information, not only on financial matters, interest rates, and how to keep your credit rating points high but on trends in the community.

Ask for a small business loan officer or vice president of the bank when you want to talk about a business loan. Try to use the same personnel when doing your banking and speak up if you are always directed to new, inexperienced people. Banking personnel don't charge for their services and can be good advisors.

BUSINESS CONSULTANT

A business consultant will advise you on major decisions, such as your central business concept, location, image development, fees, marketing, new market areas, and so on. Good, affordable consultants for small businesses are hard to find, but well worth the research time. Their fees range from $50 per hour on up.

Very good free services available in larger cities are the SCORE (Service Corps of Retired Executives www.score.org) and ACE (Active Corps Executives) programs of the Small Business Administration. These two programs will work to match you with a retired or active businessperson who answers your business questions. Their knowledge and experience can be valued resources. Many local banks, Chambers of Commerce, YMCAs or YWCAs, universities, and adult education courses offer programs to help the beginning and expanding business owner as well.

PUBLIC RELATIONS/MARKETING/ ADVERTISING CONSULTANT

The services of these three specialists often overlap, depending upon the consultant and her or his business knowledge and skills. Public relations experts specialize in letting the world know you have arrived. They use their contacts and expertise to put you and your business venture in front of the public. That may sound intimidating, but it may be as simple as being interviewed by a local newspaper or radio station. Many business people credit their success to having a public relations firm working for them at a crucial stage in their business. As nutrition practice becomes more sophisticated, public imaging will, no doubt, be more important.

Hiring a public relations firm is expensive (ranging from $500 to $2500 or more per month, often for a minimum of six to twelve months). Be careful and specific in your negotiations on prices and services. To assure that you like what is produced, ask to be involved in all stages of development.

A marketing or advertising firm usually can offer logo development, business card and brochure design, market research, and advertising savvy-marketing avenues that get your message to your target markets. Again, fees can vary greatly from a few hundred dollars to many thousands. Advertising fees can be a percentage of the cost of the ad campaign, or it can be a project fee. Most firms can create the artwork and broadcast ads.

Get quotes from several firms and be honest about what you can afford to pay. Often, if they need the business or they especially want to work with you, they will negotiate a fair price for your needs. All of the options are independent of one another so don't feel you have to buy a full package. Buy what will work best. To determine that, you can talk to people who have marketed other services in your area and to several marketing firms until you feel comfortable with the answers.

If you want to do your own marketing and feel confident you can generate the artwork or wording, look into using a local university's art department or freelance artist. All newspapers, magazines, radio, and television stations offer free advice through their sales consultants. Not only can they assist with simple suggestions, but they can advise you on the best time to run your ad, e.g., morning spots on radio or Sunday newspapers, and so on. Use the experts to help sell your products or services, or to improve your image.

FINAL WORD

The wise use of professional advisors can save you time, energy and money. Their combined expertise will enable you to enter into your business venture confident that your organization will run at its optimum. They are also an expensive investment that you need to stay on top of--don't assume the work will be done as you expect. Continue to stay involved and have checkpoints and meetings along the way. Continue to stay in touch with people you want to work with through a phone call, a card, an email, and a small Holiday gift even when their services aren't needed at that time-it's easier than starting over with someone new.

REFERENCES

1. Edwards P, Edwards S. Working Smarter. *Home Office Computing;* July 1991.
2. 2000 Dallas/Ft. worth Small Business Resource Guide. SBA; 2000.
3. Curtin R. *Mastering the Basics of Small Business.* New York: American Library; 1985.

Figure 13.1   **Business Management Team**

Attorney   Form of business structure
                            Contracts and letters of agreement
                            Office leases
                            Copyrights, trademarks, patents
                            Lawsuits

Accountant   Bookkeeping systems advice
                            Financial statements/Audits
                            Employee deductions
                            Income tax records and reports

Banker   Loans
                            Credit information
                            IRA, Keogh, and SEP accounts
                            Business checking and savings
                            Community trends

Business Consultant   Networking and contacts
                            Setting priorities
                            Management skills & decisions
                            Marketing suggestions
                            Business strategies

Public Relations/   Image development
Advertising   Business cards/brochure
                            Market research
                            Promotion ideas
                            Advertising layouts
                            Media contacts
                            Logo design

Investment Counselor   Retirement options
                            Investment advice
                            College savings plans
                            Asset management

Looking for a different kind of career in dietetics and foods?

Chef Kyle Shadix, CCC, MS, RD

What is your training and background?

I received my B.S. degree in Consumer Foods and Nutrition with a minor in Food Science from the University of Georgia, Athens. I my junior year, I lived abroad in Orleans, France where I immersed myself in the French language and culture. I graduated from the famed Culinary Institute of America in Hyde Park, New York and am a Certified Chef de Cuisine. My masters degree is in Clinical Nutrition from New York University and I completed my internship at Mount Sinai Medical Center.

What have you done with your varied background?

There have been many opportunities come my way. I have worked for Sloan Kettering Cancer Center, The Food Group New York City, Daily Soup Company, Bouley Bakery, personal chef to playwright Terrance McNally, and other freelace work. Today, I am also a contributing author to the MinuteMeals cookbook series (Wiley), a weekly columnist for Slimfast.com and a monthly columnist for *Today's Dietitian*. As an active member of the ADA, I serve on the Membership Advisoty Board and I am founder and president of the National Organization of Men in Nutrition (NOMIN), a networking group of ADA.

National Organization of Men in Nutrition (NOMIN)

Our mission and goal is to promote dietetics careers to all males and to support men who are nutritionists, RDs or DTRs to grow profes-sionally.

Membership is open, but you must meet the following criteria: be a RD, DTR or have established eligibility to write the Registration exam or have completed a baccalaureate degree and/or a CADE accredited supervised practice. You are also eligible if you have earned a master's or doctoral degree in a nutrition or food major. Membership is furthermore open to all nutrition students and Active members of the Canadian Dietetic Association.

To join N.O.M.I.N., please contact:
Kyle Shadix
E-mail: chefkylerd@msn.com
Phone: 212-280-8242
Join the discussion group by sending an e-mail to:
NOMIN-dietetics-subscribe@yahoogroups.com

Chapter 14

Money and Finance

Jan Thayer, RD and Kathy King Helm, RD

To most people the measure of success in business is to make money. Others may say a business that pays its bills, while it satisfies its clients is more successful. Whatever your definition, a business venture that doesn't make enough money is either a hobby or one that has a limited lifespan. Entrepreneurs and employees must appreciate the importance that generating revenue means to the success of businesses.

A hospital wellness program may advertise that it was created for the enjoyment and health benefit of the employees, but cutting medical insurance costs is usually the underlying reason for in-house programs. From the beginning, the consulting nutritionist should establish the financial record keeping that shows her programs are successful and cost effective. Anecdotes from successful clients can be used in marketing, but the management will want good numbers to document successful programs.

A financially successful business usually starts with sufficient capital investment, followed by fair prices, good collection of revenue, paying bills on time and appropriate record keeping for you, the IRS, and any lender. Managing money and keeping records should not be difficult tasks. The challenge is to know what needs to be done.

Before anyone will be able to help you secure a loan or set up your books, he or she will need to know what you plan to do. The information generated in the business plan will be beneficial, also knowing the type of business structure you will use and an estimation of your start-up costs (see Chapter 15).

INITIAL INVESTMENT

Good financing offers peace of mind, the option of changing your mind and freedom to create without survival being in peril. Successful private practitioners estimated twenty years ago that they invested $5,000 to $20,000 or more in their first year in business.(1) Today, start-up costs may be two or three times more than needed then. The money usually comes from savings, loans, credit cards, trade credit

(credit terms extended by sellers of products), and reinvestment of profits throughout the year.

Practitioners with well-equipped, well-staffed offices in rented space pay the higher fees. They usually develop the appearance of stability and success much sooner than low-budget small ventures. Investing more money into a business will not necessarily make it more successful. However, an adequately financed venture has a better chance of becoming a lucrative business faster.

Practitioners who either have more time than money or those who want to keep the risk and investment low make smaller investments. This is possible by sharing office space in a physician's office, or health club, or by working from home.

SOURCES OF FINANCING

One reality to face in developing a business venture is the money commitment. Financial experts encourage new business owners to try to use someone else's money for part of the capital (bank loan), instead of exhausting personal assets and credit sources. This maintains the owner's financial strength. The owner may need to contribute later during financial emergencies or expansion projects. The most common sources of financing are: (2)

- **Personal savings:** The primary source of capital for most new businesses comes from savings, second mortgages, and personal credit sources. Credit cards should be saved for emergencies, not day-to-day expenditures. High credit card debt will keep most lenders from giving you a loan. Being even a day or two late paying the monthly bill can increase your interest rate to over 20%.
- **Friends and relatives:** Often, this money is interest free or at low interest, which can be very beneficial when starting out.
- **Banks and Credit Unions:** These are the most common sources of loans. They want to be involved in successful ventures, and you must show you have done your homework and have a repayment schedule in order to attract a loan. SBA loans are usually handled through designated banks.
- **Venture capital firms:** These firms help expanding companies grow in exchange for equity or partial ownership and a strong involvement in the business.
- **Angel investors:** These are people with money who want to help small businesses grow in return for stock, but most don't want involvement on a daily basis.(3)

Your success in obtaining funding depends upon your assets, business expertise, connections, and your ability to sell yourself and your business plan.

Lending institutions are in business to make money by loaning money for an interest fee. Loaning money involves taking a risk that the new business will be successful, and the owner is hard working, honest and reliable. To be successful in obtaining a loan, you must be prepared and organized. You must know exactly how much money you need; why you need it and how you will pay it back.(4,5)

It's common for a lending institution to require you to invest a certain percentage of your own money if a loan is granted. Or, it may ask you to place your money in an account and borrow against it, or secure the loan with personal assets. If you are seeking an expansion or recapitalization loan, your financial business records for the past three years, personal credit records and business reputation will be evaluated.

Commercial Banks

Commercial banks are the most common lending institutions. They offer many services besides checking and savings accounts. Banks offer basic financial counseling and credit analysis at no cost to regular customers. Most commercial banks make short, intermediate-term and long-term loans. You may be asked to put personal property, Certificates of Deposit, savings, or other assets of value up as collateral. Occasionally, where you have established credit, you may be asked only to sign for the loan. When you use assets to secure a loan, they aren't to be sold, spent or used until the lending institution releases them. Read your loan agreement carefully before you sign.

Credit Unions

Credit unions usually offer low cost checking accounts, savings accounts and low interest loans on autos, personal loans, home improvement (to create a business office), and sometimes on larger items.

Small Business Administration (SBA)

The SBA of the United States Government is another resource alternative for a new or established business loan. The law stipulates that SBA loans can be made only to businesses that are unable to get funds from banks or other private sources. This is usually because the personal assets or type of business will not qualify for a regular loan (except at high interest rates), not because the person is a poor risk. A bank, however, will usually make the loan, guaranteed by the SBA up to as much as ninety percent. Especially with new businesses, the SBA may ask you to contribute fifteen to fifty percent of the initial investment.

Occasionally, the SBA will make the loan itself, but this is rare. Only one-quarter of the total 30,000 or so loans the SBA makes or guarantees each year goes to new businesses, so competition is tough. Less than ten percent of SBA loans go to women-owned businesses each year, although the SBA reports that women are more successful in starting a small business.(4) Interest rates on an SBA loan are attractive because they are lower than banks usually offer. As attitudes change in the federal government, SBA money becomes more or less available.

The SBA requires extensive information about you and your business venture.   You can pull the information together or hire an accountant or CPA to put the proposal together for you, or to guide you in assembling and filling out the documentation required. It used to take months for SBA loans to be approved, but now the process has been reduced to several days if the paperwork is in order.

SBA loan programs are generally intended to encourage longer-term small business financing, but actual loan maturities are based on the ability to repay, the purpose of the loan and the useful life of the assets financed.(5) Maximum loan maturities have been established: 25 years for real estate; up to 10 years for equipment (depends upon the useful life); and generally up to seven years for working capital.(5)

LOAN PACKAGE

The loan package is the finalized presentation compiled to secure a loan from a bank, venture capitalist, SBA, or a combination of these sources.(4) It succinctly presents your basic idea through the executive summary and plan. In a nutshell, it explains who you are, your financial status and how the money will be used and repaid. Usually, having an accountant or CPA provide a review of the figures presented substantially improves the chances for getting a loan. A review is less involved and less expensive than an audit and only as accurate as the figures used, yet it often satisfies bankers because it offers some limited assurance about the reliability of the financial information.(4)

Typically, bankers will request or appreciate having the following; ask what is necessary, and then use your best judgment on the other items depending on your loan needs: (4,5,6)

Loan Proposal Outline (5)

Cover letter
Table of Contents
General Information
- Business name, names of principals, Social Security number of each owner, and the business address
- Purpose of the loan-exactly why is it needed
- Amount required

Business Description
- History and nature of the business
- Business plan with its market analysis (products and competition)

Management Profile
- Personal history of each owner (resume, business experience, letters of reference)

Company Information
- Copies of contracts you already have signed, lease agreements, insurance carried, etc.

Financial Information
- Personal balance sheet and your personal income tax returns for the past three years (see Figure 14.1 Balance Sheet)
- If already in business:
  a. Company balance sheet and past three years of tax returns
  b. Company profit and loss statement (see Figure 14.2)
  c. Ages of accounts receivable and payables as of current date
- Business cash flow projections for at least one year (see Figure 14.3)
- Source of repayment
- Requested duration of loan
- Collateral to be offered to secure the loan (official appraisals of assets may be necessary when the market value is not easily determined)

What Bankers Look for in a Business Loan (5,6,7)

- **Experience and track record:** You may be new to this venture, but you must convince the banker you have been successful in your career and other projects you have managed. Use your business plan to show your expertise.
- **Personal and business credit:** Bankers will look closely at your personal credit history, credit score and how you have repaid debt in the past. Get a copy of your credit report, and make sure it's accurate.
- **Personal investment:** Banks want to see that you have confidence in your venture by investing your own assets as well.
- **Collateral:** Besides personal investment, banks usually want something to secure the loan. This could be real estate, your home, a car, Certificates of Deposit or other assets.
- **Repayment plan:** Explain how you will repay the loan from what sources of revenue. This plan must look feasible so ask for more repayment time in order to keep the payments lower.

Before beginning to prepare all of these documents, ask your individual loan agent what forms he or she needs. Most business consultants suggest the loan package be typed and bound in an attractive folder or notebook.(6)

Numerous options exist on loans so work with your loan officer and financial counselor to choose one that fits your needs. Loans termed "line of credit" are very helpful for peace of mind and yet do not usually cost anything if you don't use the money. Other loans may be set up so that during the first six months or year, you only make interest payments. A bank may request that you submit semiannual, or yearly financial status reports, but occasionally, nothing may be needed.

Credit Scores

Each person who makes purchases on credit in the U.S. begins to generate a credit report at the three big credit reporting agencies: Equifax, Experian and Trans Union. The best score you can have is 850 points, and the median score for people with the best credit is 720 points.(8) (You lose points for having too many credit card accounts, by having high balances-even if they are paid on time and, of course, for chronically late or delinquent accounts.)

Does it make any difference what your score is? It can make a BIG difference! According to Kiplinger's Personal Finance Advisor newsletter (8), for example, on a 30-year fixed rate mortgage of $250,000, having a score of 700 will cost $21 per month more in interest, or $7560 over the life of the loan. If the person's credit score is 675, he will pay an extra $112 a month, or $40,320 over the life of the mortgage.

How do you improve your score?
1) Only have one or two credit cards that you pay on in a timely manner-not just the minimum payment-keep the balances low.
2) Don't be tempted by the numerous mailed promotions for credit cards, and the 10% discount at checkout desks to start a new credit card-too many cards will hurt your credit score.
3) Annually, look at your credit reports (they are easy to find in search engines under "credit reports"), and make sure the information is accurate and no one else's credit has been merged with yours. If you shared credit accounts with a former spouse, make sure your report reflects separation of the accounts, and get bad reports removed through working with your ex-spouse and the credit agency if they were not your purchases.
4) Remember that it may take six months to a year to repair a minor flaw (8). A big blemish, such as paying bills 30 days late, will take three to

four years to be removed from your record.(8) For a free estimate of your score, visit www.eloan.com.

When the Answer is "No"

Don't look at a "No" answer as a total defeat. Ask the banker what else he or she needs, and go back several times to achieve your desired results, or until an agreement will not work out. Many loan officers make loan decisions based upon past experience with certain professions or industries; being turned down may have nothing to do with you. Move on to the next institution and improve your package presentation.

There are times when you should not accept a loan if one is offered, for example:

- the term of the loan may be too short, so the payments may be too high and stressful each month; or
- the interest rate may be too high, and the payback amount outrageous; or
- the loan may tie up all of your assets as collateral and limit your future growth instead of helping it; or
- the closing costs on the loan may be thousands of dollars more than you expected.

If you can, either try to find another funding source or do without the loan until bills are paid down more and terms improve. If you really need to use someone else's money to grow and prosper, consider the interest, closing costs, etc., as the cost of doing business.

MANAGING MONEY

Whether you decide to incorporate your business or not, when your business begins to make money, it has a life of its own. The money generated must be accounted for. Records on incoming revenue should match bank deposits into the business bank account. All business expenses, plus the owner's salary or consultant fee, should be paid by check from that account. Personal expenses for groceries or the house note should only be paid out of funds appropriately transferred to the owner's personal account.

Banks usually charge higher service charges on business accounts than on personal ones, but the charges are deductible. Large amounts of business money should not be left in a non-interest-bearing checking account when it will not be used immediately. A checking-with-interest, savings, money market, or other interest account should be used even for just a few weeks to generate interest.

A business check should be written and cashed when you need petty cash. Cash taken in as payment from clients should be recorded as income and deposited, not pocketed or used.

Good Banking Relationships

In his column in the *Dallas Business Journal,* bank executive Guy Bodine suggests that small business owners take the time to develop a relationship with their bankers before they need a loan. He gives the following eight points to help the relationship grow: (9)
1. Meet your banker for lunch and keep your banker informed.
2. Educate your banker on the type of business you run, and make him or her come to your place of business.
3. Seek counsel from your banker.
4. Build credibility.
5. Limit surprises.
6. Do your homework: Develop a business plan.
7. Submit timely financial information to your banker-good and bad.
8. Keep your money deposited in the bank.

Cash Flow

Cash flow is just what the name states, the flow of money through the business-how much money is coming in regularly, as compared to that needed to pay current bills. As a new business owner, it should be assumed that it may take six months or more before enough money will come in to cover all expenses. When planning for working capital in your start-up costs, allow enough to keep cash flowing and bills paid. Limited cash flow is not only frustrating, but if it becomes serious, more money may have to be borrowed or supplied by the owner to keep the business open. Cash flow can also be a problem for established businesses when unexpected economic downturns happen, large emergency expenditures increase the debt load, or joint venture partners back out at the last minute.

SUGGESTIONS FOR IMPROVING
CASH FLOW INCLUDE: (6)

- Request all payments at the time of the visit from patients; get upfront and interim payments for projects; and retainers for consultant positions.
- Improve collection efforts on outstanding accounts, especially the larger ones.
- Lower inventories of purchased items, including supplies, teaching materials, printed diets, and promotion materials.

Figure 14.1 Sample Balance Sheet

BALANCE SHEET

Assets

Cash in checking account	$ _____
Cash in savings account	_____
Credit union savings account	_____
Life insurance cash value	_____
House fair market value	_____
Car(s) (fair value)	_____
Furniture and personal effects	_____
Other	_____
Total Assets	$ _____

Liabilities

Balance on car loan	$ _____
	_____
Home mortgage	_____
Credit cards	_____
	_____
Other	_____
	_____
	_____
Total Liabilities	$ _____
Net Worth (Assets minus liabilities)	$ _____

- Avoid making new purchases that will increase the business overhead and either deplete savings or create additional time payments.
- Deposit temporary excess funds in a savings account or money market fund to draw interest.
- Evaluate when to take cash discounts and pay a bill quickly to save money or when to delay paying bills until the end of the pay period to conserve cash-

Figure 14.2 Sample Profit and Loss Statement

PROFIT AND LOSS STATEMENT
(DATE)

Income

Nutrition counseling	$ _____
Public speaking	_____
Nursing home consultation	_____
Book royalties	_____
Other	_____
	_____
Total income	$ _____

Losses (or Expenses)	
Rent	$ _____
Utilities	_____
Telephone and answering service	_____
Equipment	_____
Salaries or consultant fees	_____
Insurance	_____
Auto	_____
Benefits	_____
Supplies	_____
Other	_____
Total expenses	$ _____
Net income	$ _____

Other reductions

Taxes	$ _____
Depreciation	_____
Other non-cash reduction	_____
Adjusted net income	$ _____

Figure 14.3   Sample Cash Flow Planning Form

CASH FLOW IN

Jan.   Feb.   Mar.   April   etc.

1. Beginning cash balance
2. (Income sources)
3.
4.
5.
6.
7.
8.
   Total cash available

CASH FLOW OUT

Operating Expenses
1.
2.
3.
4.
5.
6.
7.
8.

Capital Expense
   1. Loan payments
   2. Income tax and Social Security

Total cash required
Cash available less cash required
Money to be borrowed
   (if negative total)
Debit payments (if positive)

Ending cash balance
Operating loan balance
   (at end of period)

outflow. Request longer pay back periods from large accounts you spend a lot of money with each year-they may give you 60 or 90 days.

TAKING CREDIT CARDS

A number of consulting nutritionists offer the use of credit cards to their clients as a means of payment. Many patients like this convenience and the fact they can then delay their payments. Credit cards help attract patients who would have delayed or avoided coming due to lack of ready cash. People who conduct group classes have found there is less resistance to the up-front fee when credit cards can be used. According to credit card experts, a business can expect from a 10 to 50 percent increase in sales and about twice the average cash purchase, when it starts offering credit cards as a payment method.(10)

A representative from your local bank can explain the service to you but check around for the best services and prices. Today, it is difficult but not impossible to become a merchant who offers credit card usage from a home-based office. However, you must have a good personal credit rating. To process credit cards you will need charge forms and a imprinter, or software for your office computer, or the automated swipe equipment to buy or rent for anywhere from $125 to $1200. You can input the charges by hand into your computer or swipe the card and get immediate confirmation the card was charged. Some programs may still accept deposited credit card forms into your bank account, just like checks. You will be charged two to six percent per bill, plus a processing fee of about $.25 to $.35 or more per item.

You can increase your fee slightly to cover the service charge cost, but that would mean that all patients are subsidizing the credit card users. Actually, the increase in business may offset the added service charge so that no fee increase would be necessary.

On-line Credit Card Payment

The newest credit card innovations are on-line and, eventually, wireless payment of bills through services like PayPal and Billpoint.(11) These two services are great ways to make payments to individuals and small businesses. Both services make their money by charging the seller (card user) a small fixed fee and a percentage of the total dollar amount sent on each transaction. PayPal is used in an estimated one-quarter of all eBay auctions. And Billpoint, which is partly owned by eBay, is used many more times. The services can be used to have patients pay you, clients pay you and you pay your bills, or send money to pay for your next printing job, instead of sending a certified check or wire transfer. To use PayPal, go to its web site www.x.com and in a secure area, fill out a short registration form, enter your credit card number, and type in the email address of the recipient-PayPal takes care of the rest.

COLLECTION

Patients should be asked to pay at the time of the visit. You can call their insurance companies, PPOs and HMOs to ask for co-pay amounts or whether your bill is covered at all. Ask patients to pay you the co-pay amount or the full amount and give them an itemized receipt or superbill. (See Figure 16.1 Sample Superbill. You can order this billing form at www.eatrightPA.org)

The older your accounts receivable grow, the less likely you will be able to collect them. In a service business such as nutrition counseling, since no inventory is lost, no write-off can be taken for bad debts (except for actual expenses such as teaching materials, computer printouts, etc.). Therefore, new practitioners must realize the money has to be collected or else the diet appointment didn't have financial value. When you sell a product like catered food, the actual expenses can be deducted, but not the lost profit if the bill is not paid.

A written contract or letter of agreement for a completed consultant job is very good proof the other party should pay you. You may have to get a lawyer and go to court to get the money. You will be able to deduct your actual expenses for the job and the cost to recover the money. But the actual cost of lost time, mental aggravation and legal fees may mean you are only breaking even, or less. Timely collection of funds should be a business priority. The purpose of establishing credit policies and setting credit limits helps assure collection of accounts, and they set limits on the risk of loss.

Contracts or letters of agreement can be written for large consultant contracts so your fee and expenses can be submitted bimonthly and paid in two weeks. Another option is to break the total expense for a project into thirds, for example, and have one portion paid upfront when the proposal is signed, another halfway through the project, and one at the end upon completion. You can always stop or slow down work if the agreed upon payment is not made in a timely manner.

Billing

If billing becomes necessary, here are some hints. Date statements as of the last day of the preceding month, rather than the first day of the current month. The customer will be inclined to pay sooner, since the statement appears to be a month older. Quickly identify delinquent accounts and speed up the collection process with a more vigorous follow-up. Accounts delinquent over 60 days should receive a pleasant, tactful phone call from you, or someone representing your business, requesting that a payment be mailed by a deadline date. If you don't receive payment or if the balance doesn't shortly follow a partial payment, a second tactful call should be made. Request immediate payment before the account is turned over to collection.

Collection agencies state that small medical bills are one of the hardest types of bills on which to collect. They state that any account over six months old, and often only two to three months, usually isn't collectible. Most agencies charge 50 percent of the bill as their fee if they collect it, and few will touch an account with under $100 outstanding.

Credit is costly if you can't collect. As an example, you provide $100 worth of services to a patient or other client, and your profit margin is 25 percent. If the patient never pays, you will have to collect $400 worth of fees just to recover the uncollected $100. When you consider how much you have invested in your business, you can easily appreciate why business people can't tolerate delinquent accounts.

BOOKKEEPING

Accounting or bookkeeping keeps track of money you earn or spend and what you own and owe, i.e., your worth. Your income (revenue minus expenses) is recorded on an income (profit and loss) statement (see Figure 14.2). Your net worth is assets minus liabilities and is recorded on the balance sheet (see Figure 14.1).

A good bookkeeping system is necessary to record all of your financial transactions, but it should be simple enough for you to use yourself. The larger and more complex the business is, the more comprehensive, but not necessarily the more complicated, the book-keeping system must be. The information generated will help you know your financial position, evaluate success and pinpoint problems. These records can also help you make comparisons from year to year and help make more accurate projections for the future.

A good accountant or CPA will be able to help you choose the system most appropriate for your business. Office supply stores have a variety of simple paper and pencil bookkeeping record systems; one of the most popular is the Dome book entitled "Simplified Monthly Bookkeeping Record."

There are a variety of low cost simple bean counting software programs available for under $100. For full-powered accounting packages for mail order and other businesses with inventories or a large number of billing needs, there are good programs for under $500.

Don't expect that accountant on a white horse to set the program up for you and you get away with knowing nothing! Read the book, learn the system and either set the system up for yourself or pay someone trained in the system to do it, while you sit there and answer all the questions and watch how it is being done.

You will need to know how to do it!

BUDGET

In his book, *Private Practice,* Jack D. McCue, MD, says "fewer than two percent of (medical) practices have a budget (13)." The number of self-employed dietitians using a budget is no doubt as small. Agreeing on a budget, forces you to examine projected expenses and agree on the gross income, hours of work and charges necessary to generate the projected net income.

Budget projections are very difficult to make during a year when a person's income is dependent upon inconsistent projects and short-term consultant jobs. In those cases, a budget for each project and good fiscal management can help assure the year is balanced financially.

Another option is running monthly Profit and Loss and Sales records to compare with the previous month's records, as well as the previous year's records, for the same period. This process makes you immediately aware of changes in income so purchases can be made or delayed, and bills can be paid or stretched out until the last of the credit period.

Cash Versus Accrual Accounting

The IRS will ask that you indicate which form of accounting you use in your bookkeeping-cash or accrual. Cash accounting is when you record income as you receive it, and expenses as you pay them. When you record income as it is earned, not necessarily collected, it is called accrual accounting. Accrual accounting is usually used in businesses that have large inventories of products where flexibility of figures and dates may be beneficial. Financial consultants usually suggest that service businesses such as consulting and private nutrition practices use cash accounting because it's simple and easy to use. Just recently, Congress passed legislation allowing many small businesses that formerly had to use the accrual method to use the cash method. The advantage of this is expenses can be deducted when they are paid, and uncollected income doesn't have to be counted, which saves on tax payments.

Record Keeping

The following list shows the typical progression of record keeping for a physician-referred private practice patient visit.

1. Record patient's appointment.
2. Obtain medical diagnosis, written or verbal diet order from referring physician, along with pertinent chemical scores.
3. Fill out initial interview sheet, assessment, history, and food analysis (or questionnaire given to patient in advance by email or hardcopy).
4. Give patient written diet handouts.
5. Give the patient an itemized bill and request payment as he or she gets ready to leave. Mark the bill paid on patient's form.
6. Give an appointment card to the patient if there is to be another visit, and make an entry in the appointment book.
7. List the payment on the bank deposit slip.
8. Mark the bill paid in accounting system.
9. Send a follow-up communiqué to the referring physician.
10. File the patient's folder.

Each day, record all income (checks and cash) on the business bank deposit slip, and credit card deposit records in the accounting system. All bills should be listed as you pay them under expenses. The check date, check number, amount, and deduction code or account should be listed also.

Monthly, all income and expenses should be tallied and totals to date brought forward. You should also know how much money is uncollected in accounts receivable and how old each account is. Send bills out biweekly to shorten the collection cycle.

Whatever method you choose for bookkeeping never lose sight of the fact that as the owner, you will ultimately be held responsible for the accuracy of the reporting system and its figures.

Record Retention

Files need to be kept on your business for important documents and records of business transactions. There isn't total agreement among experts as to the actual length of time to hold records, so check with your own advisors.

Suggested record retention schedule:

Permanent
- Audit reports of accountants, financial statements
- Capital stock and bond records
- Cash books and charts of accounts

- Cancelled checks for important payments
- Contracts and leases still in effect
- Correspondence (legal and important matters)
- Deeds, mortgages, bills of sale, appraisals
- Insurance records, claims, policies, etc.

ACCOUNTING SOFTWARE (12)
Reviewed by Home Office Computing

Easy Bean Counters	Rank (1-10)
Peachtree Office Accounting	8.5
One-Write Plus	8.1
Quicken Home & Business	7.8

Full-Powered Accounting	
QuickBooks Pro	8.5
M.Y.O.B. Accounting Plus	8.0
Peachtree Complete Accounting	7.5

- Patient files
- Corporate minute books of meetings
- Tax returns and worksheets
- Trademark registrations and copyright certificates

Seven years
- Accident reports and claims
- Accounts payable and receivable ledgers
- Cancelled business checks (see permanent listing)
- Contracts and leases (expired)
- Invoices
- Payroll records
- Purchase orders and sales records

Three years
- Correspondence (general)
- Employee applications and personnel records (terminated)
- Insurance policies (expired)

One year
- Bank reconciliations
- Correspondence (routine)

TAXES

Learn which forms to file and how to fill them out, dates to file, and tips to minimize over or underpayment of estimated taxes. Even if your accountant or CPA fills out the forms, you should be familiar with what he or she is doing.

As a self-employed person, you have a variety of tax obligations, in addition to filing the federal and state income tax forms. You will need to estimate your federal tax commitment and pay it quarterly, up to 100% of what you paid the previous year if your income is under $150,000, or 110% if your income was over $150,000. There is also Self-Employment Tax (Social Security and Medicare) at the rate of 15.3% of your adjusted income, as well as additional state or local taxes (income or sales). However, 50 percent of the self-employment tax is deductible on the 1040 form.

Partnerships must file returns and specifically state the income items and deductions, but the profit or loss is passed through to the partners, according to the percentage of ownership. Corporations must file and pay taxes on any profit and shareholders must pay tax on dividends. S Corporations do not pay taxes, but have their profit or loss reflected on the shareholders' tax returns (unless the state does not recognize S Corporations, and they are taxed as a corporation). Some states also have personal/business property tax to pay each year on the value of the vehicles, copier, desks, etc. owned by the business. For people who own their own business property, there is also property tax to pay.

Deductions

Self-employed practitioners usually deduct the following expenses:
- Office supplies, postage, teaching materials, etc.
- Rent paid for a commercial office or a home-office (if it meets IRS rule: used regularly and exclusively for your business), plus a percentage of the real estate taxes, mortgage interest, utilities, insurance depreciation, repairs, and cleaning costs, but not landscaping.
- Cost of gas, water and electricity at a commercial place of business
- Advertising and promotion
- Telephone, answering service, fax, modem, computer, and copy machine (present tax laws allow up to $24,000 deduction in the year you buy equipment without having to depreciate it, otherwise the

expenditure must be depreciated over the life of the car, copier or whatever.)
- Hire of office assistants and subcontractors
- Dues to professional societies (social clubs are usually excluded)
- Cost of operating an automobile for business: $.325 per mile in 2002)
- Furniture purchased new; used furniture can be depreciate, but not deducted
- Professional books, newsletters, journals that help you run your business or keep you current
- Usually 50 % of the cost for business-related meals and entertaining
- Job hunting expense, if not looking for first job or a position in an unrelated field
- Expenses incurred in attending business conventions; be careful, if mixed with pleasure
- Gifts to clients up to $25.00 each-buy a gift instead of a meal in order to take the full deduction
- Health insurance: C corporation-write off as a company benefit; all self-employed people can deduct 50 percent in 2000 and 100 percent in 2007.
- Disability insurance, if you have a C corporation, as an employee benefit
- Contribution to retirement accounts
- Interest on loans and credit cards, if business-related
- Bank charges and credit card processing fees on business accounts
- Professional licenses, fees
- Special uniforms
- Social security taxes: deduct half of your 15.3 percent payment

Any additional types of deductions should be discussed with your tax advisor. Personal, living or family expenses are not deductible. These would be items such as:
- Withdrawals of money from the business by owner
- Insurance paid on a dwelling house
- Life insurance premiums
- Payments made for house rent, food, clothing (except uniforms), servants, upkeep of pleasure auto, etc.

Possible Deductible Home-Office Expenses (10)

(If the IRS Criteria are met: exclusive use and principal place of Business)
- Cleaning, repair, trash collection, and maintenance of a home office
- Condominium association fees
- Household furniture converted to use in the home office

- Household supplies used in the business space
- Mortgage interest (partial)
- Real estate taxes (partial)
- Security system
- Second telephone line, if it is used exclusively for the business, and business long distance on the first line
- Utilities attributable to business use of home

Loans

Since money borrowed is not considered taxable income, repayment of the loan is not an allowable deduction. Interest paid on a business loan can be deducted.

Retirement Plans

IRA, SEP (Simplified Employee Pension), SAR-SEP, Profit-Sharing Keogh, Money Purchase Keogh, Paired Keogh, and 401 (k), SIMPLE, and Defined Benefit Plan are forms of retirement plans self-employed people can use. These plans allow an entrepreneur to invest in tax-deductible accounts that accrue interest tax-free until retirement. ROTH is an IRA funded with after tax money, but after maturity, the withdrawals are tax-free. Each option has its advantages and limitations. Before choosing the program(s) you will use, talk to your investment counselor, banker, accountant, and insurance agencies to see what they offer.

BUYING/SELLING AN ONGOING PRIVATE PRACTICE

Today, more successful dietitians own their own businesses, but with our mobile society, their businesses might be for sale. After years of working on a private practice, it is painful to think about giving it up, but selling is better than just letting it dissolve. However, determining the value of a service-type business whose success is closely associated with the personality of the owner is not easy.

Stuart Rosenblum, CPA with Wilkin and Guttenplan, made a nationwide study of how to set purchase values on various types of businesses.(14) Although he did not identify a medical-related private practice, he did mention several service businesses. He estimated that an employment agency owner could ask .75 to 1.0 times the gross annual income, equipment included, for the business (the price varying with the business reputation, specialization and client relations). The owner of an insurance agency with its policies renewed each year could ask 1 to 2 times the amount of the annual renewal commissions. A travel agency owner with good contacts but no ongoing revenue from prior sales could only charge .04 to .1 times the annual gross revenue for his business. The major determining factor in valuing a business is how much ongoing worth can be transferred to the new owner.

A buyer should consider the following factors: (15)

Profitability. What is the future profit potential of the business? Start by analyzing balance sheets and profit and loss statements of the present owner for the past five years, or however long the practice has existed. If these forms are not available, ask for copies of the income tax forms. Are the profits satisfactory? Have profits continued to grow? Ask the seller to prepare a projected statement of profit and loss for the next two months, and compare it to your own estimations.

Tangible and Intangible Assets. The most common are inventories, typewriter, computer, furniture, and teaching materials. Make sure they are in working order and not outdated. Consider whether the items are something you can use. If the asking value seems too high, call around to obtain estimates of similar equipment from dealers of new or secondhand items. Intangible assets would include the business name, any trademarks, copyrights, patents, or similar items. Make sure the seller owns the assets and can prove it. If a third party also has rights to the assets, a written consent assigning the rights to you must be obtained. The assets could be licensed to you for your unrestricted use as the buyer of the business. Also be sure the seller is restricted from adapting the trademark to use again.(11)

Goodwill. This is the dollar amount the owner is asking for the favorable public and professional attitudes toward her or his going concern. You should be realistic in determining how much you should pay for goodwill. Since it is payment for favorable public attitude, you should make some effort to check this attitude. Judge the value of this intangible asset by estimating how much more income you will make through buying the going business verses starting a new one. How much of the business will stay, and how much will be lost because of the present owner leaving? Even with the owner's best efforts, her client accounts at nursing homes, drug rehabilitation centers or physicians' offices may not choose to contract with you for nutrition services. If that is the case, the business owner can't include those contracts in her or his determination of the business' worth.

Liabilities. You should be sure there are no outstanding debts or liens on the assets. The seller should payoff all accumulated debts before signing an agreement.

Business worth. After you have researched the above variables, there is still the question of worth. Determine this through negotiation and bargaining. Are you sure local physicians and contracts will use your services? Do you have any verbal or letters of agreements to that effect? Have you carefully evaluated the lease agreement, zoning, the growing competition, and other possible factors that may affect your business? Will the seller train you in running the business or offer any other intangible services?

Some business owners have sold out, only to start a new business in competition with the buyer. Consider placing limitations upon the seller's right to compete with you for a specific period of time and within a specified area. As a safeguard against costly errors, get legal advice before signing any agreement.

Items typically covered in a contract selling a small business are: (15)

1. A description of what is being sold
2. The purchase price
3. The method of payment
4. A statement of how adjustments will be handled at closing (prepaid insurance, rent, remaining inventory, etc.)
5. Buyer's assumption of contracts and liabilities
6. Seller's warranties (against false statements and inaccurate financial data)
7. Seller's obligation and assumption of risk pending closing
8. Covenant of seller not to compete and any limitations
9. Time, place and procedures of closing

The seller and buyer must comply with the bulk sales law of the state in which the transaction takes place. The purposes of this law are to make certain the seller does not sellout, pocket the proceeds, and disappear, leaving creditors unpaid. The seller must furnish a sworn list of her or his creditors, and you, as the buyer, must give notice to the creditors of the pending sale. Otherwise, the seller's creditors may be able to claim the personal property you purchased.(15)

Payment. There are several ways practitioners have negotiated the payment for a practice. One is, of course, a lump sum of money up front. Another way is time payments with either a balloon note at the end of three to five years, or money up front followed by regular payments for several years. Another option is to pay an up-front amount, followed by a percentage of the gross income, for a period of one to five years.

When the buyer and seller can't agree on the worth of the practice, several have used the last option: up-front money followed by a percentage. To keep sales from dropping, it's advisable for the seller to train the buyer on how to run the business and market it.

INDEPENDENT CONTRACTOR OR EMPLOYEE?

The IRS is very particular about who is claiming to be a self-employed independent contractor and who is actually an employee. The self-employed person may be taking deductions, like health insurance or home office that reduce the taxes paid. The key to who is employed and who is self-employed is essentially a matter of control-who calls the shots with regard to how you work (10). IRS Publication 937 details the guidelines, but following are some major distinctions:

- An employee must comply with instructions about when, where and how to work.
- An employee is trained to perform services in a particular way; independent contractors use their own methods.
- An employee is integrated into the business; to remain independent a contractor should avoid having permanent office space on the client's site.
- An independent contractor will more likely be incorporated and have a separate business with his own equipment, tools or materials; projects will have end points and not be open-ended.
- An employee is paid by the hour, week or month; an independent contractor is usually paid by the job or on a commission.

WAYS TO IMPROVE YOUR BUSINESS

Regardless of the type of business you have and what you sell, there are common problems shared by most businesses. There are also common business practices that may improve a business or business venture:

- Use a budget, and become involved in the regular evaluation of your business's output and financial status.
- Keep accounting systems relevant and effective-reevaluate regularly. Take calculated, well thought-out risks.
- Use prosperous periods to reduce your firm's debts and strengthen finances.

Many businesses and financial consultants encourage new business owners to use their first year in business to become established in the marketplace, while keeping overhead minimized. The second year should be used for gaining stability and becoming financially secure. The third year on could be used for expansion and calculated risks. To be rewarded with longevity, a business must first have a stable income generated from clientele support.

REFERENCES

1. Leonard R. *Private Practice on Your Own.* Washington, DC: The Community Nutritionist; July-August, 1982.
2. Sundlund C. The Golden Egg. *Entrepreneur;* May 2002.
3. Evanson D, Beroff A. Heaven Sent. *Entrepreneur;* January 1998.
4. SBA Conference: *Finding Money.* Dallas, TX; May 1990.
5. *2000 Dallas/Ft. Worth Small Business Resource Guide.* SBA; 2000.
6. Wexler H. *A Businesswoman's Guide to Working with Professional Advisors.* Denver, CO: Mid States Bank; 1980.
7. *Get the Advice You Need Before You Start Your Business.* J.P. Morgan Chase & Co.; 2002. www.Chase.com. Accessed July 2002.
8. After a certain point, higher credit scores don't win lower interest rates. *Kiplinger's Personal Finance Advisor;* June 2002.
9. Bodine G. Grow a Banking Relationship. *Dallas Business Journal;* 1991.
10. Edwards P, Edwards S. *Working From Home.* NY: Penguin Putnam; 1999.
11. Cohen A. Pay It Forward. *TIME;* November 13, 2000.
12. Dunlap LB. Accounting Software. *Home Office Computing;* March 1999.
13. McCue J. *Private Practice.* Lexington, MA: The Collamore Press; 1982.
14. Pollan S, Levine M. Playing To Win. *The Atlantic Monthly;* Fall 1988.
15. *Starting and Managing a Small Business of Your Own,* U.S. SBA, 4th ed. Washington, DC: U.S. Government Printing Office; 1982.

Chapter 15

Startup Decisions and Costs

The cost of starting a business venture can vary greatly, depending on the region of the country and the tastes of the practitioner. Some feel if they are going to start a business, they are going to do it right. Others try to see how little they can spend to make the venture fly. Both can be successful, but both also have failed.

Investing a large sum in overhead each month to cover prime office space, extensive advertising, a secretary's salary, and new furnishings can create a successful, stable image right from the start. This should logically attract more business---eventually. Eventually is the important word. There is a point where adding more money to create a good business will not necessarily bring in more clientele faster. However, an equally bad error can be made by not investing enough to give clients the feeling you will there next week.

Before trying to guess how much you are willing to spend on this venture, first decide what kind of office, furnishings, services, staffing, and marketing you would ideally like to have. Then estimate the cost to see if you can afford it. Compromises may have to be made. It may be that initially the office must be shared with another professional to cut the rental fee, the computer leased, photocopying sent out, or a typing service called in as needed.

As mentioned earlier, most business consultants encourage new business owners to buy only the essentials, look for affordable quality, and keep the overhead low, especially the first year. During the second year, try to increase the profit and savings and wait until the third year to expand and invest in more expensive ventures. The years involved are not as important as the business and financial growth that should logically take place first.

It's a well-known fact in business the more metropolitan the area and the more ideal the rental space, the higher the cost, unless the area is over-built. This is especially true on the East and West coasts, compared to rural America. You must pay more for office space and services when competition drives up the costs. Consultants' fees can reflect these higher costs. The figures that follow are just rough estimates of the costs involved. Call around in your local area to get more accurate figures.

IMPORTANCE OF WORKING CAPITAL

Up-front money is initially invested to buy or rent the essentials to start your business, for example, office space, printed materials, business cards, scale, calipers, insurance, telephone, answering service, furniture, and so on. The money that maintains these essentials and your salary are the working capital. Therefore, when estimating your expenses, recognize there are two categories: up-front money to open the doors and maintenance money (working capital) to sustain the business. When planning a business, these two categories don't include the money being generated by clients.

The working capital should be readily available, but it does not have to be in your checking account. It could be a prearranged line of credit from your bank that isn't used unless it is needed—or any one of a number of choices mentioned in Chapter 14. As a reminder, arrange to have six months of working capital.

OFFICE SPACE

Choosing the correct office location, along with good marketing, may decide your ultimate success in business more than your nutritional expertise. Your office space can be instrumental in conveying stability, credibility and success to patients and clients---or just the opposite.

Novices to business often don't know what to look for. Some choose office space that costs very little but, unfortunately, they sometimes get the quality they paid for. Others sign high dollar leases that destine them to work just to pay the rent. Some practitioners have found that sharing office space with a physician or even renting space in the same building as an influential or controversial physician may keep other physicians from referring patients.

Knowing that some practitioners work successfully out of their homes, others try it, but have dismal luck. You can avoid most of these problems with a little research and objective evaluation.

Rental Office Space

The ideal office location is convenient, accessible and presents a good image. Clients will be more tolerant of inconveniences such as limited or paid parking, no elevator service, and little waiting room space, as your relationship with them grows. However, you can avoid these problems by anticipating them and seeking a better location.

It may take several years before your business will attract clients from very far away. Practitioners suggest that offices be located near prospective clientele. Market research should help identify that area of town.

If you want to counsel patients, choose office space in a medical complex instead of an office building. You may find you will attract more patients, if the physicians in the building are good referral agents. Fewer patients may get "lost" between being referred and actually scheduling a nutrition consultation.

Although "store-front" businesses in shopping malls or corner retail centers can do very well, private practitioners are not known for choosing these locations---yet. As emergency medical centers and daytime outpatient services become more prevalent in retail areas, maybe dietitians will opt to be there too.

There is one final point on a rental location: Before signing the lease, closely evaluate your neighbors, the surrounding businesses in the area and the landlord. If you are signing a long-term lease, it is important to know if the area is going downhill, if neighboring renters are disruptive, or if the landlord maintains property well.

Seeing Patients at Your Home

Before starting a private practice out of your own home, realize the home environment can be a blessing or a big mistake. The home setting should be as professional as any private office. That means no interruptions or phone calls during patient interviews, and a comfortable, clean and uncluttered setting. If the home does not have an appropriate waiting area, it may be necessary to allow more time between appointments.

A positive benefit of working out of one's home is patients and clients seem to relax more quickly. This eases counseling sessions, interviews or business work at odd hours. Also, it is convenient for you, requires no travel and overhead is reduced; therefore, profit per hour can be higher.

On the negative side of using the home: It may be an intrusion into your family's privacy, patients or physicians may be hesitant to use your services, and you may feel tied to the work setting. Some dietitians report they do not work out of their homes because they are concerned their business' image would not appear as established and successful. It's usually a poor business decision to use your home to see patients/clients when it's difficult to find in a large apartment or condominium complex.

If a den or other room is used exclusively for seeing patients or as your office, a percentage of the square footage and a portion of the related expenses or a rental fee may be a business tax deduction. A multipurpose room, such as a living room or den with the family TV can't be used as a deduction. Consult with your financial advisor on your specific situation.

Zoning laws for your neighborhood should be checked before starting to see patients at your home. The laws were written to protect the neighborhood quality of life from any undue disruption, excessive traffic or commercialism. Practitioners who already work quietly out of their homes and have only one or two patients per hour have not found that zoning was a problem. If it becomes one, it may be possible to obtain a zoning variance for your business. Unless the zoning is correct for a business at home, an outside sign is usually not permitted.

Home Visits

Private practitioners in both rural and affluent areas have had success when visiting patients in their own homes. Patients enjoy the convenience.

For the practitioner, home visits are not an efficient use of time, if they pull him or her away from the office where other patients could be seen. If, however, the practitioner does home visits instead of renting an office, the savings could make it a good option.

It's advisable when scheduling home visits to require a 24-hour notice of any cancellation, or a fee will be charged. This is especially applicable when working with very affluent, busy individuals who want your services but they have lots of changes in their daily schedules. For these people,

---

Sample Start-up Cost Estimates

Working Capital
  Have six months of capital available before starting.
Lease
  Deposit: Damage and last month's rent?
  Monthly rent: $6 to $30+/square foot/year.
  Nameplates: $5 to $150 (be sure to check).
  Parking: Is staff parking included in rent? Is cost high for clients?
Utilities
  Deposit: Amount varies.
Telephone
  Deposit: Amount varies, but may run from $100 to over $400.
  Installation: $100 to $800.
  Phone: buy or lease a phone system (2-line about $50/mo.).
  Monthly rate for business line: $15 to $65+/line.
  Yellow Pages listing: One line is free; everything else is extra.
  White Pages listing: Listing is free, but boldface is extra.
  Long-distance service: $5/month, plus phone bill.

Services
Answering service: $7 (from phone company) to $100 month.
Answering machine: $40 to $300, depending on features.
Call Forwarding: $2+/month.
Call Waiting: $5 or less/month.
Accountant fees: $75 to $175+/hour.
Attorney fees: $125 to $300+/hour.
Temporary secretarial service: $12 to $24.00/hour.
Typing service: $10 to $24/hour.
Receptionist-secretary Salary varies, but the best are expensive.
Cleaning service: cost varies.

Insurance
Office liability, theft and fire: $250 to $1250/year (you own the building).
Malpractice: About $90-175/year, depends on company and coverage.
Disability: $20 to $40.00/month.
Health: Amount varies, probably $170 to $300/month.
Life: Amount varies.

Office Supplies (many office supply stores offer nice products for laser printers)
Announcements: $15 to $65/100.
Business cards: $65+/1000.
Letterheads: $25 to $60/100.
Envelopes: $18 to $65/1000.
Brochure: Varies greatly; get several quotes. Range: $.15 to 3.00 ea.
Logo: Artist fees vary greatly.
Bookkeeping system: $40 to $500 to establish.
Copying and printing: Price around; prices vary with quantity printed.
Postage and miscellaneous: Keep supplies in modest amounts.
Handouts and teaching materials: Keep in modest supply.

Equipment and Furniture
Medical scale: $200+.
Typewriter/Word Processor: $250+.
Copier: $75+/month to rent or $1500+ to buy.
Calipers: $175 to $450.
Computer and software: $1000 to $3000 to buy new; used or leased.
Fax machine: $200+; may be answering machine and fax.
Furnishings and carpet: Amount varies greatly.
Advertising: Experts suggest 15% of the budget for advertising first
    year.
Incorporation: $300 to $3500; cheaper legal fees online, same filing
    fees.

seeing a nutritionist at home is like seeing a personal trainer-it works well, but scheduling can be a problem. It should not be at your expense.

Travel time, gas and other related costs must be figured to help decide home visit fees. Some practitioners charge their patients a flat rate while others charge according to the total time involved.

As home visits become more commonplace or when insurance coverage more readily applies to home rehabilitation, this option may be very viable and popular.

Office Layout

If you can afford it, it's always a nice touch to have a receptionist or secretary--even one shared in common with other offices--to greet patients as they arrive. Patients expect to have a place to sit and wait and a more private place for the diet consultation. Except for group meetings and large families, there seldom will be times when the waiting room will need more than four chairs and your office more than two.

Most practitioners decorate their offices to fit their own tastes, not as a medical clinic. Patients seem more at ease with warmer surroundings and the break from what is traditionally medical.

To establish credibility immediately, practitioners' certificates, diplomas and awards should be framed and displayed in their offices. Patients do notice and read these items.

Office Safety

For the sake of safety, it's advisable to have an office fire extinguisher, flashlight and smoke alarm. A diagram of the exits should be attached to the back of the main door. The furniture and decorations in the waiting room and your office should not be obviously dangerous or fragile. Any steps or stairways should be well marked and lighted.

When clients are being seen in the evenings, it's best to ask group members to leave together or to call the building security person to make sure the client or you get into your cars without problems. When you are working before or after normal business hours (when few people are around), keep the office door locked. This precaution also applies whenever working out of your home---do not just let people you do not know walk into an unlocked house. With a little care, potentially negative situations may be avoided.

OFFICE AGREEMENTS

Rental or Lease

The following guidelines may be helpful to you when renting space:
• Do not accept the stated rental fee at face value. Virtually all rents are

negotiable unless there is a shortage of office space in the area.

- Be on the lookout for especially attractive bargains caused by the economy or overbuilding. Some property owners may be strapped for cash and be willing to make attractive offers.
- Look for ways to operate with a minimum amount of space. Should your business be successful, chances are good you will be able to find additional space when it is needed.
- When the business is growing and expenses are covered, practitioners seeking to serve a larger market area should consider renting two smaller offices at different locations (for example, one close to downtown and one in the suburbs), rather than one large one. This doubles the business's exposure and convenience to clients, while holding down the cost of doing business, if it's planned well.
- Be aware many leases have additions that boost the rental costs well above the base price per square foot. Maintenance or management fees may not have limitations on escalation. Compute these costs into the amount of the lease before signing.
- In negotiating for consulting space, be sure to mention that your business will not need special plumbing, extra electrical outlets or private lavatory facilities--this will mean less expense and fewer problems for the building owner, and rental could begin sooner.
- Be sure to ask what the rental fee includes, such as, shared waiting room, receptionist, utilities, insurance, carpeting, and so on. Discuss who will own any shelving, carpeting or other additions you may pay for in your office--usually the landlord takes ownership if it is "installed," unless another arrangement was agreed upon. If you want to cover the floor but not leave the carpet, use an Oriental or Southwestern-style rug.
- Will any months of free rent be offered to you as an enticement to rent?
- Check to make sure you can sublease your space in case the need arises.
- Most leases run a minimum of one to three years, but occasionally special concessions can be made for new or small businesses. Realize the shorter the term of the lease, probably the sooner the rent will go up.
- Have a lawyer review the terms of the lease.

The major advantages of having a rental space of your own are you can control its use, you can decorate it to your tastes, materials and records are readily available, and a business phone can be permanently installed. All of these elements help contribute to a more smoothly run operation and the appearance of order and prosperity. In a food management or similar practice, the office locale can be more flexible, especially when clients seldom come to the office.

Deposits. Before moving into rented space it may be necessary to pay not only the first month's rent, but also the last month's rent and a sizable damage deposit. In all, it may amount to three or more times the monthly rent! Ask your financial advisor about local state laws governing the money held by the landlord and your rights to interest, early payback and so on.

Rental fees are quoted in two basic ways: a monthly rate, such as $350 per month, or as cost per square foot. The cost per square foot is usually for one year unless indicated otherwise. It may range from $6 per square foot in some locales to $30 or more in others. To figure your rent, first determine the total number of square feet to be rented, then multiply that figure times the cost per square foot to arrive at the total cost per year; divide by 12 months to arrive at your monthly rent.

Co-leasing

Co-leasing takes place when two partners or other people agree to rent an office jointly. This is often an advantage when the square footage is too large for one and it is useful to share the cost. If the office space is only large enough for one person at a time, the days are alternated.

It is not advisable to co-lease with another nutritionist, unless you are partners and working for the same goals. Otherwise, trying to advertise two businesses selling the same or similar service under the same telephone number, and handling "walk-in" patients without intruding on each other's territory could prove too troublesome.

It is again extremely important you choose a co-lessee well, and that a lawyer reviews the lease agreement. The agreement may hold you both equally responsible for damage or theft that your co-lessee or his clients inflict. It may leave you with the full responsibility if the other person moves or leaves and does not fulfill the entire lease agreement. No doubt, if you and the other co-lessee present yourselves as "one" to the landlord, he or she will expect you both to be responsible for the property and the terms of the lease. You could therefore agree that each of you is responsible for any damage that happens during your rental time; and each co-lessee owes half the rent for the term of the agreement. Again, make sure you can sublease the space if necessary. Read the agreement carefully, change terms as necessary and make additions, and then submit it back to the landlord.

Subleasing

Sharing office space is an alternative for those who want all the amenities of a nice office and locale, but at less expense. In addition to the office telephone, copy machine and receptionist may be shared. Again, all agreements should be in writing and reviewed by a lawyer.

An office may be subleased from a speech therapist or psychologist who only needs the office several days per week or who has too much space for his or her business. The office rent and expenses can be split according to the percentage of the week each uses the office, or for whatever amount you agree upon. Be sure to negotiate and get the best deal for yourself as you would with any landlord.

Office space can be shared with a physician or clinic. Several different options are possible in this instance. The private practitioner could remain independent and do her own billing, marketing, printing of materials and scheduling of her own appointments while subleasing or renting space.

Another option would be to give a percentage of the consultant fee in return for the use of the office and its amenities. A third option is to negotiate a retainer fee, where you see patients for the physician or clinic during a designated time in return for receiving a retainer fee--this is a good option when your services are sought after but the patient load is variable. A final option that some practitioners are still able to find is office space for free so that nutrition services are more accessible to the patient.

As you negotiate rent with a physician or clinic, private practitioners warn that office managers and doctors sometimes overestimate the number of persons you will see. Agree on a financial arrangement you can afford, not one based on ultimate expectations.

Close association with other professionals can provide numerous benefits. Several very successful practitioners report that much of their success when they first started in business came from having one or more "mentor" physicians who promoted them. Some physicians charged for the space, but others offered it for free out of friendship and respect for the practitioner and to aid patients.

Depending upon your individual situation, some important questions need to be discussed with the physician: Will you be able to see other doctors' patients at the office? Who will schedule, pull charts and bill patients? Can you use the copy machine? Who will market you and how? Remember the more services you request, the more you may have to spend. Write down all agreements and have a signed copy for each party. A simple letter of agreement will work. A termination/separation clause is advisable. When a contract is coming up for renewal, you should start negotiating at least a month in advance to work out all differences.

Parking

In some locations, parking space is at a premium, especially in downtown or medical center areas. If a parking lot is owned by your building, does the lease include spaces? Can they be added when negotiating the lease?

Name Plates and Floor Directories

Most office buildings have some kind of directory outside the building, in the lobby, or on each floor, in addition to door nameplates. Seldom will a landlord of a medical building allow you to print your own--they like them standardized. This again could be a lease option to negotiate. Don't assume anything; one practitioner had to pay up to $26 per line for four partners on six floors.

Utilities

When utilities are not included in the lease, the utility companies can give you an estimate of your monthly bill. For electricity, they will need to know the number of watts of each light and how many hours per week it will be used, in addition to the estimated usage of other equipment, such as air conditioning, a typewriter or computer. For gas heating, the square footage of your office can be used in determining an estimate. A money deposit or a letter of credit may be necessary to obtain new service. If you live in the area, try to negotiate using your established good credit at home.

Telephone

The ongoing changes after the break up of AT&T will necessitate that each practitioner checks on the best telephone coverage available locally. To survive, a business must have good telephone service and coverage.

A new business phone system may cost $100 to $800+ to install with new wiring, DSL, and multi-line equipment. Converting an existing private line in an office or at home is usually only a fraction of that cost. If you have never had a business line, the telephone company may ask for a deposit; call for an estimate. The monthly fee for the business telephone line will range from approximately $15-$65 or more per line.

Other services you may consider for your phone are call waiting, call forwarding, conference lines, and a limited service line. Call waiting will allow you to accept a second incoming call while keeping the first call on the line. Call forwarding allows you to transfer your incoming phone calls to another phone number where you or your answering service can answer it. Limited service lines are not available everywhere, but the line allows a limited number of outgoing calls to be made each month for a reduced rate. Calls above the limit are charged extra; in-coming calls are not counted. The rates and availability of these services vary-so call your local company for more information.

Whenever you pay for a telephone line, business or personal, you will be given a listing in the white pages for free; bold print is extra. To have a Yellow Pages listing, you must have a business line. One listing under the most appropriate heading (probably "Dietitian" or "Nutritionist") will be given to you. Additional listings, bold print, extra lines, logo, a large ad, and so on will cost extra and will be billed monthly or however you arrange. If you share office space with someone who already has a business phone, for an added fee you can have your name added to that line. It then will be in information and in the Yellow Pages.

Answering Service

When you begin your business, the phone should be answered during normal business hours, Monday through Friday. An answering service or recording machine can give you coverage when you are away from the phone. An answering service with live operators that receives your call through call forwarding, but does not answer with your company name, is the most inexpensive, while giving a personal touch.

A telephone answering machine or voice mail can give you coverage. The public is familiar with talking to a machine. Callers will use it if the message is clear, creative and of good quality.

Administrative Assistant/Secretary/Receptionist

There is little doubt that a small business owner would enjoy using the services of a secretary/receptionist, however, there are ways to have the duties covered without the full cost of an employee. According to surveys conducted by popular women's magazines, a good, experienced secretary is usually paid as much as a good dietitian with years of experience. Some alternatives are to hire someone part-time for several mornings per week, set up your office so that you can handle it yourself, use a secretarial service at peak times of the year, or find office space where a secretary's services are included.

INSURANCE

Malpractice

Call The American Dietetic Association to find out the most current malpractice carrier and policy information. Prices vary according to the number of hours worked, the desired limits on coverage, and whether media work is covered, as well as traditional services. There are several companies with different types of coverage available.

Office Liability and Furnishings

When clients or patients visit your office, there is always the risk that someone will get hurt on the premises. In rental space, the landlord usually carries liability coverage, but the coverage is often limited. Insurance for office contents in case of fire, theft or other loss is easily acquired, along with the liability coverage. When sharing space at a physician's office or clinic, good liability coverage may already be available to you under their policy--check. When working out of your home, home insurance companies ask they be notified so coverage can be increased. Some insurance companies are reluctant to offer home office coverage for expensive electronic equipment like computers, laser printers and so on. Check around to find a good policy.

Disability

Disability insurance will provide a certain level of limited income while you are ill or disabled. The most expensive coverage begins after only 15 days of illness and lasts 5 to 10 years up to life. To reduce premium cost, choose coverage that starts after 60 or 90 days of illness and lasts for only one or two years. You may feel this insurance is an unnecessary added cost, but statistically, more people get ill or disabled by an accident, chemo treatments, chronic diseases, and so forth than get killed. If you are your sole support, or you have family that depends on your income, this insurance can keep your life stable while you recover.

The premium and disability coverage are dependent upon your age, health and present income. Unfortunately, self-employed individuals have a more difficult time qualifying for this type of insurance, according to most companies. Check with several insurance companies, including ADA, to see what they have to offer and compare costs and coverage. If you are still employed, start the coverage before you quit your job.

Health

Health insurance is a necessity with today's health care costs. One hospital stay for one week or more could wipe out an uninsured person's savings and business. To help reduce the cost of a policy, try to join under a spouse's policy, contact local HMOs or PPOs, or join a group policy (through The American Dietetic Association, executive clubs, rural cooperatives, small business owner groups, local chambers of commerce, or local insurance brokers). In some cases, if you have two or more employees in your business, you can qualify as a group. Another way to keep premium payments lower is to choose major medical coverage instead of a comprehensive policy. You would have to pay the first $1000 to $3000 of a bill, but then coverage may be 80 percent after that. Prices and coverage vary so greatly you will need to take the time to get several quotes and discuss the coverage in detail with the agents. Do not go uninsured.

Life

Life insurance to pay off your loans and debts, as well as to help support your family is an important consideration. Term life insurance is the least expensive for the amount of coverage if you are younger and in good health. However, as the person grows older, the yearly premiums may increase quickly, unless you choose a policy with a guaranteed premium.

Variations of whole life policies are readily available today. This type of policy is more expensive from the beginning, but eventually can act as a savings account to be borrowed against. This type of policy has a definite total price; therefore, premiums do not continue indefinitely as with term insurance.

OFFICE SUPPLIES

Business Cards

Before ordering cards make sure your address and phone number are stable. A graphic designer can design your cards or you can choose from the layout options at a quick print store. For times when information will be changing, cards can be printed from the business supply store can be laser printed a sheet at a time, as needed. Allow two weeks to have cards printed. Because of the cost savings, most businesses order 500 or 1000 cards at a time. Cost for printing depends upon the layout, paper, ink, embossing, and the number of different colors of ink. The first time the cards are run, there may be typesetting and layout fees. When the ink color is changed, there is an ink clean-up charge.

Letterheads

If the letterhead paper or ink is special, it is more economical to print a larger amount, because of the one-time charges for ink clean up, embossing, imprinting, and so on. Paper that is standard stock can be printed easily on a good printer when more is needed. When the letterhead is on special paper, it can be more economical and time efficient to order the paper by the ream and keep it on hand.

An economical way to send out a large mailing or form letter on your letterhead is to produce an attractive, clean master copy, and reproduce it on good paper (logo, your name and address, letter, and all). Do not use heavily textured paper, as this interferes with the ink attaching to the paper. A 24# weight paper at 90+ brightness of laser or inkjet quality works great.

Plain paper should be purchased to match the letterhead for additional pages of a letter. Business letters are usually sent on 8 1/2" x 11" paper, but notes can be on any size with the appropriate size envelopes.

Brochures

Good quality brochures are assets to a business; typesetting or desktop publishing is highly recommended. To save money, the brochure could be a self-mailer, but for times when the best image is required, use an envelope. Before printing your brochure, have several people read it and offer suggestions. Make sure it's copyedited and free of errors before it's printed.

Bookkeeping System

A beginning bookkeeping system with an appointment book, cash ledger, receipts, file folders, and yearly ledger can be purchased for under $40. Simple software systems are available for under $75 to $100. Your accountant or CPA may request that you purchase a definite kind but most are reasonable. It may be to your benefit to use Quicken, QuickBooks Pro, Peach Tree, or another system (prices vary between $75 and $500) that can be emailed to your accountant for monthly or quarterly reports and review. (See Chapter 14.) You can easily convert the final year-end tallies into an income tax return or send the file to your accountant. Don't purchase a more complicated or expensive system than you need. Upgrade the system as your needs mature.

Diets and Handouts

The most important criteria for patient or client materials are to write them in simple, clear language on impressive paper with an easy-to-read layout. Also, don't load the patient down with every free booklet available on a subject--pick the best ones, free or not.

EQUIPMENT AND FURNISHINGS

Medical Scale

If a scale is used, a good balance beam medical scale is suggested. A waist high balance beam is not suggested because it is awkward for very heavy patients to stand on the scale without touching the beam. Spring scales are not always accurate.

Skinfold Caliper

For consultants who work with weight loss, sports nutrition or nutrition assessment, calipers are a must. They range in price from approximately $.50 for the plastic ones to $175-$250 for the metal ones to $450 for the computerized ones.

Typewriter

If you decide to buy a typewriter for the fill-in-blank forms and envelopes you don't know how to do by computer, look for one with pica size type so that elderly patients can easily read it, not script style, which is not appropriate for business writing.

Computer

A computer, its components, printer and software are becoming necessities in business for e-mail, word processing, nutrient assessment, desktop publishing, scanning, and so on. Systems may be leased for a minimum number of months but prices have become so reasonable most people buy their systems. For businesses where you write manuscripts and letters, search databases and communicate with other businesses, a computer, modem and fax are standard office equipment.

Copier

When the volume warrants it, consider buying a photocopier-new or rebuilt. Practitioners state having a plain paper copier to reproduce forms, bills, bulk mailings, instruction materials and so on saves tons of office time. At the start of a business, it may be more economical to share a copier or find a convenient quick copy store. Used, rebuilt copiers are available for reasonable prices. Also, consider buying an all-in-one machine that scans, photocopies, and acts as a fax.

Office Furniture

Prices vary with personal taste. Make the setting comfortable for yourself and the client. For dietitians who will be seeing very large patients, buy sturdy chairs without armrests or with a wide area between armrests, and not so soft that standing up becomes embarrassing.

For practitioners who will be meeting with executives from large corporations or when image is important to clients, consider buying pre-owned (used) office furniture from a reseller or business auction house. Since the furniture is used, it costs less but the quality is usually superior to new fiberboard furniture at the same price.

MARKETING

Advertising

Business consultants suggest that at least fifteen percent of your budget be allocated to cover the cost of the first year's kick-off campaign in marketing, such as newspaper ads, business lunches, brochures, and direct-mail letters. Also, allow ten percent or more of each additional year's budget for on-going marketing.

MISCELLANEOUS

Although we like to feel that we have anticipated all of the applicable expenses, we, of course, haven't. Memberships and subscriptions will need to be budgeted. A dependable car may have to be purchased. A "cushion" needs to be planned to cover petty cash expenses and unexpected larger expenses.

Good preplanning makes the evolution of a business an anticipated pleasure, instead of a crisis management seminar.

Chapter 16

Fees and Reimbursement

VALUING YOUR TIME

An important element of managing money is knowing the value of your time and effort. Too often we spend countless hours doing $10 per hour secretarial work when we should be doing "boss work" like making public presentations or negotiating contracts. If you have something more important that you could be doing and you have the money to pay for it, don't sit around doing work that can be easily delegated.

PRICING STRATEGIES

One decision you must make about each service or product you offer is its price. There is an image associated with a product, as compared to its competitors, that makes it very attractive to its target markets or turns them off. The level of service, or the quality of the materials and workmanship in the product, must warrant the price being asked. Historically, dietitians have charged very little for their services and products, but that is slowly changing. We still tend to underestimate the size of the market willing to buy a "Cadillac" option. Perhaps we have worked with limited budgets too long.

The six common pricing strategies are: (1)
1. **Demand oriented:** you set the price according to what you think the market is willing to pay, all the strategies use a little of this method.
2. **Skimming:** you charge a very high price to reach a small, elite and profitable market.
3. **Trading down:** you add a lower priced, less prestigious service to your existing elite service; this is used to expand to a less elite or affluent market segment.
4. **Trading up:** you introduce an elite expensive service to increase the status of other generally lower priced services and to attract new buyers.

48

5. **Cost plus:** you start with what it costs you to have the service or product and then add mark up according to institution policy (commonly used on books, clothing, etc.).
6. **Under bidding:** you set the price with a low profit to be more attractive than competitors; this is a very common method used by dietitians, but it often makes you work very hard with nothing to show for your efforts.

COMMON QUESTION

Q: There seems to be great variation in the cost of nutrition services. As a new consulting nutritionist, I am struggling to create an image and become known. How do I charge?
A: In any transaction, each party gives up something to obtain something else. Price must reflect the perception of a fair exchange by both parties.

Even when no money is exchanged such as with free public health services, donation of time to dietetic or trade organizations, giving free speeches, and the like, there is still an exchange of something valued. If you don't feel the exchange is fair, you usually won't continue doing it.

In addition to monetary value, price may reflect the value of your time, effort, personal services, caring, loyalty, power or prestige, goodwill, and many other nonmonetary components. A higher price generally connotes more value placed on the product or service a client receives. Unless there is some advantage to your service as compared to the competition, you will only be able to compete on price.

Traditionally, dietitians have not been very good at playing the pricing game. Their fee-for-service is often based only on speculation by the dietitian, rather than on what the market would bear. It appears that the nonmonetary variables such as the uniqueness of the knowledge we share, the highly individualized care, and the initial program development time often has not been considered. Many dietitians jeopardize their ability to give time-consuming higher-quality services because their prices are so low they must instruct many more people to make a living or to make the clinic profitable. There is a current trend toward change.

No matter the price you charge, the "perceived value" felt by the buyer must be equal to or higher than the fee to continue to attract customers. The best way to justify your worth is through measuring the outcome you produce through your consultation.

(Answered by Marianne Franz, MBA, RD, Louisiana Tech)

Establishing Fees

It's illegal (price-fixing) for us to discuss what charges you could ask for your services. It's also illegal for you to call around your area to ask the going rates of other health professionals. You decide for yourself what you need to charge. We can, however, discuss the factors to evaluate when you establish fees for your work:

- How much expertise and experience does the work require?
- How difficult or demanding is the job?
- How much total time will the job, paperwork and follow-up take?
- How much direct overhead cost (handouts, teaching materials, travel expense, hiring another consultant to help, secretarial time, computer use, etc.) and indirect overhead (to maintain office, telephone, insurance, etc.) will be expensed to this job?
- What will the market bear, so that you don't price yourself out of it?

After you have considered all of the variables in establishing fees, charge whatever you want since it's your business and your decision.

Fees are a curious item. If you charge a small fee, sometimes, not always, patients, physicians, and clients think that you aren't as good as the competition. If you charge a fee that your reputation, years of experience, or expertise can't support, no one will pay it. Arriving at "correct" fees for different types of jobs is more a process of negotiation and learning from experience. As a practitioner becomes known for quality work and a good reputation, new business will come his or her way. The fee will become less important because people are willing to pay for what they feel is the best. According to Harry Beckwith, marketing consultant, your fees aren't too high until 25% of your clients complain (2).

FEE STRUCTURES (3)

Flat Rates The same fee is charged for the same service to any client. Used when selling the same service again and again because you have a good idea of the time and expense involved. Easy to use for speaking engagements, routine clinical consults and group classes.

Per Hour Rates The hours of work are variable or may be unknown in advance so a fee is charged only for the hours worked. Used for subcontracting, long therapy sessions and consulting projects. Clients are most comfortable with an approximate time frame or maximum number of hours.

Per Head Rate This rate charges according to the number of individuals who participate. This rate is often used for workshops, teaching or speaking to groups who "pay at the door." It does involve some risk, but if attendance is good you can do very well. You can couple this rate with a flat rate to charge for a minimum number with each extra person at an added fee.

Project Rate This rate covers the development of a project like writing a series of educational booklets or comparing bids from contract food service companies for client accounts. Clients like project rates because they are easy to compare and unless you have an agreement otherwise, you usually cover cost overruns. This rate includes your expenses, overhead, profit and some room for miscalculations or unexpected delays. If the client is at fault for the delays, your agreement could make him responsible for any added costs. If the project is cancelled through no fault of yours after the agreement is made, you should have agreed upon some compensation for your lost income. To protect yourself from nonpayment, consider asking for your fee in thirds (1/3 upon signing an agreement, 1/3 midway and 1/3 at the end upon completion and approval) or half the amount up front.

Retainer Fee You can ask for a retainer fee when you are asked to be "available" by a consultant account, physician's office, or for a Board of Directors of some organization. The amount you charge may be based on your normal hourly rate or whatever you feel your availability is worth. A retainer should be tied to a limit (such as one eight-hour day per week or forty hours per month or whatever) and anything over that amount should be charged extra.

If you presently work at a site on commission where you take all the risk and the client-load is inconsistent, and you feel the clinic people want a nutritionist's services, you might negotiate to have the job changed to a retainer so you could depend on a more stable income.

Contingency Fee or Commission Payment You are paid only if the project is successful or you work somewhere like a clinic and you take the full risk on whether patients pay. Writers are sometimes asked to work on speculation, and employment recruiters or many salespersons work on commission. The risk is high because a lot of time and overhead may be invested without any promise of income, but the income is usually hefty when it does come. If someone asks that you work on commission, make sure the reward is worth it either financially or professionally.

FEES IN DIFFERENT SETTINGS

Diet instruction fees should be consistent so that patients feel that they are charged fairly. There is no standardized way of charging for nutrition consultations. Some practitioners charge by the hour, but charge a minimum fee for very short appointments. They give their patients an estimate when asked how much the fees are. Other practitioners charge by the visit and then try to keep the appointment within a certain time range.

Several practitioners have programs where the diet consultation "package" takes three to eight or more visits. Printed diets are given out only after much education and assessment has taken place. The program commitment is made clear in the beginning. The fees are either paid in cash or credit card up front, or paid as they go, or payments are heavily weighed up front.

Following this same way of thinking, many practitioners automatically include several follow-up visits in the fees charged to clients. It's commonly agreed that a one-visit instruction rarely changes behavior. By paying in advance, patients make more effort to attend appointments.

Group classes for weight loss, gourmet, "natural, " or heart healthy cooking are very popular with the public. For the private practitioner group classes represent challenge, a creative outlet, and the possibility of making more income per hour because of reaching more people at a time. Here are two hints that may be helpful to a practitioner thinking about doing group classes: First, preregister attendees instead of letting them show up at the door, so that you can cancel if attendance will be poor or adjust your room and handouts if a large number plan to come. Second, collect the fee for ongoing classes at the first session, or when preregistering so that attendance will be better and your budget more stable.

Public speaking or speaking to professional groups can be very satisfying and fun. It should be financially rewarding. Organizers often work harder to have a better audience turnout when they are excited about the speaker and there is a fee to cover. Occasionally, there will be times when you choose to give a free talk, but at that time let the organizers know that you are waiving the normal fee, so they don't tell everyone you work for free. If the organization is nonprofit, either asks for a receipt showing that you donated your fee, or ask that they write you a check, which you will deposit, and write one back to them. Check with your accountant, they don't always agree on what is necessary for tax deduction purposes.

When you first begin public speaking, you may not be familiar with what organizations are willing to pay. The best way to find out is to ask the person who calls to set up an engagement. They know what their fee boundaries are, and most people are very willing to share and negotiate with you. If the fee is low, try asking for more; also ask that your travel and handout costs be covered, or include an extra amount in your fee to cover local travel expenses. Always take your business cards and brochures to pass out and let everyone know where to find you. An easy alternative is printing the information on the handouts for your presentation.

As you become an established and sought-after speaker or an author of some note, your fees can reflect this. Travel and accommodations will be included for out-of-town travel. However, although the fees will be much higher, when you consider the travel time to distant speeches and any lost income while away from the business, the actual net income may be modest. Speakers often look on the opportunity as one to grow professionally, to travel and meet new people, and to sell books, products, consultative services, or whatever. With the cost of air travel today, many program planners schedule their meetings so that speakers and attendees can stay over a Saturday night.

Consulting to business, media, or sports teams usually comes after years of specialized training or experience in the field. However, young practitioners with expertise in nutrition assessment, wellness, and other emerging areas are also being asked to consult at this time.

If you are stumped on how much to ask for a consultant job, ask the client to make an offer, like a daily rate to make a media tour. At least then you would know the ballpark they are in, and you can then negotiate if it is too low. Don't answer too quickly and agree to a figure without doing your own calculations first. Clients are often hesitant about mentioning a fee first, in case you would have been willing to work for much less.

If you set the fee yourself, use your best calculations on what it will cost you to do the job, estimate your hours, supplies, computer usage, secretarial time, telephone, FAX, mail, travel and needed profit, and then estimate more hours to do the job by approximately one-fourth to one-third. Most often the problem is not that we set our fee too low, but that we underestimate how long a job will take. Coming in under budget is always acceptable, if it happens. More negotiating suggestions are found in Chapter 17.

Charging commercial clients is different than charging a patient in a private consultation because what you produce, like a menu, video script, article for publication or whatever will potentially bring in revenue to the client. You can always negotiate to arrive at the final agreement. What you want to avoid is coming in too low so you don't make money or coming in so high that you sour the client on using your services. You are looking for a well-thought-out beginning asking price with room to negotiate.

The factors to consider in pricing your services are:
- The popularity and recognition factor of your name and reputation. How the product will be used and the profit potential for the client.
- Your best estimate plus a cushion on the number of hours and other resources this project will cost you.
- Consider asking for a royalty for as long as the item is in use. Ask for editorial or revision rights to up date the product as needed or yearly. And finally, if the client wants to state that you are a staff member or consultant, ask for a retainer fee and have a letter of agreement on your rights and liability limitations. Talk to your professional advisors concerning your protection, proposal, fees, and before signing anything.
- Have your agreement on fees, expected outcomes, review process, project aborting, etc. down in writing and signed before you start work.

- Ask for a nonrefundable portion of your fee up front to cover some expenses in case the project plans change.

COMMON QUESTION

Q: What can I use for arguments to substantiate why as a consultant, I should be paid $75 per hour? I am competing with dietitians who are willing to work as an employee for $18 per hour.

A: First, realize we are in a state of transition from being somewhat passive to more assertive nutrition experts who ask a competitive fee for service or as a wage. Each of us is making the transition according to our own timetables and by what our lifestyles dictate. If someone loses a job to a more flamboyant peer or suddenly becomes the family's sole support, awareness and attitude changes evolve more quickly.

Next, not every client or consultant position is willing to pay the higher fee, no matter how good you are. In other words, you won't get every job, nor will you want every job. Some jobs aren't worth more than $18 per hour.

In some instances if you really want the position, your only other option is to negotiate to do all of the required work in fewer hours for the same total income. For example, if there is $2000 budgeted for nutrition consultation each month, sell the client on the idea that the money is a flat fee paid to have the job completed and not tied to being on the job physically for eighty-seven hours per month or whatever. You will complete all the group classes, counseling, assessments, documentation, menu review, or whatever is required, and be at the job thirty-five to forty hours per month or more often if needed. You will have to use your time well and produce for the client, but the pay is better and you didn't lose the job. The client will have her or his nutrition needs met and still be within budget.

If a prospective client is comparing your consultant fee against an $18 per hour employee, there are some good points that may help your case, but the client must believe you are worth that fee or no amount of logic will sway him otherwise!

Possible selling points are:

- As a consultant, you can bring your own teaching materials, films, weight loss program, and previously successful seminars. The client doesn't have to pay for development time and hit or miss programming.
- When the cost of fringe benefits and Social Security, etc. are added to the hourly wage, the amount increases by one-third to one-half.
- If you have been marketing well and using the media or other exposure to build recognition of your name, this is a selling point that may help attract more business to the client.
- If you have expertise in computers, culinary skills, kitchen marketing, eating disorder programs, or you know people who could be beneficial to the client's programs or staff, try sharing enough to the client in the additional benefits you could bring to the job.

Once a "sell" is made to the client, realize that your arguments can't be just campaign promises if you want to keep the position. You promised short-term excellence and the client will expect you to deliver.

REIMBURSEMENT

When someone other than the patient pays your fee for nutrition counseling, that is called third party payment. That "other" party is usually an insurance company or government program. At this time independent private practitioners report inconsistent coverage of their fees by third party payers, but it improves when the practitioner takes the time to work with payers on behalf of the patients.

The American Dietetic Association's 1995 publication, *Nutrition Entrepreneur's Guide to Reimbursement Success,* clearly explains the steps to improving your chances for insurance reimbursement: (4)

Step 1 Identify, define and describe your services so you will be able to code and charge for your services.

Step 2 Establish a rationale and implementation plan for charging for MNT. Do your homework and find the research and articles that establish the beneficial outcomes of MNT.

Step 3 Establish fees or charges. Based upon your overhead, expertise, quality of services and so on, determine what you will charge.

Step 4 Become a Preferred Provider. Before you reinvent the wheel, call your State Reimbursement Chair and find out what has worked in your state and which providers have already started covering MNT. Find out the present reimbursement rates and whether some companies pay too little to be worth the pursuit. Then call each area provider, especially if you have a patient with that insurer and send your letter introducing your services, the research on the benefits of MNT and ask for a provider application.

Step 5 When patients call for an appointment, remind them to get their physician's referral in writing. Ask for their insurance company's name, their policy and group numbers, and the 800 number to call to find out about whether nutrition consultation is covered. Call the insurer and find out if nutrition therapy is covered, what the co-pay amount is and how many visits will be covered. Make the phone call even if there is little chance of coverage in order to increase awareness of your services. Usually, obesity must be complicated with other problems to be covered by insurance.

Step 6 Code your services. (5)

MNT CPT Codes:

97802–Initial Assessment and Intervention (15 minute unit)
97803–Reassessment and intervention (15 minute unit)
97804–Group (2 or more individuals @ 30 minutes/ unit)

Please contact the Pennsylvania Dietetic Association at
www.eatrightPA.org to order this form in quantity.

Figure 16.1 Sample Superbill

MEDICAL NUTRITION THERAPY STATEMENT

SUBSCRIBER'S NAME _____
PATIENT'S NAME _____ PATIENT'S DATE OF BIRTH _____ DATE _____
ADDRESS _____
INSURANCE CO. _____ POLICY NO. _____ GROUP NO. _____

Sample

ICD-9 Codes

- 783.1 Abnormal Weight Gain
- 783.2 Abnormal Weight Loss
- 285.9 Anemia, Unspecified
- 307.1 Anorexia Nervosa
- 716.90 Arthritis
- 493.90 Asthma
- 414.0 Arteriosclerotic Heart Disorder (ASHD)
- 564.1 Bowel, Irritable Syndrome
- 307.51 Bulimia
- 574.20 Cholelithiasis
- 585 Chronic Renal Failure
- 749.2 Cleft Palate with Cleft Lip
- 428.0 Congestive Heart Failure
- 564.0 Constipation
- 555.9 Crohn's Disease
- 277.00 Cystic Fibrosis

- 722.6 Deg. Disc Disease
- 715.90 Deg. Joint Disease
- 648.8 Diabetes, Gestational
- 250.01 Diabetes, I
- 250.00 Diabetes, II
- 648.0 Diabetes, Pregnancy
- 250.4 Diabetic Nephropathy
- 558.9 Diarrhea
- 562.11 Diverticulitis
- 562.10 Diverticulosis
- 787.2 Dysphagia
- 307.5 Eating Disorder, Unspecified
- 646.1 Excess Weight Gain, Pregnancy
- 783.4 Failure to Thrive/ Physical Retardation
- 693.1 Food Allergy
- 535.4 Gastritis

- 558.9 Gastroenteritis
- 530.81 Gastroesophageal Reflux
- 271.3 Glucose Intolerance
- 579.0 Gluten Sensitive Enteropathy
- 274.9 Gout
- V08.0 HIV Infection
- 042.9 HIV Specified Infections
- 272.9 Hyperlipidemia
- 401.9 Hypertension, Essential
- 251.2 Hypoglycemia
- 244.9 Hypothyroidism
- 646.8 Insufficient Weight Gain, Pregnancy
- 271.3 Lactose Intolerance
- 263.9 Malnutrition

- 627.2 Menopausal Syndrome
- 412 Myocardial Infection
- 278.0 Obesity
- 733.00 Osteoporosis
- 332.0 Parkinsonism
- 533.0 Peptic Ulcer Disease
- 270.1 PKU
- 564.2 Post Gastrectomy Syndrome
- V22.2 Pregnancy, Normal
- 593.9 Renal Disease
- 780.5 Sleep Apnea
- 556.9 Ulcerative Colitis
- 269.2 Vitamin Deficiency
- Other _____

Services

MNT CPT Codes, if applicable
- 97802 Initial assessment & intervention, individual, face-to-face _____ Units
  Each unit = 15 minutes
- 97803 Re-assessment & intervention, individual, face-to-face _____ Units
  Each unit = 15 minutes
- 97804 Group (2 or more), each 30 minutes _____ Units

Other CPT Code, if applicable
- Initial Eval. & Consultation
- Follow-Up Consultation
- Nut. Assess, Comprehensive
- Phone Consultation
- Instructional Material
- Diet Instructions
- Other: _____

Total Charge _____
Amount Paid _____
Balance Due _____

RD Name _____ RD Signature _____ Date _____
RD # _____ Provider # _____ Phone # _____
Address _____

WHITE - Office Copy   YELLOW - Insurance Copy   PINK - Patient Copy

© 2002 Pennsylvania Dietetic Association

PROS AND CONS FOR BECOMING A PROVIDER

Pros
Provides coverage for needed services
Improves professional recognition
Increases income
Covers patients who need it most

Cons
Low fees for private practitioners
Increased paperwork
Must accept Medicare payment
(no additional fee can be charged)

Consider using the Superbill from Pennsylvania Dietetic Association that you can order in quantity at www.eatrightPA.org. (See sample Figure 16.1.)

Step 7 Document the effectiveness of your services. Let referral agents know how well patients have responded and improved chemical values, etc.

Step 8 Track whether patients and you get reimbursement and at what percentage discount.

Medicare Coverage for MNT

For many years ADA, its leadership and state members have been working very hard to get Medicare Part B coverage for Medical Nutrition Therapy for diabetes and renal disease. It finally became a reality in January 2002. It allows dietitians and nutrition professionals to receive direct Medicare reimbursement. The coverage is a wonderful new opportunity for many practitioners, especially those employed by hospitals and skilled nursing facilities. Private practitioners will have a hard time covering their overhead with the low pay scales and required paperwork.

Criteria for coverage was published by The Centers for Medicare and Medicaid Services (CMS): (6)

- The RD credential will be proof of education and experience.
- Dietitians in states with licensure or certification must have that credential. If the dietitian practices in more than one state, the credential must be obtained in each.
- The RD must enroll, and submit CMS Form 855 I, Individual Medicare Provider Enrollment Application. The form can be obtained from either:
  CMS' Web page   www.hcfa.gov/Medicare/enrollment/contacts
  ADA's Web page   www.eatright.com/members/statecarriers

Another resource to help you pursue reimbursement is: *Money Matters in MNT: Increasing Reimbur$ement Success in All Practice Setting$, 3rd edition* by Mary Ann Hodorwicz, RD, LD, MBA. E-mail: hodorowicz@aol.com.

REFERENCES

1. *Competitive Edge,* Marketing seminar notebook. The American Dietetic Association, 1987.
2. Beckwith H. *The Invisible Touch.* New York: Warner Books; 2000.
3. Kelly K. *How To Set Your Fees and Get Them.* NY: Visibility Enterprises; 1984.
4. *Nutrition Entrepreneur's Guide to Reimbursement Success.* Chicago, IL: The American Dietetic Association; 1995.
5. Farr L. Medicare MNT Payment Schedule by Geographic Area. *TDA Today;* Spring 2002.
6. Farr L. CMS Issues Final Rule for Medicare Part B MNT. *TDA Today;* Winter 2001.

Chapter 17

Negotiation and Contracts

Historically, negotiating was an arena where one person was the victor and the other was the victim. Stronger individuals used negotiations to control the opposition. As a result, the final agreement usually heavily favored the victor. The victim accepted the agreement, but later often either did not follow through in good faith or learned to manipulate or sabotage to gain lost ground.

WIN-WIN NEGOTIATING

In the last twenty years or so, a new era of negotiation strategy has evolved in business called win-win negotiation.(1) With this strategy, both parties feel they benefit from the agreement. Now everyone can become quite adept at representing themselves and their points of view, while expecting the other party to negotiate in good faith. Some compromise may be necessary by both parties.

When negotiations stall on an unbalanced or unfairly weighted agreement, it's not uncommon today to hear the "victim" try to nudge the other party into a win-win agreement. He or she might say, "I can't see how I will benefit from this agreement as it stands. Would you be willing to compromise on...?" Or, "We have tried to be very fair and negotiate in good faith. You haven't offered any inducements or compromises that show you feel the same."

Successful Negotiations

There are many good books published on the art of negotiation. In reality though, after you know a few guidelines, the only way to gain expertise is through experience. One negotiation prepares you for the next one. One often learns as much by a session that went poorly as by one easily won that lacked challenge. Your confidence will grow.

Negotiation should be seen as a game of minds, each vying for its needs to be met without having to give up too much in return. When taken in this light, negotiation can be fun and challenging, worthy of thorough research and time to develop the strategy.

When negotiating:
- don't share all of your information up front;
- clarify each point during your discussions;
- document each concession as each party makes it, so parties can't renege later; and
- determine who the other party's leader is as soon as possible; it may not be the person speaking.

Consider the following points to avoid: (2)
- Don't be overwhelmed by the successful position or status of the other party. You are there to negotiate as an equal, not kiss their boots. Don't start off by creating the wrong business relationship.
- Don't worry about the results. Walking away should always be an option.
- Don't negotiate over the phone. Don't oversell and push too hard or far.
- Don't appear too up tight, but don't relax!
- Don't "lose your cool" and get angry, unless it's needed for dramatic effect.
- Don't allow the other person to intimidate or manipulate you with dramatic posturing, anger or "Drama Queen" tactics.

Advantage Points to Remember: (3)
- Try to set up the negotiations on your own ground or somewhere neutral where you feel comfortable. The other party's home ground or office may be intimidating.
- Wear your "power" outfit so you feel comfortable and in control. Overdressing in business attire may prove to be successful in some instances.
- Don't say something you will be sorry about later. Don't quote figures and offer services until you have a chance to think about them, because once spoken, they may be difficult to change. If you don't know what to say, try, "I am very interested in what you're suggesting. Let me research it and get back to you tomorrow."
- Be aware of your body language. Sometimes it gives information that may be to the other party's advantage. Nervous movements may sabotage an otherwise strong presentation.
- If you aren't comfortable with negotiating for yourself, hire a qualified lawyer or other business advisor to go with you to help carry the session. Or, have them coach you before you go into the negotiation session.

STEPS IN NEGOTIATING

Step 1: Qualify the other party.

Is the other party a "middle man" who can only pass on information or the one in charge? Are the businesspersons who want you to write restaurant menus truly solid and well financed? Does the fitness center have any intention of contracting with you after you share your nutrition proposal with them? How do you know the other party is worth your investment of time, effort and money?

The best answer to all of the above questions is to ask tactful, straightforward questions of the other party. Don't be so caught up in trying to impress them, you fail to evaluate them! Another method of qualifying someone is to ask for references or a financial statement (when appropriate). The reputation of a business or its owner can give a clue whether they are credible and honest. Call the Better Business Bureau to see if there are any charges against the company.

Step 2: What are the other party's "needs," and are they "over a barrel" for some reason?

By knowing as much as you can about what the other party "needs" from the negotiation, you have a better negotiating position. Examples could be the Health Department has given them a 30-day ultimatum to clean up the food service, or that business is poor and your name and reputation will draw more clients.

Use this information to your advantage, but don't always share the fact that you know their problems. One of the greatest challenges in negotiating is to evaluate the other party and decide how open you should be and how much not to share.

Step 3: Are there any "desires" that are strong?

In some instances, people or businesses may be motivated more by what they would "like" than what they need. They may want to be the first hospital to offer corporate wellness in the city and may disproportionately allocate funds to it. Or, the team coach may want a nutritionist to work with the players, so they can win "state" this year. Or, a restaurateur may want his menu to appeal to more clientele by offering nutritious menu items.

Step 4: Determine how low you can go.

What do you need and want from the negotiations? Determine your financial breakeven point and the amount of profit you will need to make the project worth your time. Develop statistics, illustrations and logical arguments to support and defend your views. What can you ask for, but be willing to give up as a concession? Never ask for the minimum you will accept. Ask for more, and then expect that the final agreement will probably be a compromise.

Step 5: Do you have a "Sears Plan" ready? Jean Yancey, a former small business advisor in Denver, Colorado, encouraged people to offer the "Sears Plan" (good, better and best alternatives). If the other party doesn't like one alternative you offer, have another ready to go. The best offer would be the most comprehensive and costly. The better offer is a good compromise. The good offer will at least get your foot in the door or provide an option in case negotiations stall.

Step 6: Determine what other items besides money you will ask for in the agreement. What interim payments and reports will you want? Ask for regular monthly payments, or for some projects, one-third up front, a third at midpoint, and the final payment upon completion. What about royalties for as long as your materials are used? What about editorial or revision rights when programs become dated? Are travel, office, mail, and phone expenses included? What staffing or support services will you expect? What marketing support will you request?

SELLING

A sale takes place when a client or patient agrees to pay for a service or product, or more globally, when someone agrees to do what you want done. To survive in business, sales must happen. Of course, everyone wants to offer products that are in such demand they "sell themselves," but that is a rarity.

Dietitians can increase their sales by improving their presentation skills and by taking better advantage of sales opportunities. Constantly be aware of instances where your nutrition services can be appropriately sold.

Getting Your Foot in the Door

Often before you can sell a physician or corporate leader on your services, you must first get past their secretaries. In a corporation, go as high as you can to give your sales presentation. You want to reach the decision-maker(s), but you may have to start several levels below.

Some tricks of the trade shared by Barry Wishner, RD, are to make the client feel like he or she is special, part of an exclusive club. Say, "I have heard that your OB practice is one of the most progressive, patient education-oriented practices in the area. I have a nutrition service that OB patients love, which will generate increased revenue for your practice. Can I have five minutes of Dr. Johnson's time to explain it to her?" It also works to appeal to their human nature by saying something like, "I had a baby five years ago. I am a dietitian, but I know how difficult it is to keep your weight gain under control. Do you offer a nutrition seminar to your patients? I have my brochure and sample patient education booklet, could I have five minutes of Dr. Brunson's time to explain my program?"

Sometimes it works to stop by a physician's office, and ask to schedule an appointment that day to talk to the physician. If he or she is unavailable, then ask to talk with the head nurse. If the nurse will talk to you and your message sounds interesting, you may be scooted into the physician's office in between the next two patients.

Try using someone as a referral to get to see the top person. Once you have established good rapport with a businessperson or physician, it is not out of place to ask if he or she knows of other CEOs, wellness directors or physicians who might be interested in your program. Ask if you could use their names as referrals.

A-B-C Accounts

In any business, no matter what you sell there will be some people who use your services or buy your products more than others. Sales experts suggest many different numbers, but everyone agrees that the majority of your time and resources should be spent maintaining and keeping your "A" accounts happy. "B" accounts use your services on an irregular basis, but given good service, or added attention, some might become "A" accounts. "C" accounts rarely, if ever, use your services. They might be contacted yearly in a mass mailing.

All three accounts could be in the same medical practice or may be very cordial to you at local Chamber of Commerce meetings. Some will be major clients and some won't. The important lesson to learn is that you spend your time and resources where they are most effective. Take the time to identify who supports you. Keep your "A" accounts happy!

The Sales Presentation

The sales presentation includes four major components, each with a specific purpose (3):

1. Introduction. The purpose of the introduction is to establish with the prospective client how you are different from all the others waiting to sell the same product. You do this by making statements that focus attention, specify direct benefits or warn of danger. For example, "From your year-end report, I saw that your company spends more than $2,500 per employee on health insurance. We have a wellness program that reduced medical expenses at the Reed Company by twenty percent last year."

2. Investigative Phase. This phase is one of the most important in the modern-day sales process. Get the buyer to define his or her other needs, wants and expectations. Do this by asking open-ended questions and by listening to the answers. The information obtained in this exchange will help you personalize your presentation and perhaps think of new products to sell. For example, "Have you ever tried any employee education seminars, and did they work?" Or, "What are your company's three worst employee health problems in your opinion?"

3. Presentation Phase. During this phase, carefully choose facts for their effect on your client. Show how his or her needs will be met by what you have to offer. Buyers base their decisions on fact and emotion. Garner emotional support for you and your services. If you see that the buyer is drifting or does not appear to understand, go back to the investigative phase and refocus attention by asking more questions. You need to be flexible. The outcome of this phase should be a natural progression to the close.

4. Closing. This is the time to bring the presentation to closure, either by asking for a sale or other commitment. One way to accomplish this is by summarizing the client's needs and identifying solutions you have to offer. Ask when you can begin, or how you can provide more assistance, or when you can provide more information. Your purpose may have been to introduce yourself and explain your services. Several ideas for closings might be: "If we have an agreement next week, how soon can I get started?" Or, "What more can I give you to help you make your decision?" Or, "Is there any reason why you wouldn't want to offer a weight loss program to your employees, given all the possible benefits?" Or, "Can I count on your commitment to this program for the coming year?"

Even if the client is not interested in your services at this time, leave the session as friends and on a positive note. If the client isn't ready to give an answer, ask when you can call for his answer. Don't give up. After the sales call, drop a note into the mail thanking the prospect for his or her time.

PROPOSALS

A proposal is a comprehensive marketing tool used to present the selling points of an idea. One could be used to interest a corporation in using you to create their nutrition wellness program. Or, sell an obesity seminar to a clinic director, or to interest a financial backer in a new product or business venture.

Proposals can range from a simple one-page typewritten information sheet to a typeset, bound presentation containing a volume of pages, along with a slide show and taste session. The scope of the proposal is determined by what is expected, what is used by the competition, and what will be impressive enough to make the sell. The experienced practitioner is not the only one to use a proposal. The novice may find it to be the very marketing boost to build her or his business more quickly.

Proposals should only be long enough to interest the client and make the sell. Care should be exercised so that explanations are not so detailed that clients can carry them out themselves without you.

Proposals usually represent many hours or days of research of the market and the client so the proposed item is "positioned" correctly. It will fit the client's needs. A proposal may include:

- An introduction or explanation of the scope of the proposal
- An overview of the market and its potential
- A short analysis of the competition
- Background information about the client and his needs
- Your answer to fulfilling the client's needs
- Why you are best for the job (include resume and references)
- Estimates of costs and potential income
- Any final selling points

A proposal should build in excitement and interest, as it leads to the answers you have to offer. Which points you use and their order are at your discretion. You want the client to feel they can't live without you and what you have to offer.

Whenever possible, the proposal should be made in person to the entire staff of decision-makers. Questions and any confusion can be handled immediately. An experienced negotiator may choose to paraphrase the proposal and offer a shorter written copy.

However, instances may arise when a proposal must be mailed or left at an office. When you are not there to give the introduction and to promote the concept with tact and enthusiasm, a letter of introduction and the written document must do it for you. A phone call should be timed to coincide with the day the person receives the document. If the contact person must sell the concept to others, when preparing the proposal enlist his help. Ask what selling points, statistics or other information he feels will be needed to impress the others. The answers you receive may give you great insight into the client company and its real interests.

There is always some fear of risk in giving a potential client the opportunity to see a truly unique, clever idea, such as an invention or new business concept. A proposal should never be detailed on how you will do your job; in most proposals, you are selling the client on using you, your creativity and expertise. It's fairly standard to ask before the proposal is offered the ideas be considered privileged information or to have "Confidential" stamped on the proposal. As an added safeguard, if you are very worried about controlling the concept, it is acceptable to bring another person with you as an associate (and witness). Finally, you can ask that the client sign a Non-Disclosure Agreement (see Chapter 12). However, some people will take offense to being asked, or will refuse to do so on legal grounds (they may have already had plans to pursue the idea). For example, you may be one of several people presenting a proposal on being a nutritionist for a new food company.

If an agreement is never reached, but your unique idea is used by the client, you could sue if your case is strong enough (a witness or written agreement may be necessary to do so). You will have to be able to prove the unique idea was owned by you through copyrights, trademarks or patents.

A proposal provides a perfect opportunity again to offer the "Sears Plan" to a client: the "good, better and best" approach. Anticipate that the client may be hesitant to buy the most comprehensive plan you have to offer. Be ready to promote the contingency plan of lesser cost, in case the first one doesn't sell. A third "at least you got your foot in the door" plan could be either offered initially, or you could wait and use it if all else fails.

Presenting a proposal may lead to other new ideas or ventures between you and the client. Or, it may only help your client decide what he doesn't want to do. Whatever the extent of the agreement to work together, it should be outlined, signed and all parties should have a copy.

Assertiveness in Business Grows in Time

As Herb Cohen states in his book, *You Can Negotiate Anything*, we actually negotiate several times per day every day of our lives. Whether we need a refund on poor service, a package delivered on time or the secretary to answer the phone more pleasantly, we are trying to have our wishes met. We sometimes have to become more assertive to do it.

To be more effective in your work and to negotiate better contracts and consultant fees, it helps to know when and how to stand your ground. For persons who are not used to being assertive, finding a happy medium between being passive and being overbearing or stubborn is a necessity. Finesse will develop in time. Consider how you would handle the following situation:

Business Negotiations
Two businessmen called the nutritionist to ask if she felt she had expertise in menu development for their proposed natural food restaurant. They told her they had heard good things about her professionally and wanted her services. They also mentioned they were well financed and planned to start a concept that could be franchised

nationwide. A meeting was scheduled for the three on the coming Thursday.

The nutritionist was very excited about the concept. At the meeting the two men asked verbally for her confidentiality, and she agreed. They then explained in general terms what they planned to do, where, when, and how successful it would be. The two men were dressed in business suits and were apparently successful, if appearances can be trusted.

The two men asked to see some of the nutritionist's work in menu and recipe development and she agreed (she had brought her restaurant portfolio on her past client accounts). The businessmen were impressed. They told the nutritionist they might even have a staff or consultant position for her at a very good salary, if she would consider taking a chance with them by working in return for a "piece of the action".

The nutritionist was always willing to pursue new, exciting concepts, but she had heard too many similar proposals before to go blindly into another one. She knew it was her turn to start asking some questions: Who was backing the venture? What experience did the two have in the restaurant business; if it was very little, who was going to be hired to develop and manage the concept? What did they want her to do besides menu and recipe development, some marketing, personnel training, ongoing updating, and testing of food items, or whatever? How many hours per month? Also, what did they propose would be her fair share of a "piece of the action"? Would it mean she would be a partner or shareholder? Legally, how would it be set up?

The reason for this battery of questions was the fact they had first said they were well financed, and then asked her to work without pay, at least initially. The questions were probing, but the businessmen were asking her to participate in their business venture in return for nonpayment of her services. She had every right to find out as much as she could before calling her own lawyer and other business consultants to discuss the offer.

Too often less assertive or business-wise nutritionists accept appearances as the truth and unwisely believe that other people always have their best interests at heart. The businessmen were there because they wanted something they thought the dietitian could supply (good reputation, recipes, expertise, credibility, or whatever). It is always better to try to find out up front if a business relationship is honest and open, than to assume everything is okay. You risk not being paid, or being professionally burned by people who misrepresent themselves and their capabilities.

AGREEMENTS

Agreements, or exchanges of promises between two parties, can take several forms. The more common are a verbal agreement, a bid, letter of agreement, or contract. Some forms do not offer the business novice much protection, in case the other party does not perform as expected. Contracts are more detailed, but are sometimes too complex and expensive to be useful. The best agreements are between two reputable people who have adequately discussed their expectations of the other person.

Verbal, or Gentleman's, Agreements

Verbal, or gentlemen's, agreements for fees and services are usually considered legally binding in most states and are very common. Professional consultants and advisors often quote their fees for certain services and we agree to them verbally. We may agree to consult at a physician's office or a health club on a handshake. Verbal agreements are fine when you know the other party, and both of you know what is expected and perform accordingly. In cases where there are misunderstandings or one person does not produce as expected, a verbal agreement can prove to be inadequate protection.

COMMON QUESTION: Keeping a Successful Account

Q: I am negotiating with a physician to offer nutrition consultation in his office. I am willing to work hard, take a financial risk and build the program. But what guarantees do I have that when I become successful financially, I won't be replaced? How can I protect myself before I make the investment?

A: If the physician is a fair and honest person, there are ways to avoid problems. If she or he is not, the situation probably will be out of your control. First, realize that it is only a good deal if you both feel you have been fairly compensated for what you have each contributed. So get out in the open what each of you is offering the other. You may be offering time, effort and some money, and the physician is offering client referrals, facilities and some money. Later on as you become successful, the possibility of being replaced is reduced if the following have taken place.

- You have a working relationship with the physician and the staff and you are considered an asset.
- You are closely identified with the nutrition program and, if you go, so will the program and client load.
- Each of you feels fairly compensated. Also, incentives should be built in so that extra work or effort on your part is rewarded.

- You developed the teaching materials on your own time and copyrighted them. The programs can only be used as long as you are a consultant there.
- Finally, before beginning, you and the physician should put your agreement in writing. At this time, try to add a simple partnership buy-out agreement in case the physician wants the program, but wants to replace you.

You may be surprised; it may be the physician who fears you leaving more than the other way around.

Bids

A bid, or cost estimate for a job, is legal. It can be a good agreement if it's specific as to quality and date of completion, and both parties agree to any changes in writing. The most common shortcomings of bids are too little shared information. To help remedy this, bids may be accompanied by an explanation or sample of a similar finished product or a proposal (see Figure 17.1).

Figure 17.1 Sample Bid

SMITH & JONES NUTRITION SERVICES, INC
2530 Ridgeway, Tucson, AZ 85728

BID

For development of a diet manual for EARTH GROWN FOODS on lacto-ovo vegetarian diets for the following limitations:
- Low Calorie
- Low Cholesterol
- Diabetic
- Low Salt

The manual will include sample menus, nutrient charts, references for recipes, and a brand-name food guide. The finished manual will contain approximately 100 pages.

Completion date: One month from the acceptance of this bid.

Project cost: $10,000.

Earth Grown Foods   Date

Letter of Agreement

A letter of agreement is also legally binding, but less formal and complicated than a contract. For many people a letter is also less intimidating. To be good, this form of agreement must be comprehensive and may include the following information:
- What the agreement is for, i.e., services, product, etc.?
- Who is providing it?
- When?
- Where?
- For how much?
- How often?
- Who is paying for it, on what schedule or by what process, i.e. billing, monthly fee, etc.?
- Any additional provisions?
- Terms of the agreement?
- Termination clause by either party?

A letter of agreement may be written in the form of a short exchange of promises (see Figure 17.2). It may be in the form of a business or personal letter that outlines what the agreement is as the writer understands it. It's suggested that both parties sign the agreement. However, courts of law will often stand behind a letter that was sent by certified mail (return receipt requested) when no rebuttal was made, and the work was allowed to progress as if the agreement were accepted.

It's highly suggested that you consult with your lawyer concerning the provisions you should include in your letters of agreement to cover your particular business. After you're more familiar with this type of agreement, you will seldom need legal input, except in cases of higher risk.

Contracts

Contracts are used when the risk is greater, the money higher, and when more control is needed. Legal input is highly recommended for the development or review of all contracts before one is signed.

A contract may have any number of provisions and limitations. Don't be hoodwinked when someone tells you, "You can look it over if you want. It's just a standard contract." Take the time to read every word and ask questions about clauses you don't understand.

Parties to a contract exchange promises. These may be expressed (i.e., communicated explicitly and clearly, either in verbal or written form) or implied (i.e., deduced from actions or behavior).(4) Proper contracts involve the following ethical conditions: (5)

Figure 17.2 Sample Letter of Agreement

THE WOMAN'S HOSPITAL
7600 Jones Street
Atlanta, GA 30303

January 19, 2003

Ms. Stephanie White, R.D.
Nutrition Consultant Services of Atlanta, Inc.
7800 Fannin, Suite 203
Atlanta, GA 30310

Dear Ms. White:

This letter is to confirm our telephone conversation of January 18, 2003. As agreed in our conversation, your firm will provide its services to this hospital according to the following provisions:

1. The hospital agrees to pay $75 per outpatient consultation to Nutrition Consultant Services of Atlanta, Inc. No other benefits or privileges are offered or implied.
2. This agreement shall be for six (6) months and automatically renewable at the end of each six month period.
3. Appointments will be coordinated by the Food Service Department and Nursing Service. Initially, a nutrition therapist will be available Tuesday, Wednesday and Thursday from 9 am to 5 pm. Lunch break will be from 11:15-12:00 noon.
4. A copy of each patient's interview sheet will be sent to each referring physician and a copy put into each patient's chart by the nutritionist of Nutrition Consultant Services of Atlanta, Inc.
5. A super bill will be given by the nutritionist to each patient to file with his or her insurance company, and payment will be expected at the time of the visit at the clinic cashier's desk.
6. This agreement may be terminated by either party with thirty (30) days written notice.

Thank you for your assistance. If you have any questions concerning the agreement, please do not hesitate to contact my office.

Sincerely,

Cary D. Henry
Administrator

1. One party makes an offer, which is accepted by the other party.
2. Each party must offer the other consideration (i.e., something of value) in return for what it is to receive from the other party.
3. Both parties must act of their own free will, free of duress and undue influence.
4. The agreement cannot include fraudulent representations or violate the law.
5. Certain types of contracts must be in written form (e.g., real estate).

One item of great concern to consultants, employees and subcontractors is the **non-compete clause** in a contract. If one is used, it must be reasonable. Most non-compete clauses state clients provided by the contractor or employer are not to be taken or approached for a period of time after the consultant or employee leaves. Recently, courts of law have said that special training or proprietary information must be taught to the employee or consultant by an employer in order for a non-compete clause to be used. Check with a lawyer in your state before signing an agreement with a non-compete clause.

Generating a contract can be expensive and time consuming. Your legal bill will be less if you know what you want. Write a bulleted list of what you have agreed to do, what the client wants, and any special provisions, such as who will pay for what up-front or who has final edit on the materials. Tell your lawyer to make the contract: practical, easy to understand, and complete, in order to protect your reasonable interests. Unless cautioned otherwise, some lawyers produce very expensive documents that are so detailed and overwhelming no one will sign them.

CONCLUSION

Underlying this discussion on negotiating and agreements should be the awareness that the outcomes work best when both parties are honest, open and work in good faith. No written document can make people work together well if the relationship is poor. Learning how to "read" the other party and keep control of your advantage points becomes easier with experience, becoming better known, and trial and error.

REFERENCES

1. Warschaw TA. Winning By Negotiation. New York: McGraw-Hill; 1980.
2. Negotiating Tricks. Report No. 200, 1978 by Chase Revel, Inc.
3. Cohen H. You Can Negotiate Anything. New York: Bantam Books; 1989.
4. Sobel M. The 12-Hour MBA Program. New Jersey: Prentice Hall; 1993.
5. Wiesner DA, Glaskowsky NA. Theory and Problems of Business Law. New York: McGraw-Hill; 1985.

Chapter 18

Computers in Nutrition Practice

Computers are not new to the field of dietetics, however many of us are just learning to appreciate the functions they can perform. According to Ellyn Luros-Elson, RD, President of Computrition, Inc., her company now has software that can do everything she did (nutrition-calculation wise) in her internship and first two years of work. Recipes can be calculated for cost and nutrients in minutes. A patient's allergies and food preferences can be allowed for on menus. Drug and nutrient interactions are caught before the patient is served. Computers can easily handle repetitive tasks.

This could scare some practitioners. It will replace some. However, for most dietitians and dietetic technicians, it will free them to do more care, do more creative things in food service, help them publish e-books, do desktop publishing, or easily remain aware of the latest research.

WHAT CAN A COMPUTER DO FOR A PRACTITIONER?

Before investing in the expense of a computer, software and training on how to use the system, research what you want the computer to do. Too many small business owners buy a computer because they think they must need one. But they have no idea (other than for bookkeeping and nutritional analysis) what to do with it. What an expensive investment!

Nutrient Analysis

Nutrient analysis of recipes, menus and food intakes is probably the most familiar computer function to dietitians. Before the use of the computer, it was so time consuming to analyze foods for nutrient levels that it was not done with any regularity, except perhaps in research settings.

Today, practitioners use nutrient analyses while working with individual patients, corporate clients, athletes and restaurants. Clients are impressed and curious about computer printouts that show "scientifically" how nutritious their diets are. The truth, of course, is the results are only ballpark figures.(1) Plus, the menus analyzed may not be representative of the client's normal eating patterns. The amounts and ingredients of foods may even be thirty percent or more wrong, because of the guesswork involved in a layman's food diary or recall. And, finally, the database used to analyze the foods may not be complete enough, so entire foods are left out of the calculations, or their approximate recipes are estimated. To help avoid these pitfalls as much as possible, a practitioner should instruct the client on how to measure foods (ideally by weight). A week's record could be recorded with three representative days chosen for analysis. Take care to find analysis software that has an accurate and adequate database, and where new research was used to update the government figures.

Nutrition Histories and Assessment

Nutrition histories, fitness and lifestyle computer questionnaires can be developed or purchased for use by the patient or you in your office. The questionnaire results can be used to motivate the patient by showing specific areas for needed improvement, or where the person is doing well.

Handheld and portable laptop computers make nutrition assessment and enteral and parenteral or BEE (basal energy expenditure) calculations available at a patient's bedside. These tools are crucial to critical care dietitians, and for outpatient consultants who also use the diabetes, renal or exchange programs.

Word Processing and Desktop Publishing

Word processing capabilities of a computer are well known. Articles, menus, newsletters reports, letters, individualized diets, and other written items can be typed, viewed on the screen, corrected or changed, and then printed. If the item is stored on the hard drive or software, it can be recalled and reused or corrected as needed. Lists of names and addresses of patients, colleagues or customers can be sorted and then merged with a letter to give a bulk mailing that individualized look. Labels or envelopes can be printed to match the headings. By preprogramming nutrition care plans onto software, a practitioner can individualize, or adjust a plan for each patient and then print it for a personalized presentation. If you have a computer with adequate memory and a laser printer, there is software to produce as good quality printing as produced by print stores. Color printouts also are possible for a fraction of the cost of ten years ago.

With the right software, books can be loaded onto the Internet and sold as e-books. There are companies that help you publish, market, and fill orders (see Chapter 27 The "Write" Way to Get Published).

Business Management

Business management is greatly simplified through use of software with financial spreadsheets and accounting capabilities. More detailed and complete records can be maintained of customers' buying habits and sales figures. The computer can calculate food orders, cost analysis per vendor or menu item, inventory control, employee scheduling and paperwork and, of course, many other bookkeeping functions. Detailed records can be prepared more regularly and compared with past incomes, expenses and forecasts.

Bookkeeping records can be sent by telephone using a modem and your computer to your accountant for auditing and tax preparation. Software is available that will turn your computer and its modem into a facsimile machine (FAX). You can then send or receive printed material over the phone line and communicate more quickly in the business world. (See Chapter 14 Money and Finance.)

Email capabilities are possible through cell phones, computer terminals, laptops, and other newer communication devices. Along with a cell phone, email has become an essential business communication tool. It can also be a waste of time, if too much effort is spent checking out the spammed messages, jokes and unnecessary business banter.

The World Wide Web is making advertising, promotion, sales and information sharing history. It is beginning to change the way people live, buy goods and services, learn, and handle business. (See Chapters 21-23 for more detailed uses.)

Teaching

Teaching nutrition to patients, clients or students can be carried out on a computer. Topics such as energy balance for weight control, sports nutrition and menu planning, plus diabetic or other clinical diet guidelines or behavior change lessons, can be programmed onto software in an interactive, self-instruction format. It's expected in the next ten years that as much as 30 percent of students will take courses online for their advanced education.

A computer may be used for evaluating the effectiveness of your nutrition counseling sessions. By pre- and post-testing a patient in a non-threatening environment, the patient and you will be able to tell whether the patient and his family understood the most important points.

Researching Literature and Reports

Researching is another function that can be carried out on a computer. Through use of a modem and the appropriate software through your telephone, you can access information in much larger databases at libraries, government offices, and banks. Companies in the business of placing journal reports, medical literature, media articles, stock reports, and so on, on databases for sale to subscribers can be accessed for a fee. When practitioners want to write an article or book on a subject or appear on the media, they can have the most recent information at their disposal. (See Chapter 21 Using the Internet.)

COMPUTER ADVANTAGES

Computers require time and commitment to work well but the effort is worth it. Most of us are not born "computer-friendly." It's an acquired skill. The major advantage computers provide is greater volume of quality business output. In today's market, computers can help give you an edge in offering more information and service than your competitors.

Chapter 19

Office Policy and Dealing With Clients

Kathy King Helm, RD and Alanna Dittoe, RD

There are other factors besides your knowledge and nutrition information given to clients that influence their opinion of your services. Clients usually expect their association with you and your office to be courteous, organized, efficient, reasonable in cost, and timely. Actually, our clients' expectations are no different from our own.

CREATING AN EFFECTIVE OPERATION

Competition is growing for the consumer's dollar, and a business owner can't afford to turn clients off with inadequate service. Personalized care of clients should begin when they first call to ask about your services or schedule an appointment. Attempts should be made to impress clients with the non-dietetic functions of your operation.

Establish office hours and days and try to follow your schedule as closely as possible to help develop an image of stability and continuity. As long as clients can leave a message for you, it is not necessary to be available in the office, in person, five days a week. In the beginning, try to condense your patient instructions and interviews with other clients to only a few days per week. The remaining days can then be used to hold down another job while you start your business, or give you time to market your business, write or whatever.

Telephone coverage for your business is extremely important. The telephone is your clients' major link with you. During normal business hours Monday through Friday, clients should be able to either reach you by phone or leave a message with a secretary, answering service or voice mail machine. If you can't answer the phone yourself and you don't want to give out your cell phone number, be sure to take the time to instruct the secretary or answering service on what to say and what information to ask for. Check your messages regularly and have someone call to check for you when you are out of town. Messages on telephone answering recorders should be well prepared--keep trying until you record a message that people will not only listen to, but also respond to. A higher level of service is perceived when calls are returned promptly.

Some hints that may be important to you concerning your telephone answering service include the following:

1. Don't allow your services and fees to be given over the phone by someone, unless the person is trained to properly "market" your business. Have them say, "I will be happy to take your name and number and have Ms. Buckmaster, the nutritionist, call you back."
2. Caution your answering service or secretary about giving out your private home phone number and address.
3. When you are out of town, instruct your answering service to tell people that "Ms. Buckmaster will be in the office to return your call on Monday, July 10; can she call you back at that time, or is this an emergency?" If you have another dietitian who knows your practice, you might have the answering service say, "Mary Jones, RD, is covering all calls and I can have her call you if you wish." If it is an emergency, have the number of the covering dietitian or the local hospital clinical nutrition department. In case you need to be reached, leave a number where your secretary/answering service can reach you or leave a message.

When scheduling appointments with new patients, use the conversations as opportunities to "market" your services. Take the time to ask questions about the patient and his or her nutritional needs, pertinent lab values, and referring physician's name. Request that the patient bring a copy of the most recent lab results and, if available, the physician's written referral for the appointment. Explain what the patient will receive in the way of individualized care and information. State approximately how long the appointment will take and how much it will cost. Make sure the patient knows the directions to your office, the suite number, where to park, if it's a problem, and the date and time of the appointment. Request that the patient give 24 hours notice if the appointment has to be changed or cancelled.

The office setting should be quiet, comfortable and professional. The office furnishings usually are not as important as the atmosphere, hospitality and service provided. However, because of the image they want to portray and their clients' expectations, some private practitioners spend extra for more affluent looking office space and interiors. One practitioner reports that in a survey of her office patients, the majority mentioned the office coffee as the best amenity. Offering tea, coffee, water, or a snack in an office setting can be "that little extra" that make patients feel more at home.

The chart system for your office can be as expensive as a computer system or the color-coded system, or as simple as a manila folder for each patient. Because of the importance of documentation of a patient's progress, it is best to have the patient's nutrition chart available for all visits. The patient's medical chart is usually only available when you work in a medical office.

The information to include in the patient's chart is name, address, work and home phone numbers, their physician's name, the referring physician's name (if different), and a copy of the diet prescription, if available, pertinent lab values, a diet evaluation, action plan, and goals. The follow-up sessions should have any changes in lab values and other objective measurements. After the initial instruction and when something significant happens to a patient, the referring physician should be notified, and the contact documented.

Publications for your clients to read enhance the service and contribute to the positive positioning and image of your practice. Any booklets, programs, etc., you write should definitely have the copyright notice added to them. Include the cost of handouts and diets in the fee for the instruction. Many consultant nutritionists keep a supply of books, booklets and other educational items they know patients want to buy. In most states, sales tax must be collected, and a sales tax, or even vendor's license, may be necessary.

When preparing printed diets, the typeface should be easy to read, not script, as some people with poor eyesight also have trouble reading single-spaced 10-point font.

Information overload is a common problem. Avoid giving clients too many publications. Start with one or two at the initial visit and assess what each person needs or wants. Patients and their families can only absorb a small amount of information on a new subject at any one time. Save the less specific material and the larger number of booklets for the few clients who want them.

Many practitioners report their patients are impressed when they use folders to hold take-home materials. The folder usually has pockets on the inside to hold the diet and any booklets. On the outside of the folder, print the company name or logo for easy identification of the contents and for advertising purposes or attach a business card to the folder to provide your address and phone number.

Diet manuals are readily available to all practitioners today. In writing your own diets, you may choose good ideas from several manuals and from your experience. If you are unaware of your local medical community's nutritional biases, try to purchase diet manuals from the local hospitals, or make an appointment with a hospital dietitian to discuss them. Pages should not be photocopied directly from a manual, unless it was designed for that purpose or you request permission from the copyright owner.

In private practice, it is not necessary to have a large variety of different diets, such as in the hospital. Practitioners report the most common nutrition therapies are the following: weight loss, diabetic, hypoglycemic, low salt, low cholesterol, hyperlipidemia diets, allergy, high potassium, normal pregnancy, and good nutrition for the healthy individual. Specialties in your medical community may dictate that other diets be developed.

DISTINCTIVE SERVICE

Private practitioners and outpatient counselors know their consultative sessions and handout materials need to be different and better than those provided by free hospital clinics or by physicians' nurses or secretaries. Practitioners must create this difference, or patients and clients will balk at paying the fee. The keys are "quality," "individualized" and "personalized."

Many dietitians, though not all, think it is important to use different terminology in private practice from that used in acute care settings: "diet" could be "nutritional care plan" or "food plan," and "diet order" could be "nutrition prescription." Some practitioners call the people they instruct "clients" instead of patients, especially in more wellness-oriented settings. Always remember, care should be taken to differentiate patients from their illness. In other words, a person is not a diabetic or a hypertensive but, instead, a person with diabetes or hypertension.

Whether a consultant wears a white jacket or lab coat is a personal choice. Some patients appear to feel intimidated by the authority signified by the white, while others expect the white jacket or lab coat, which shows you are the nutrition authority.

COLLECTING FEES AND ENDING A SESSION

The end of the interview is a good time to talk about rescheduling a visit, or to discuss why it is not necessary. This is a good "ending" subject and lets the client know the visit is over. As you are winding up, be sure to incorporate some system to collect the fee. You may simply state, "I will make out your receipt now--how do you want to pay for your instruction?" or "The fee for the initial visit is $___ and revisits are $_____ . I will give you an itemized receipt that you can attach to your insurance company's form, along with a copy of the referral slip from your doctor. Depending upon your policy, you can submit these materials to get reimbursed for our visit." If you have a office assistant, be sure to train her or him on how to collect fees as well.

If a patient continues to linger after the closing of the session and you have other commitments, you can either relax and take a minute longer, or you can try standing up and walking slowly toward the door to show him out, and simply state, "I want to thank you very much for coming. I am sorry to rush, but I have another patient waiting."

COMMON QUESTIONS

Q: *I can't get physicians to refer patients to me, and the patients who call me from my brochure and newspaper ad don't show up. What can I do?*

A: Your services could be so new that physicians and prospective patients haven't learned how to use them yet (even when you try to tell them). Or, there could be some more painful answers like you haven't, and don't know how to, establish credibility (check Chapter 4), your appearance or personality may not meet the expectations of your target markets, or you could be saying the wrong things or "right" things in the wrong way.

Before you change too many things on your own, I would talk to a business consultant. Long-term this could save you a lot of time and money. You can usually find a person like this in the Yellow Pages, through contacts in professional or business groups or the SCORE through the SBA. Talk to the person over the phone and if you like him or her, get an appointment.

In preparation for the appointment, write down what you say to prospective patients over the phone and to physicians when you interview with them. Go over your marketing strategies like the prices, promotion, products and location(s) you use for your business. Take copies of your brochure and ads. Listen to what the person suggests as solutions and try them out, since you have nothing to lose. Don't get discouraged! We all have things to learn.

One Maryland dietitian who had this same problem had to work on lowering her voice because she sounded like she was twelve years old over the phone, instead of twenty-nine. An advisor told a short, young looking woman to buy suits, instead of wearing such feminine dresses in pastel colors that lacked any "power." Similarly, a male dietitian who consulted to major hospitals and corporations for very big fees found that he was most successful in landing the accounts when he dressed in expensive suits and shoes like the successful corporate president he was (virtual corporation-one person with temporary help as needed).

One experienced clinical dietitian opened her business charging the same higher fees as a practitioner who had been in business in the area for many years and was very well established. It took a while for the new dietitian's business to grow because there was price-resistance, since she was new and unknown in the community. Does this mean every dietitian should start with low prices as a marketing strategy? Of course not! It just means it takes time for a business to become established. If the level of service matches the price asked, and the target market needs the service or product and can afford it, the business will grow.

Once you try a few new ideas and they seem to be working, go back to see the physicians who have not been referring to you and start building a rapport with them and their office staff. Use some of the ideas mentioned in Chapter 20 on Promotion. Good luck!

Q: My patients aren't returning after the first visit. What might be wrong? What can I do?
A: There are many reasons why patients don't return. Some reasons are in your control; others are not. The reason physicians overbook and some dentists and psychiatrists charge for no-shows is because a certain number of patients will not keep appointments. This point known, there are still professionals who do not have a problem with no-shows, and there are times when each of us experiences it more frequently.

After allowing for bad weather, business advisors will tell you it is significant whether patients don't show at all or they call to reschedule. Not calling or showing up is, of course, more symptomatic of a problem.

Some of the more obvious reasons patients do not return are:
- They feel no commitment to the care plan because you did not involve them enough in developing it, or it did not fit their true lifestyle.
- It was not their choice to make the appointment and they only gave lip service while there.
- The patients did not understand the importance of follow-up and how it would improve their chances for successful behavior change.
- They followed your suggested guidelines and did not get results--or they got results without following it.
- You did not impress them with the consultation, your manner or something about the office visit. (Some patients will not take advice from traditional-thinking, or young, or inexperienced counselors.)
- The fee was too high for what they felt they received, or for their present income.

- The consultation style and approach may have been too threatening, embarrassing or too familiar to suit the patient. (We do not always hit it off with every patient.)
- The instruction materials may have been too confusing.
- The patient may believe his present habits fit his needs better, and he is not willing to change. Maybe the suggestions weren't reasonable--or maybe they were, but not at this time.
  Areas you may want to evaluate and improve if you deem them a problem are:
- Are you marketing and describing your services well over the phone when the patient calls for an appointment? Fees should be mentioned up front, along with what you have to offer and what commitment you expect from the patient. The patient should feel he knew what to expect.
- Do you impress upon your patients the importance of follow-up visits?
- Is the patient's visit a pleasant one? Is he greeted and given good, timely service?
- Are you up-to-date and knowledgeable in nutrition and counseling? Can you offer a variety of solutions, and are you flexible enough to make changes when they are needed?
- Are your counseling sessions organized and professionally handled?
- Do you have the appearance of a credible, competent stable professional? Can you change your appearance to look more like what is "expected" by your clientele?
- Are your fees too high or low for what you offer or for your local community? Could you offer more or package it better?

Two of the best ways to take the mystery out of this process are by sending a note to remind patients a week in advance and by calling all patients a day ahead to remind them of the appointment and to ask how they are doing. Calling a patient can serve several purposes: the patient may feel more at ease about stating a problem, he may decide to make a greater commitment because of your apparent interest, or he may cancel future appointments on the spot.

EMPLOYEE CONSIDERATIONS

If you decide to budget an office employee into your business, there are several considerations to think about:

1. Administrative assistant is the term used for secretary in most business settings.

2. How will the person spend her or his day--write a job description.
3. In the beginning, can she/he work mornings or a short week to help keep overhead lower.
4. Decide how much you can afford to pay. It may be worth paying a little more to keep someone who speaks well on the phone and is courteous and efficient in the office.
5. Decide what skills are most important for the running of your office before you start to interview applicants.
6. Talk to your financial advisor about what "perks," if any, to offer as present or future incentives to your employee(s).
7. Discuss with your accountant or CPA the difference in costs to you for an employee versus leased or temporary labor (payroll taxes, social security, worker's compensation, added paper work, pension plan, etc.).

To assure the person represents you well, take adequate time of your own to train the new assistant. You should decide whether to teach her how to market your business on the phone or just to take messages. Office policies need to be determined and procedures established to carry out the daily routines. A poor employee can harm your business so do not hesitate to terminate someone who does not work out.

Although there is added expense in having an employee who can perform such duties as typing, mailing, screening, confirming patient appointments, scheduling new patients, collecting fees and greeting clients, they can be as valuable as your right arm.

Several private practitioners have hired Dietetic Technicians in their offices to cover the secretarial duties, as well as conduct initial interviews with patients and fill out the needed medical, laboratory and nutritional data. They are very happy with the DTRs and highly recommend that other dietitians consider hiring them too. It may take time to find the right person(s), but it is worth it, if in the future you generate more income and have a better-functioning business.

CONCLUSION

Other than having a good background in nutrition, it is just as important that a consultant have good management and business skills in order to succeed. A practitioner should strive to produce distinctive service and provide up-to-date information with flair.

——Taking Your Ideas—— to Market

Words of Wisdom:

"Every job is a self-portrait of the person who did it. Autograph your work with excellence."

"Quality is never an accident; it is always the result of high intention, sincere effort, intelligent direction and skillful execution; it represents the wise choice of many alternatives."

Willa A. Foster

Chapter 20

Promoting Your Venture

A commitment to advertising and promotion is essential in any business, small or large. Lack of sufficient promotion is one reason so many businesses stagnate or fail to attract customers. When economic times get tough, advertising is one of the first budget items cut, which often makes sales even worse-it can be the wrong thing to do!

MARKETING A SERVICE:
COUNSELING, MANAGEMENT

Marketing is concerned with getting and keeping customers. Product intangibility has its greatest effect on the process of trying to get customers. How do you propose to sell something, like nutrition counseling or management consulting, that a customer can't hold in his hand, feel or see?

Intangible services can seldom be tried out in advance. Prospective buyers are generally forced to depend on surrogates to assess what they probably will get. They can look at before and after pictures of weight loss patients. They can talk to current users of your services. They can see and hold your elegant calling card, brochure or business proposal in its attractive binder. Service marketing expert, Harry Beckwith, states there are four keys to successful service marketing: (1)

1. Price: The more it costs (to a point), the better it seems. If customers come to you because you are the lowest price, they will leave when someone else's price is better, if that's all they care about-work to offer more.
2. Brand: It creates a powerful barrier to entry for aspiring competitors. When people think of nutrition-you want them to think of you. Choose a memorable business name-not initials, not frivolous, not commonplace. To entice our memory the name should be "unique, short, sensory, creative, and outstanding." Your personal name may be good. Spend the time and money to have your logo and name in front of potential customers, but back it up with good service.

56

3. Packaging: When you are timid about investing in your brochure, office, business cards, presentations, and so on, you're saying you lack confidence and passion for your enterprise. Usually, timid marketing doesn't work.
4. Relationships: Business is personal, especially in a service where you are sitting across from the person. Show clients you are interested in them; offer them a beverage and remember what they chose; remember important details about them (write notes), and ask how they want something done. Don't work with "toxic" clients and employees-get rid of them. They will drain you and run off other productive client relationships. The eight keys to lasting relationships are: (1)

- **Natural affinity.** Work with people you like and who like you.
- **Trust.** Mutual trust is the basis of a good relationship.
- **Speed.** Answer the needs of your customers in this computer age with overnight delivery; people now expect things to be done fast.
- **Apparent expertise.** Look like you are well respected in your profession (mount certificates on the wall), look successful, and keep current with the newest research.
- **Sacrifice.** Bend over backwards to please the customer by meeting an earlier deadline, or calling to find out the answer to a client's question on a food product.
- **Completeness.** If you want to be known as an expert in nutrition, don't become an expert in only one disease; if you design kitchens, you must know about equipment, ventilation systems and building codes. Be complete!
- **Magic words.** Know the magic words of relationships--the client's name, "Thanks," "How are you doing?" and "Welcome."
- **Passion.** Passion will attract people to you and make them want to return. If you love what you do, it will show. Passion is worth billions!

It is easy to understand why banks build large, sturdy buildings and hire articulate consultants in business suits. Also, why proposals are in "executive" typeset and leather bindings, and why architects laboriously draw renderings of buildings. It explains why insurance companies offer "a piece of the rock," put you under a "blanket of protection," or "in good hands."

PUBLIC RELATION'S ROLE IN MARKETING

Public relations programs are designed to create a positive climate in which a company or group can do business, earn recognition and gain acceptance. Marketing programs set forth strategies for selling or promoting products and services for which funding is sought or consideration is to be gained. Such strategies define an organization's competitive edge and its position within the marketplace. (2)

Public relations (PR) is primarily a communications tool, whereas marketing also includes needs assessment, product development, pricing, and distribution. PR seeks to influence attitudes, whereas marketing tries to elicit specific behaviors, such as buying, joining, etc. PR defines the image of an organization, whereas marketing defines the organization's goals, business mission, customers, services, and so on.(2)

Selling products or services, or soliciting funds should take place after public relations and marketing campaigns have opened the doors, creating a favorable climate for success. (2) Effective public relations do not necessarily require costly expenditures. It does require a clear understanding of an organization's image, products and marketplace.

Elements of successful PR and marketing campaigns: (2)
- Planned, not left to chance
- Continuous, not single shot
- Proactive, not just reactive, to events and problems
- Clearly focused with well-defined goals, timetables and specific assignments
- Well-managed, evaluated and revised regularly

PROMOTION

Promotion is the communication you use to help others become familiar with you, your services or product. Promotion has become more important to dietitians than ever before because of the changes in the marketplace.

First, consumers are now shopping around to find the best nutrition services and products for their money. Second, there is confusion today in the public's mind about who to believe in the nutrition field. Finally, dietitians aren't the only legitimate players in the nutrition arena. We may have had ownership in the past in some market areas through default but today that is no longer the case. Nutrition is in demand by the consumer; it's therefore a competitive area of business. (3)

Dietitians often neglect to plan and oversee adequate promotion for programs, not realizing poor attendance or lackluster promotion reflects back on the program. Actually, it shows lack of foresight and follow-through if a practitioner devotes total attention to the development of an excellent program that could produce client satisfaction, and yet fails to insure the program's success through adequate promotion. (4)

Promotion will attract far more clients to our doors than any form of legislation. Because the health-care focus is evolving to more health promotion and to attracting the "well" individual, we must accept that our services are among the many nutrition options available to each consumer. Therefore, dietitians must learn how to promote themselves and their products.

PROMOTION TOOLS

There are many tools that can be used in promotion. The target market, your budget, the degree of competition, and the image you want to project usually determine which technique you select. Some promotional tools are far more effective in reaching the target market but may also be very expensive (like television or color ads in magazines). Other techniques may better meet the expectations of the target markets, for example, tasteful brochures and business cards at a one-on-one meeting. Medical professionals have been slow in using less traditional promotion tools, such as billboards and neon signs, but sending a bouquet of balloons or Holiday deli tray to top referring physicians' offices have been very effective.

When trying to evaluate which forms of promotion to use, public relations experts suggest you go down a list of the promotion options, and hypothetically try to fit the service or product to it. Look for ideas that are creative, unique and in good taste.

Promotion is most successful when a plan is designed for multiple exposure of the name or message to the target market over an extended period. For a weight-loss program at a fitness center, promotion could include newspaper and radio ads, free media publicity, direct mail promotion, and in-house newsletter promotion to members. You could give gym bags printed with the program name and logo at registration, and program T-shirts when fitness goals are met. These are just a few promotion ideas; there are dozens more.

There are advertising and public relations firms and individual consultants that can create promotional campaigns for a fee. For most dietitians with many projects, that is not always an affordable option, but it may be a wise investment for selected projects. Promotion costs should be seen as part of the necessary expense and investment made to create demand for what you sell. The challenge is to choose wisely, and be cost effective when investing in promotional programs.

BRIEF OVERVIEW OF PROMOTIONAL TOOLS

One-on-One Communication

One-on-one communication can be your most effective form of promotion. It affords the opportunity to speak, hear, see, and exchange viewpoints face-to-face. As the promoter, you have the opportunity to read the body language and expressions of your listener and then adjust your presentation for best impact.

Satisfied customers are walking promoters of inestimable value. Through word-of-mouth advertising, listeners may be more influenced to try a dietitian's service, because the promoter lends credibility as a satisfied customer.

Public Speaking

Speaking to individuals and groups is considered the most efficient way to market, according to surveys of small business owners. It lets you get your messages across and establish your credibility at the same time to large numbers of people.

Speaking does not come easily for some people, but there are Toastmasters groups and others to join that allow you to practice your skills in a supportive atmosphere. You can also hire a speaking coach to help you with slang, organizing your ideas and the dramatics of entertainment through speaking.

Whether speaking to a woman's club, a state dietetic association, or a large national Chef's association, the following are some suggestions that will make speaking more predictable and enjoyable:

- Ask for an appropriate speaking fee. When you are paid to speak, you place it as a higher priority, and you get more excited and rehearsed. Your enthusiasm is often contagious. The fee should cover your honorarium, travel, preparation time, handouts, food samples, or whatever. As you become better known, your fee will greatly increase. Local speakers usually make $50 to $500 for presentations. National speakers can make $500 to $3,000 and keynote speakers often make $1,500 to $10,000. Writing a best selling book helps increase your fees, as well. If a speaking engagement can't afford your fee, negotiate. Ask to sell your books, or at an all day meeting, offer to do a second presentation (since you will be there anyway) and ask for 1½ times your normal fee for both speeches-it makes the trip more profitable for the same amount of time. (It saves the sponsor money by not having to pay for travel and honorarium for a second speaker.) You can handle all of these arrangements yourself or hire an administrative assistant or agent to do it for you.
- Find out as much as you can about the audience, its needs and any human interest facts. What specifically do they want you to speak on? Who will be in the audience, and how much do they know about the proposed topic? What are the educational backgrounds? Have they heard other speakers on this subject? Will there be questions, debate, etc. afterwards?

- Find out about the logistics: physical building, room, audiovisual capabilities (PowerPoint?), and whether they will reprint handouts. Request a letter of confirmation with the date, time, place, topic, expenses that will be reimbursed, and honorarium. Be sure to request a cancellation clause of at least 30 days or more, and for professional speakers, a partial payment if cancelled within that timeframe.
- Be sure to mark your calendar and get the name and phone number of the person who called.

Logo

A logo is a symbol. If it is used to identify a product, it is called a trademark. If it is used for a service, it is called a service mark. Logos can be fun, or highbrow and sophisticated, or somewhere in between. Logos are used to identify the business and draw attention to whatever they are used on, such as stationery, posters, business cards, brochures, or billboards (see Figure 20.1).

Business Owner

Private practitioners are potentially their own best marketing assets. Your personality, image, communication and business skills, and expertise in nutrition will be ultimately responsible for attracting and keeping clients.

Business advisors suggest business people use at least the following four practices to help promote their business:

First, use the phone and its marketing potential, talk to clients regularly, confirm appointments, and respond to referring physicians. Call back people who want to know about your services. Take the time to show an interest in their needs, to tell them briefly what you have to offer, to let them know what you will expect from them, and to discuss an appointment time and your fees. By taking time to market your services instead of just scheduling an appointment, the client will become excited about the expected personalized care.

Second, use your writing skills to correspond with people on a timely basis and to publish. For those who feel weak in this area, there are adult education classes, books and editors to help you.

Third, use public speaking to make yourself more visible in your community and to interest people in nutrition. Speaking to clubs, community groups, PTAs, and at conferences, will make people recognize you as a nutrition specialist.

Fourth, become involved in several local or national organizations that could benefit you personally or professionally. Attend meetings,

Figure 20.1 Logo Samples

A Selection of Logos

(*Source:* Reprinted by permission of the business owners.)

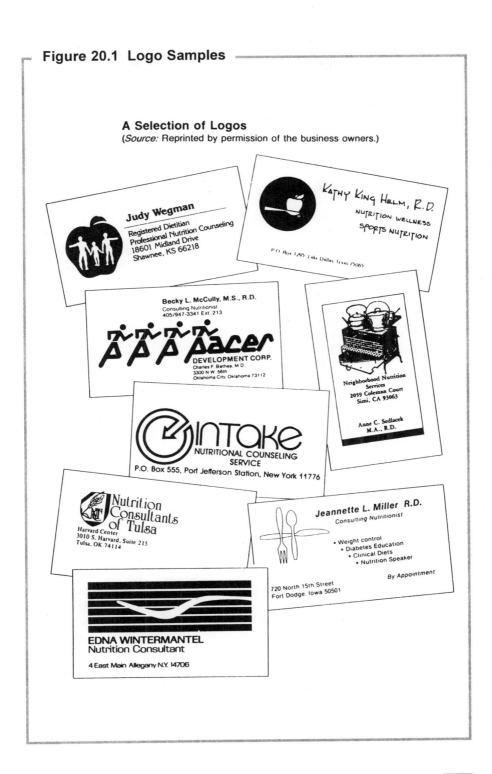

support activities, and run for offices. Dietetic organizations, including Dietetic Practice Groups, need input from active, assertive dietitians on their way up. Small business owners' groups, executive clubs, Toastmasters, and local political groups offer opportunities to become involved.

Writing for Publication

Writing is an ideal medium for practitioners to distinguish and promote themselves by communicating with the public or their peers. Writing for lay periodicals or books provides the opportunity to reach a potentially large audience, to share your views, to be paid for your work, and to become known.

Writing for publication in professional journals does not pay directly, but it helps establish you as a knowledgeable, qualified professional and excellent resource. Articles may also lend credibility to your programs and services. This type of promotion also may attract more business in the form of referrals or consultation opportunities.

Business Cards

Business cards should always be carried and handed out. They can be powerful marketing tools and one of the least expensive. Other peoples' cards should be saved and used the next time you want to network or you need some information. Business cards should list your name, credentials, business name, phone number with area code, e-mail or website, and full address.

Some considerations to think about: Do you want to print appointment information on the back of the card? Does the card look too cluttered as it's laid out? Can everyone read the typeface (script and Old English are difficult to read)? Since card sizes are fairly standard, will choosing another size card make your card stand out, or be thrown away? How can you best use color, style, paper, and design to attract attention to your card? (See Figure 20.2.)

Letters

Many business people have boosted their careers through well-written letters. All too often, we overlook the contribution that impressive correspondence can provide. The neatness and grammatical correctness is as important as the content of a letter. Letters with numerous corrections or misspelled words are poorly received (see envelope address layouts in Figure 20.3).

Busy people will often refuse to read obvious mass mailings, such as those addressed to "Dear Sirs," or "Dear Philadelphia Physicians," or those that are poorly photocopied. Due to having access to a PC, it

Figure 20.2 Sample Business Cards

Sample Business Cards
(*Source:* Reprinted by permission of the business owners.)

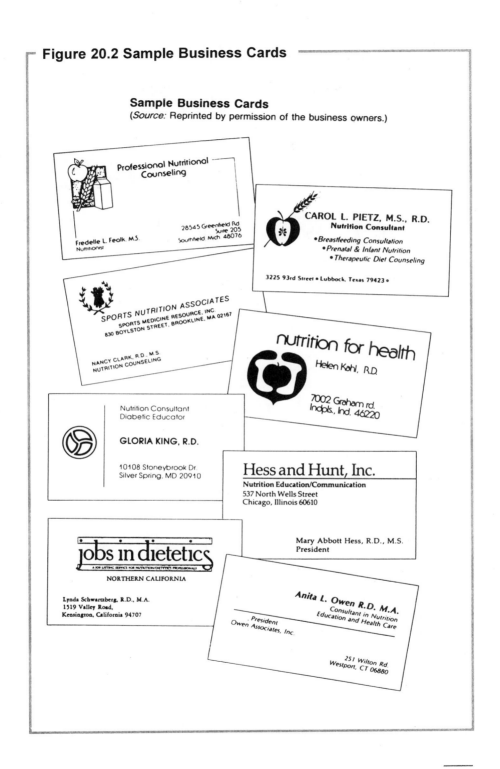

Figure 20.3 Sample Envelope Layouts

Sample Envelope Layouts
(*Source:* Reprinted by permission of the business owners.)

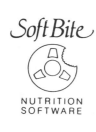

NUTRITION
SOFTWARE

P.O. Box 1484
East Lansing, Michigan 48823

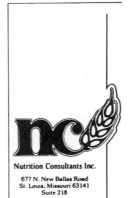

Nutrition Consultants Inc.

677 N. New Ballas Road
St. Louis, Missouri 63141
Suite 218

111 S. Tremont Street
Kewanee, Illinois 61443

KATHY
SCHWAB
R.D.

NUTRITION
CONSULTANT

1 0 1 1
S. W. Curry - 4
Portland
Oregon
9 7 2 0 1
503/295-1119
503/233-4567
EXTENSION 194

 SMITH AND MANTERNACH
NUTRITION ASSOCIATES

One Dubuque Plaza • Dubuque, Iowa 52001

 Nutrition & Diet Counseling of Rockland

24 South Main Street, New City, N.Y. 10956

NUTRITION SPECIALTIES,™
INC.

The Nutrition Experts™

St. Paul Business & Technology Center
245 East Sixth Street
P.O. Box 905
St. Paul, Minnesota 55101

should be possible for you to send out an original letter each time. Creativity, time, effort, and money must be invested to ensure that your letters are read. Business consultants suggest that even on mass mailings, the signature and heading should be individualized whenever possible.

Direct Mail

Direct mail is used when you know specifically whom you want to contact (usually either potential clients or referral agents), and when you want to increase your chances of attracting a higher-percentage response.

Personalize the mailed piece as much as possible to increase the readership. To increase the chance of having the direct mail piece read:
- put a return address with the sender's name or business, on the outside;
- add a question or statement to make the reader curious; and
- add a photo or drawing on a self-mailer to make the sender seem more familiar.

Direct mail is used for marketing surveys, announcements of a new office location or new services, and to acquaint potential clients or referral agents to your services. Postcards have become more popular, since the anthrax fiasco. Membership lists from your local medical society or national dietetic practice groups, the Yellow Pages, and shared business cards are good sources of names and addresses. Many organizations ask for a fee and an explanation of how the membership lists will be used before use is granted.

Resume

A resume can be a very effective marketing tool. It should highlight your aspects and experience that best qualify you for the position you are seeking. In other words, you may need several different resumes. It can either be chronological (listing your experience in reverse chronological order) or functional (highlighting your skills and responsibilities). Resumes also can be used along with letters of introduction, to open doors for you, or to establish credibility in a proposal, or to help introduce you at a speaking engagement.

A variation of the resume would be a curriculum vitae or vita (an expanded version that includes published books and papers). The biographical sketch (in paragraph form) often is used for introduction purposes at speeches.

Laser printed resumes look impressive. Word processing can make updating a resume very easy. However, the most important qualities are that it's free of any typographical errors and it's interesting and accurate.

Letters of Reference

Letters of reference written by prominent people who know you and your work are impressive. They help establish credibility and may help open doors for you. Keep the original on file, and use good photocopies.

Brochures

Brochures are used to introduce and promote. It's not imperative a private practitioner have a brochure, but many have found that attractive, clever ones attract business and easily pay for themselves.

The most important things to remember about a brochure are:

- Write the information with the customers' needs utmost in mind; talk about "benefits." How will your product or services make the customer happier, healthier, more fulfilled, and so on? Don't just list what you have to offer!
- Make the brochure attractive, simple to read, and interesting. Leave open space and use bullets to make scanning easier.
- Your readers may be interested in seeing a good picture of you.
- Add statements from satisfied customers.

Brochures seldom list fees because it dates them and sometimes makes them poorly received. If insurance sometimes covers your services or there is an employer co-pay program, it could be mentioned in the brochure. Your name, business name, address, and phone number should be highlighted. It is highly suggested that brochures be typeset and printed on good quality paper. (See brochures in Figures 20.4 and 20.5.)

Portfolio

There are times when dietitians want to show the scope of their creativity and samples of their work, such as creative menus, educational materials, media work, or catering ideas. When a business is new and its reputation and yours are unknown, a portfolio may be the marketing tool you need.

A portfolio is similar to a scrapbook or a slide show designed to show graphically what you have to sell. The portfolio may be in a commercially available portfolio folder, on a tripod display with charts, on slides or on audio or videotapes for dietitians who do media work. Presenting a portfolio to the client helps make the intangible promise tangible, enticing and clearly defined.

The cost of a portfolio can vary greatly, depending upon what is included. Items may range from professionally produced food photos or renderings to just copies or samples of educational materials, authored articles, menus, snapshots, letters of reference, and newspaper coverage. Occasionally, it is worth paying a professional artist or calligrapher to add a special touch. Unfortunately, many of us never use samples of our past creativity to help us win the next contract.

Posters

Using posters to promote seminars and classes has proven to be successful for some practitioners. To save money on printing costs, a large number of poster shells (ones with only partial information) can be printed at one time with the artwork, logo, business name, and phone number. The date, place, time, and event can be added as the posters are used. Sometimes a pad is attached with tear-off cards to send in for more information.

If the posters are not too large, most stores, health clubs, beauty shops, and so on that allow posters are willing to let you have display space to solicit their customers. When you use this type of marketing and you want to use the locations more than once, call or stop by when the event is over, and take the posters down and thank the owner.

Press Kits

Press kits are commonly used to interest the media in writing or broadcasting a story to help you promote your services, product, book, or speaking engagement. The kit may include a variety of items:
- A cover letter addressed to the person
- A press release on the service, product, or book you wish to publicize
- A sample of the product or book, or a copy of newspaper articles, or critical reviews
- A resume and short biographical sketch, or media bio
- A 5" x 7" black and white glossy photo of you or the product

Press kits should be descriptive, attractive and to the point. They should explain why the public would be interested in the topic. Although press kits can be very elaborate with printed covers and numerous photos, they can also be as simple as several of the above items placed in a large folder with pockets.

Banners

Banners draw attention and create name recognition. They can be used at "fun run" finish line, in a lobby during a Wellness Festival, or over the cafeteria door to promote the new line of "Light and Natural" foods. Banners can be made with paper and paint; however, they can be reused

Figure 20.4 Sample Brochure Cover

Sample Brochure Cover
(*Source:* Reprinted by permission of Judy Wegman, 1983. No portion of this brochure may be reused without permission.)

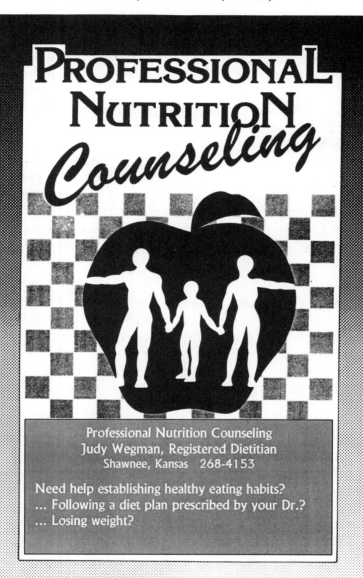

Figure 20.4 Sample Brochure Cover

Sample Personal Promotion Brochure

(*Source:* Reprinted by permission of Hess and Hunt, Inc., 1984. No portion of this brochure may be reused without permission.)

Hess and Hunt helps the foodservice and health care industry and its agencies. . .
- Meet the needs of consumers who have health concerns.
- Promote nutritious products by providing responsible spokespersons and developing publicity materials.
- Educate the public and health professionals by making presentations and teaching courses.

Hess and Hunt helps foodservice organizations. . .
- Write menus and expand current offerings of light, healthful items.
- Create effective nutrition promotions.
- Sell products to markets with specific health needs.

Hess and Hunt helps social service and government agencies . .
- Develop innovative nutrition education materials.
- Improve services to the community by teaching staff and client groups.
- Formulate food specifications, menus and evaluation tools to improve program quality and meet federal requirements.

Hess and Hunt helps print and electronic media . . .
- Obtain responsible nutrition information.
- Inform the public about popular nutrition topics by writing articles and appearing on radio and television programs.
- Translate scientific jargon into language that ordinary mortals can understand.

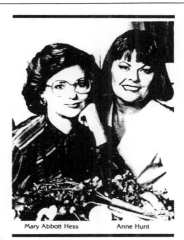

Mary Abbott Hess   Anne Hunt

Since 1979, **Hess and Hunt, Inc.** has provided insightful, professional nutrition expertise for business, industry and government. The firm brings together the broad knowledge of Mary Abbott Hess, a registered dietitian and associate professor of nutrition, and the communication background of Anne Hunt, a food public relations specialist, formerly food editor of *Sphere* (now *Cuisine*) magazine. Hess and Hunt with a support staff of experts in nutrition education, foodservice, marketing and graphic design offers nutrition communications that are both creative and dependable.

many times if they are made from cloth or heavy plastic. Banners are great promotional tools for a large area where crowds are gathered, and they also create a festive mood. (6)

Give-Aways

Give-aways (T-shirts, notebooks, mugs, gym bags, etc.) with the program name or logo are popular promotion items. The more useful and practical the item, the more it will be used and the name or logo displayed. (These items are sometimes sold as fund-raisers, rather than given away.)

FREE PROMOTION

Media

Working with the media-radio, television and newspapers-gives free marketing exposure to practitioners. One can do years of public speaking and not reach a fraction of the number of people who watch one television program or read a newspaper.

Nutrition, fitness and health are "hot" topics right now and probably will be for several years to come. Experts in these fields who have a flair for that type of work and have something unique to say are sought after.

Media people are looking for stories and information that will interest their public. It can be classified as controversial, human interest, new research, exposes, practical, or a scoop story, but it has to have a "hook" or a "handle" (some unique element to attract the audience). Working with the media is discussed in Chapter 28.

Many practitioners got their first start with the media during National Nutrition Month. We sometimes forget there are eleven other months to work with also. We do not have to wait until we are invited to contribute. If you plan to have a successful business, it is imperative people know about you. Through a phone call, introductory letter, over lunch, or at an office interview, however possible, try to talk to the local media program directors and newspaper writers. A private practitioner in Chicago reports she has been quoted or consulted on articles over fifty times in the last year in local newspapers. She sent her card, introduced herself, and offered to act as a resource person. Eventually, she was credited with a by-line, or in the article, for what she contributed.

Public Service Announcements

The media inconsistently welcomes PSAs. The PSA can announce a new series of diabetes classes or discuss childhood obesity for an hour on the radio. It can be printed in a newspaper, read on the air, or it can be a live interview. Obvious commercial promotions for your business or to sell something are not permitted unless you pay for commercial time or space. The lead-time for PSAs ranges from three to eight weeks, so call ahead and plan accordingly.

Radio and television stations support PSAs because of the service they provide to the community and because it looks good on their record when they reapply for their broadcast licenses. Newspapers usually feel PSAs increase readership.

It's become common for commercial food and beverage companies to hire dietitians as media spokespeople to offer PSAs. The dietitians are trained to provide interviews on an educational topic relating to food or nutrition and to interject the information about the company's product.

Publicity

Publicity is free media coverage of some newsworthy story, program or event. It is easily recognized as the media coverage of a local Health Fair or of the local school children during National Nutrition Month. In a recent newspaper article, it mentioned that a man named Lawrence "Herkie" Herkimer was going to be in the Sports Illustrated magazine for the second time in forty years talking about cheerleading and cheerleading camps. "I've got a soft spot in my heart for SI," says Herkie. "Back in the mid-'50s, they did a story on me and it really helped establish my company." That is what good publicity can do for you.

Practitioners can call or write the media with their requests for publicity. For planned events, such as the beginning of weight loss classes for teenagers or a sports nutrition conference, the media should be contacted several weeks in advance. When planning a special event, consider including a local celebrity, or co-sponsorship with a philanthropic organization, to improve the possibility of media coverage and to attract a larger attendance.

Publicity comes at no cost, but it may be sporadic or completely upstaged if a bigger news item breaks the same day as your story.

In an article by Peter Miller, "Be Your Own Publicist," he suggests the following references if you want to reach the media yourself, many libraries will have these resources and they may be available online: (6)

- *Bacon's Publicity Checker.* Lists over 18,000 newspapers and magazines, as well as 100,000 media contacts. (800) 621-0561.
- *Broadcasting Yearbook.* Covers radio, TV and cable and their staffs. (800) 638-7827.
- *Gale Directory of Publications.* Information on 25,000 newspapers, magazines, journals, and newsletters. (313) 961-2242.
- *Hudson's Newsletter Directory.* A listing of 4,000 newsletters by subject. (914) 876-2081.

Small companies can compete with large corporations with megabucks for media coverage, if you follow some very basic premises tested and proven by publicist Peter Miller: (6)

- Write about a topic, not about yourself.
- Be factual.
- Include your name, address and phone number at the top of the page.
- Be brief: Limit the news release to one page, but also include a cover page addressed to the individual reporter or editor, there may be a brief biography of yourself, and a short history of the business or product.

- State on the news release "For Immediate Release," which means use it anytime.
- Describe your material as a "news release."

Using this approach, Miller helped a small contact lens company in Washington, D.C., go from five employees working in an apartment to a forty percent increase in sales, and offers from all over the world to buy the firm. The publicity program cost approximately $200 over a period of seven months. (6) The money paid for printing, postage and photocopying. His time was donated because he was using them in his master's thesis. They were able to generate exposure in Newsweek, the Washington Post and in the UPI (United Press International).

PAID ADVERTISING

It's ethical, professional and highly recommended you consider using advertising. The U.S. government encourages professionals to advertise, in hopes of producing more competitive services and better values for the public. Professional organizations are recognizing it's becoming a fact of life for their members, and stress it be done tastefully.

Most practitioners use advertising as an ongoing budget item used to attract clients. Others use it only at times for special events, for new program announcements and at the beginning of seasonal peak periods (for example, September and January for weight loss). Whenever it is used, there are two guidelines that should always be followed:
- First, make it clever and distinctive.
- Second, plan to have a campaign, not just a single ad. Estimates vary that the average person must see or hear an ad between five and eleven times before he or she remembers it, so repetition is necessary. (7)

A good rule of thumb to determine how much to spend on advertising is five to ten percent of the gross annual budget. This is after the initial expense of fifteen percent for the first year. Another way would be to divide the cost of the advertising by the cost of the product you are selling or initial consultation fee. Evaluate if the number of new clients needed to break even on the advertising is reasonable (it's too expensive if you have to see twenty new patients per month just to pay for advertising). There is a point where putting more money into ads will not bring more clients or profit to your office. When you first begin a business, budget an amount you can afford to spend, and look for other previously mentioned ways to market yourself for less cost.

Most dietitians cannot afford to compete with the amount of advertising purchased by commercial weight loss and other nutrition programs. Where we spend our advertising money and the distinctiveness of our advertising are all the more important because our funds may be tight. To help determine what works for you, ask clients and patients how they heard about your business.

The Yellow Pages and the media all have free sales personnel that can assist clients in determining the best way to use their advertising dollar and help with ad ideas on a limited basis.

If a practitioner wants help on an overall advertising strategy, plus artwork and a slogan, an advertising agency or public relations firm can do it, as well as students and professors at your local colleges and universities. Obtain estimates before you agree to have work done because good firms are usually expensive.

Fees often range from $2,500 to $15,000 on up (advertising not included) to set up an advertising campaign with a logo and slogan for a small business. Fees are less if you come up with the ideas yourself.

Yellow Pages

The Yellow Pages offer a business the opportunity to advertise to everyone who owns a telephone, for a year. Most businesses find this type of advertising very productive.

Patients and clients know to look under "Dietitians" or "Nutritionists" to find a consulting nutritionist listing. Occasionally, practitioners also list under such titles as "Reducing and Weight Loss," "Physical Fitness," "Catering," or along with a contract clinic or spa. One listing in the Yellow Pages and white pages is offered when you have a business phone. All other listings, display ads, extra lines, or bold print are an extra charge.

It's recommended a Yellow Pages listing include the words "Registered Dietitian." The telephone company does not police their listings, so anyone can be listed under a title we, and the public, assume to be ours alone. Choosing a generic business name without reference to having a professionally trained dietitian involved may cause business to be lost. Examples would be "Big Pines Consultant Services" or "Moore & Associates, Inc."

To save money but still have a good size ad and several listings, buy only one larger ad and refer the other listings to it, such as "See ad under 'Nutritionists'." Put the ad under the listing where you think it will be seen best and where clients would look for your name first (see Figure 20.6).

The Yellow Pages closing date for ordering your ad is usually three to five months before the books are available. Plan ahead and call for assistance. Evaluate your listings each year and try new ideas that might work better. Ask new clients how they heard about your business to see if the ads really work.

Figure 20.6 Sample Yellow Pages Advertisements

Dietitians- Cont.

MCCULLY REBECCA L MSRD
CONSULTING DIETITIAN
MEMBER AMERICAN DIETETIC ASSN
HOURS: BY APPOINTMENT
5300 N Meridian

Nutrition Counseling Service
106 Preston Forest Village
Therapeutic Nutrition
308 E Main St

WEIGHT PLACE THE
NUTRITION CONSULTANTS
● REGISTERED DIETICIANS
BY APPOINTMENT ONLY
3400 NW Expwy

ALICE ZIMMERMAN NUTRITION LIFELINE

REGISTERED DIETITIAN
CONSULTATION FOR
● WEIGHT REDUCTION
● DIABETES
● HIGHBLOOD PRESSURE
● HEART DISEASE
● PREGNANT WOMEN
PUBLIC SPEAKING

Zimmerman Alice
8140 Walnut Hill Ln

Nutritionists

Banister Carol A RD MS
4200 W Memorial Rd

CHEHAK ANASTASIA MARIE RD
Consulting practice in nutritional
science related to health,
medical disorders and prevention
2912 Persimmon Creek Dr Edm

Nutrionics Health Systems
510 24 Avenue SW Nrm
Nutrition Consultants
1621 Oakwood Dr Nrm

NUTRITION CONSULTANTS OF TULSA

WEIGHT CONTROL - DIABETES EDUCATION
THERAPEUTIC DIETS - PRENATAL COUNSELING
INFANT NUTRITION - NUTRITION SPEAKERS
CLASSES
JUDY M. CORRELL, R.D.
CECILIA L. DAVIS, R.D.
GEORGIA W. KIMMEL, R.D.

3010 S Harvard

NUTRITIONAL COUNSELING CLINIC
2140-A S Memorial Dr

Newspapers

Dietitians use newspaper ads with varying degrees of success. The wording and placement of the ad are critical. It must be distinctive enough to catch the reader's eye. The competition to attract attention is very stiff in a newspaper, especially a large daily one. Ads should run on a regular basis in order to be remembered. Scheduling ads regularly also makes the cost of each individual ad more reasonable.

Large daily newspapers have good exposure, but have a lot of clutter and are only partly read by most people. Readers go to the sections that interest them most and skim the rest. Fortunately, newspapers know what sections are read most and by whom. Advice columns, horoscopes, cartoons, letters to the editors, sports score pages and, in small towns, the obituaries are usually read closely. Although women's sections usually are read well, on coupon day that is often not the case. Request the ad be placed on a page that is mostly writing, so your ad will stand out and not be lost between the huge furniture display ads.

Small newspapers and weekly papers are usually read more closely and have a loyal but smaller readership. The cost of advertising is more reasonable. The preferred placement guidelines for an ad are the same as mentioned for large newspapers. Also, smaller papers are usually more open to the idea of a nutrition column written by a local person, or articles that are contributed locally.

An ad should catch your attention with a catchy word, phrase, graphic design, photo, or something. It should be easy to read and understand, plus be clever. The phone number should stand out. It's not necessary to condense your brochure or calling card into an ad. In fact, you will attract more attention with the headline "Ready for Bikini Season?" than with "Nutritional Consultation by a Professional." If you can't think of an idea you like, check the ads other businesses are using and see what you like and dislike about them. If you have an idea but need artwork, go to a graphic artist. If you don't see a good idea, budget in an advertising firm or advertising student for the creation of the ad.

Radio

Radio advertising can be geared to a very specific group of the population, depending upon the type of music played and the time of day. Radio stations know from surveys their listeners' average ages, the percentages of men and women, their approximate income, and educational levels.

To be remembered, radio ads must be repeated. Sales people from stations will offer several "packages" of ad lengths and airing times to make the campaign more reasonable. They often will help with writing the ad and have a station person record it or read it live. Smaller stations have lower advertising fees because fewer people listen to them. In fact, it's the listenership that determines how much a station charges in a given market, but all fees are negotiable. The longer you decide to commit to their station, the lower the rate you will be charged. Don't accept the first figures you are quoted. Take your time and check for the best air times and prices for the target market you want. Classical stations are sometimes a very good choice to attract affluent patients for private consults, and "easy listening" for the over 40-year old group, and so on.

Businesses that can afford regular radio advertising report it is very successful. Smaller businesses with lower budgets and irregular use of radio advertising report hit or miss success. According to business consultants, if you plan to use advertising, you need to commit enough financial support to produce results or you should not do it at all.

Television

A television ad is extremely expensive to produce and to show on the air. Again, it must be repeated to be effective, and the types of programs being shown determine who the audiences will be. Television advertising reaches a large number of viewers, but is so expensive it would be very difficult for a consultant working alone to breakeven on the number of added customers it would attract. One person usually doesn't generate enough income in one hour to support this expenditure and other overhead, too. It may be possible that several consultants working together, or working for one person, could generate enough added income to warrant television advertising, but exhaust all avenues for getting free television exposure first.

A reasonable TV ad can be produced for $2,000 to $15,000, depending upon whether you hire someone to act or speak or you do it yourself. The airtime varies greatly, depending upon whether it is a small, local cable station or prime time on a major network. The better the viewership and time slot for the ad, the higher the cost-from $1,500 to $50,000 or more per week for a daily ad.

One private practitioner did invest with a partner in TV advertising to promote their quick weight loss program in the fall, during the popular afternoon talk shows. The ads cost $30,000 per week for several weeks and they did fill 50 weight loss classes with 12 people each at about $400 per person up front (plus a weekly fee for meal-replacement beverages), or over $1/4 million in gross income in 30 days. Figuring the cost of the ad, the airtime, the meeting rooms, the secretarial time, the educational materials, and the instructors to handle all those people, there was still a good profit-but very high risk if it had not worked.Infomercials can also be very lucrative (selling 10,000+ products in a day), but you would need to work with a company that already has the phone banks, credit card capabilities, staffing, actors, and video production ready to go.

INTERNET

The Internet has high reach (worldwide access) and high impact (audio and video, stereo and color, as well as animation, are ideal for product demonstration). (7)(See Chapters 21 to 23.)

There is extremely low cost for the number of potential customers who can be reached, although it may cost thousands to design and maintain a web site. At first glance, there seems to be low selectivity (who can access your site), however, through skillful use of meta tags and key phrases, you can greatly increase the chances of search engines finding your site and bringing the right customers.

KEEPING CUSTOMERS

After you have successfully attracted customers, it's important to keep them. Experts suggest it costs businesses five times more to attract a new client than to sell another item to a former customer. Customers are assets for more than just a source of revenue. They are "walking promotion" of your services and an advertising medium of great value. Each person has a sphere of influence that reaches far beyond his immediate family and business peers to a potential of several hundred people.

There are numerous ways to strengthen relationships with clients or referral agents that can be carried out with a minimum amount of effort on your part, once the system is established.

- Phone calls
- Personal notes
- Rapport established by showing genuine concern
- Newsletters (by mail or e-mail)
- E-mail communication
- Gifts and cards around holidays and special events
- Coffee or luncheon appointments
- In-services for staff

CONCLUSION

Attracting and keeping clients is necessary to survive in business. Selling and promotion should always be major priorities of any business, whether new or established. Private practitioners soon learn to carry a supply of calling cards wherever they go. Stepping forward to shake hands, and introducing themselves, becomes second nature. Although many things seem awkward at first, after so many hours and days are invested, it becomes very easy to share your enthusiasm.

REFERENCES

1. Beckwith H. *The Invisible Touch.* New York: Warner Books; 2000.
2. O'Connor JP. Presentation *O'Connor PR & Marketing,* Washington, DC.1990.
3. Rose J. Helm KK. *The Competitive Edge.* Chicago, IL: The American Dietetic Association; 1987.
4. Helm KK. Chapter: Promotion Strategies. In: *The Competitive Edge.* Chicago, IL.: The American Dietetic Association; 1995.
5. Edwards P, Edwards S. *Working From Home.* New York: Penguin Putnam; 1999.
6. Miller P. How to be Your Own Publicist. *Home-Office Computing;* December 1990.
7. Sobel M. *The 12-Hour MBA Program.* Paramus, NJ: Prentice Hall; 1993.

Practitioner Perspective

Nadine Braunstein, RD

Why have you stayed as an entrepreneur? What strategies have been your most successful in business?

I love the variety and flexibility that being an entrepreneur provides. Currently, I see private clients, supervise dietitians in a School-Based Health Center, write a nutrition column for a newsletter, give workshops and presentations to dietitians at state meetings as well as worksite wellness programs. On top of that I like to help other people, I serve as the chair of an advisory committee for a local Eating Disorder Association, and provide nutrition consultation to special needs adults, and probably a few other things.

As I look at this list I see that most of these consulting positions came as a result of a colleague recommending me, or someone saw something I did several years before they contacted me. Nurture your current clients. If they are satisfied they will return and bring you more business. It is easier to keep a current client than it is to find a new one.

What mistakes do you see new private practitioners making?

I think that people starting out don't realize how much time it takes to develop a successful business. In some ways they are some of the same issues that our clients have when it comes to changing eating habits. Looking forward a year or two seems so long, yet looking back time just flies! Also, pricing services either too high or too low happens in the beginning.

In your opinion, why are some practitioners more successful than others?

It depends on how you define "success." Longevity, reputation, and income all come into play here. I think that being attentive to your customer's needs and exceeding their expectations help you be successful. Being successfully self-employed is all about relationships. Those who are successful understand how to nurture those relationships--be it the food editor who calls you for quotes, your clients who return and happily refer others, the organization who hires you to create its wellness program, the physicians whose patients you counsel, or your colleagues who think of you when they need a good nutritionist for a project.

Chapter 21

Using the Internet

Teresa Pangan, PhD, RD and Julie M. Horner
Owners, Puttin' on the Web

The Internet is not just for those who have a website. Following are several ways to use the Internet in your professional work, regardless of whether you or your company has a website.

E-MAIL or EMAIL and ON-LINE or ONLINE ALL ARE CORRECT SPELLINGS

Equipment. To have e-mail capability, you need:
- Access to a computer with a modem, in order to use the telephone line;
- An Internet connection service, which is available in different forms: an Internet Service Provider (ISP--local dialup connection), online service (AOL, CompuServe, etc.), or a local phone company program (the service will provide the software for you to use the system);
- An e-mail name, which is selected when signing up for your Internet connection service.

Common Uses of E-mail

With the increased use of computers and the Internet by individuals, e-mail can be a convenient and inexpensive mechanism for communication. It can aid the health care delivery process by allowing written follow-up on instructions, quicker test results and dissemination of educational materials to patients. It is a means for business clients and consultant dietitians to easily communicate with each other. At the same time, issues of privacy, confidentiality and security must be addressed to ensure the efficacy and effectiveness of e-mail.

Individual Therapy

There also are an abundance of uses for e-mail in professional work beyond a simple communication vehicle. E-mail has been used as part of therapy with patients, both in one-on-one and group settings. It also can be useful for surveying clients or members.

A study with eating disorder patients found that e-mail therapy looks promising in treating patients.(1) The study evaluated the effects of a three-month e-mail therapy program for people with bulimia nervosa. Twenty-three patients were asked to e-mail a daily diary of their eating habits and feelings. Psychiatrists responded with advice, encouragement and other comments. The therapists said it took them a maximum of ten minutes to read and respond to a patient e-mail communication. Researchers found there was a significant reduction in depression and symptoms. These results do not diminish the value of face-to-face therapy. Instead, the patients' treatment may be enhanced with the combination of e-mail and office visits. Further studies are needed, but results look promising.

Group Therapy

E-mail can be effective in a group support setting; people connect when they aren't involved in a face-to-face encounter. E-mail is famous for drawing out people who have difficulty expressing themselves in face-to-face settings.(2) An online discussion group or a listserv does not require a website. Also, patients often feel more comfortable expressing their feelings in the comfort of their own home, or own pajamas. E-mail affords them this benefit. Also, with the crazy schedules of people today, e-mail can be squeezed in between activities or left until winding down at the end of the day.

There are several companies that will host a listserv for a monthly fee or on a per e-mail sent basis. The advantage of a listserv is you can have closed membership or limit that has access to the group. You can limit the group to 5, 12, 25, or any number of individuals. Also, messages to the group can be read or posted at any time of the day from anywhere.

E-mail group support can be most effective for those groups of patients where issues outside of food need to be addressed during treatment. Eating disorders come immediately to mind, newly diagnosed individuals with diabetes, cardiac rehab patients, and weight management patients are a few of the many other opportunities.

Discussion Groups or Listservs

Other reasons for forming an online discussion group are for a joint work project, or for coordinating an annual dietetic association meeting, requiring lots of planning and support from many members. An online discussion group could keep all members who are involved updated on progress and unforeseen difficulties. Preparation for a JCAHO inspection starts several months ahead of the actual inspection. A listserv could be used to help keep communication open and deadlines on target.

To find a company to host a listserv, search using the keywords < listserv + hosting>.

Surveys

Surveys are easy to setup through e-mails. E-mails can include a "hot" link that takes participants directly to a survey by merely clicking on the highlighted address. Survey results can be viewed at any time from a password protected website area, where only specified individuals have access to view results of the completed surveys. Possible uses are:

- Customer satisfaction or feedback
- Employee satisfaction with company
- Input for a new member service or project
- Opinions of customers regarding a product or service
- Input for an upcoming meeting
- Feedback on effectiveness of a meeting

Results of surveys can be viewed in spreadsheet format, graphs or placed into presentation software. Results can provide insight for making informed business decisions.

Many sites that specialize in surveys offer a free survey version to assess. The number of questions and participants may be limited, so determine your needs before you buy or commit yourself. Following are sample sites to begin your search:

http://www.supersurvey.com/
http://www.freeonlinesurveys.com/
http://www.surveymonkey.com/
http://www.zoomerang.com/

To locate other sites use the keywords <surveys + online>.

INFORMATION THERAPY FOR PATIENTS

Heading the "Information Therapy" movement is the Washington, DC-based Center for Information Therapy (http://www.informationtherapy.org/). It is a nonprofit division of Healthwise that aims to support information therapy programs and conduct research to assess impact on healthcare quality. The nonprofit organization defines information therapy as the "prescription of right information to the right patient at the right time to help people make appropriate decisions of care". The right information, person and time refers to:

- information: evidence-based, void of commercial interests or advertising, up-to-date;
- person: patient or caregivers who are involved in the decision or behavior change;
- time: just in time to help make a better medical decision or improve a health behavior.

Possible Information Therapy Scenario

Sheila has been hospitalized for a heart attack. Before she is discharged, she will be issued an electronic prescription via a secure message system for "information therapy," an Internet-based patient education tool.

First, Sheila receives an e-mail that contains links to specific, physician-approved online information relevant to her diagnosis and post-discharge needs. By the time Sheila arrives home, her e-mail has arrived. When she is ready, she can sit down at her computer and visit all the links in her "information therapy" e-mail. In Sheila's case, the links listed are links to "heart disease development overview" information about "treatment for heart disease" and "how to prepare for a visit to a Registered Dietitian and exercise physiologist."

The e-mail begins by explaining to Sheila this information is part of the process of care for her heart disease, and encourages her to read and study it. By the time Sheila meets with her Registered Dietitian for the first time; she will have completed three days of food and activity records and read an overview of medical nutrition therapy for heart disease. This initial visit preparation will help dietitians in assessing and working a patient through the pre-contemplation, contemplation and preparation for action stages of behavior change.

Taken from About Information Therapy on the Center for Information Therapy's Website (www.informationtherapy.org).

Pilot tests are being conducted on information therapy with positive preliminary results and feedback. Information therapy makes patients aware of the intricacies of their health and any diseases that affect them. It takes them into the pros and cons of their care options. It helps people share in medical decisions and come closer to self-care and self-management model of health care. Information therapy can be delivered in three ways: (3)

1. Physician-prescribed - the physician can directly select and prescribe relevant online information sources and education tools. In time, the prescription process will occur with the use of a hand-held computer.

2. System-prescribed - a health system automatically prescribes information prescriptions based on what it knows about that patient's decision needs and any ongoing management of lifestyle and medical factors. Trigger for a system-prescription could be:
   - referral to a specialist (e.g., Registered Dietitian)
   - scheduling of procedure
   - new medication prescription
   - new public health concern (e.g., anthrax exposure)
   - call to a nurse center regarding an injury
   - new diagnosis
   - scheduling of a lab or other test

   The information therapy can also be offered as a value-added service to members.
3. Consumer-prescribed - an online information therapy system has a searchable body of accurate and up-to-date information geared to help patients make informed decisions.

Currently, there is no reimbursement for information therapy. According to a survey by the American Medical Association, the biggest barrier to therapy is lack of compensation.(4) However, inroads are being made with payers and policymakers to reimburse providers for information therapy services.

The concepts of information therapy are not new. Hospital librarians, consumer health librarians and patient educators already provide these kinds of services. The intent is to standardize this information service into the treatment process for patients.

Dietitians can become involved in shaping information therapy to improve its effectiveness. A valuable addition to the initial "information therapy" e-mail could include links to content on why it is important for heart disease patients to visit a Registered Dietitian and content to erase some of the myths associated with Registered Dietitians - we can teach you how to eat your favorite foods, not take them away. On the negative side, there could be the scenario that diets are prescribed over e-mail instead of referring patients to dietitians.

Potential for Future Developments

The advantage the Internet has over handing a patient a booklet on "management of heart disease" is individualization. A user can read only what they want and skip over what they already know or are not ready to internalize. Advanced individualization can ask for users' input, and base returned information on their input. This goes back to the stage of change example. The stage of change a user is in can be assessed from their input information, and the resultant information can be focused on their stage of change needs.

Other "information therapy" benefits include the ability to track content users have visited. This enters into steep privacy issues that need to be resolved first, but the potential is for a Registered Dietitian to know what content and education tools a patient has viewed, the length of time they spent viewing the information and where they exited the "information therapy" site before their visit. The Registered Dietitian can potentially gain an insight into the patient's interests, barriers and what level of lifestyle change they are ready to commit to. It is all very exciting to look into a crystal ball and take a glimpse of what lies ahead in the future.

PROFESSIONAL SEARCHING PROGRAMS

Searching on the Internet today can be compared to dragging a net across the surface of the ocean. While a great deal may be caught in the net, there is still a wealth of information that is deep and, therefore, missed. The reason is simple: much of the Web's information is buried far down on dynamically generated webpages.

Dynamic Webpages

Dynamic webpages are created based on a user's input. A simple illustration is a search engine. When a search is performed with keywords, the search engine uses the words entered into its query form (box) to search its database (index) that is stored offline. It matches the user's words with words in its index. The results are assembled together onto a "dynamic" webpage based on the matches it found in its database.

Another example of the use of a dynamic webpage is MEDLINE. MEDLINE is a database filled with information from 4300 biomedical journals. When looking for medical information in MEDLINE, a user enters an author's name, search term or journal title. A search engine searches the MEDLINE database and returns a list of results. The list of results the user views is a dynamically generated page. Additionally, the user will click on a result that closely matches the topic they want to locate. The link they click on will initiate the process to create another dynamically generated webpage. The journal title, article title, abstract, authors, date, issue, full-text, and other information is retrieved from the MEDLINE database to be displayed on the dynamic webpage. The webpage the user views (with the journal article information) is not a webpage that a web developer created and posted on the Internet. It's created on the 'fly.' This should clarify why there is a huge amount of valuable information that standard search engines never find.

Search Programs

Search programs work well and are cost-effective for researchers and professionals who specialize in a topic area. A searching program can be set up to search on a specialty area regularly and add in new results each time the search is repeated. Over time, a well-refined search can act as a bibliography on a topic. Professional searching can be an effective way to keep on the cutting edge of a specialty. These programs work well on narrowly focused areas, not broad topics. Their prices range from free to over $200 per year (most programs actually are a one time cost, and updates are an optional cost). Popular programs include:

- Copernic (www.copernic.com)
- BullsEye (www.intelliseek.com)
- Lexibot (www.lexibot.com)

To find more professional searching programs, use the keywords: < Internet searching tools >.

The Deep Web and Surface Web

Traditional search engines create their indices by spidering, or crawling, surface webpages that are all linked together. To be discovered, the webpage must be static and linked to other pages. Traditional search engines can't "see" or retrieve content in the deep Web. Those pages do not exist until they are created dynamically as the result of a specific search into an online database. Because traditional search engine crawlers can't probe beneath the surface, the deep Web is hidden to them.

The deep Web differs from "surface" Web in the way it obtains its indexed data. The "surface" Web uses search engines and subject directories for finding information. Subject directories obtain its information from authors submitting their own Web pages for a listing. And search engines "crawl" or "spider" documents by following one hypertext link to another. Simply stated, when indexing a given document or page, if the crawler encounters a hypertext link on that page to another document, it records that incidence and schedules that new page for later crawling. Like ripples propagating across a pond, in this manner search engine crawlers are able to extend their indexes further and further from their starting points. On the other hand, the deep Web has systematic information entered into a database that is below the Internet surface and not accessible to search engine crawling. Examples of deep Web sources are: National Climatic Data Center (http://lwf.ncdc.noaa.gov/oa/ncdc.html)

- US Census (http://www.census.gov/)
- NIH PubMed - this has the MEDLINE database (http://www.ncbi.nlm.nih.gov/entrez/)
- US Patents (http://www.uspto.gov/patft/index.html)

6ι   Deep Web sites tend to have content that is narrower and deeper than "surface" websites. Also, more than half of the deep Web content resides in topic-specific databases.(5) With proper searching techniques, deep Web searches can turn up very valuable information.

The deep-Web is very large. Public information on the deep Web is currently 400 to 550 times larger than the commonly defined World Wide Web. The deep Web contains nearly 550 billion individual documents, compared to the 1 billion of the surface Web. (5)

Professional search programs are searching assistants to help access resources inaccessible to a traditional search engine. They obviously can save you library time. They are akin to search engines on your PC that have the ability to search the "surface" Web and deep Web. Some are more like meaty search tools and others are able to go far below the Web's surface into its deep waters. (6) Some of the time-saving and valuable features of searching programs are: (5)

- Assembles results from several search engines and automatically eliminates broken links;
- Ability to perform a sub search within search results;
- Automatically performs queries at intervals specified by the user, and notifies you by e-mail of new results;
- Searches specialty databases organized by categories;
- Organizes search results by concepts and finer filtering techniques;
- Creates reports;
- Converts results to HTML, so they are ready to post on the Internet as a webpage;
- Tracks information on a site or webpage;
- Saves queries to repeat at a later date and denotes any new content with a new graphic;
- Highlights keywords from search query in web pages retrieved from a search; and
- Utilizes a scoring system to display results.

OTHER INTERNET SEARCH HELPERS

There are two additional Internet search helpers for keeping up-to-date in your area of specialty: e-mail news services and Webpage change notification software.

E-mail News Services

These services are offered by medical and news websites. They are daily or weekly e-mails to announce breaking news on a medical topic or topics that you select. Headlines and abstracts with links to the full-text articles are e-mailed according to the frequency you setup. They are a good way to keep abreast of hot topics in the media. Frequently, the writers are medical journalists and may or may not have any experience or formal training in the topic they are writing on. Also, the content is typically targeted to consumers and may have little informative value to a health professional. However, it is an easy method to keep on top of breaking news stories. Scan the top news sites and medical portal sites for e-mail services. To find e-mail news services, use the keywords: < health e-mail news>. ADA initiated it's own e-mail news service in August 2002 for its members. Check www.eatright.org for more information.

Webpage Change Notification

Webpage change notification software is a program set up on your computer to connect to the Internet, and check whether content on webpages you specify have been updated. This tool is excellent for monitoring valuable webpages in your area of specialty. The program can be set up to check daily, weekly or monthly. There are several programs that will do this. They are free to less than $100. To find a webpage change notification program, go to a download or software site like www.download.com or www.cdnet.com/downloads/ and use the keywords: < web page notification>.

WEB CONFERENCES

Equipment

Web conferencing refers to technologies that allow people to communicate or "conference" over the Internet. Web conferencing is based on tools that most of us use on a daily basis--PC, telephone and the Internet.

To conduct a Web conference, all that is needed is a computer with a Java-enabled browser, a phone and an Internet connection of 56 kilobits per second or better. The different technologies for Web conferencing include stream audio (downloading sound data onto the user's computer so it is processed and performed at a steady speed to avoid pauses in the sound), stream video (downloading video data onto the user's computer so it is processed and performed at a steady speed to avoid pauses in the picture), VoIP (voice-over-IP), and web-based chat.

Voice-over-IP (VoIP) is a two-way audio transmission over an Internet connection through computers. Both users must have microphones and speakers attached to their computers, and a VoIP software program. Then the users can use VoIP to talk to one another, similar to talking on the telephone, but through microphones. Many e-conferencing solutions include a VoIP component.

A presenter can present content over the Internet using a form of slide show presentation, web-based chat and streaming audio and/or video. Attendees view the presentation by logging into the web conference, and communicate with the moderator either through their phones or through web-based chat. The moderator can interact with participants, view a list of who attended the conference and manage the communication during the event.

Many e-conferencing solutions offer meeting tools that allow you to poll participants before, during or after the meeting or presentation. Results of the polling can be tabulated in real time and can be incorporated into the conference.

Purchasing options include:
- "renting" or licensing web conferencing software that is hosted on the vendors server;
- purchasing the software retail or from a reseller, and hosting it on your own server; or
- working with a full-service vendor who will supply the planning, marketing and production of your event, as well as the web conferencing software.

Web conferencing hosting solutions include the following:
egenda http://www.e2c.com/
erooms http://www.erooms.com
genesys http://www.genesys.com/
RainDance http://www.raindance.com
e-conference.com http://www.e-conference.com/meeting.htm
Placeware http://www.placeware

A list of web conference vendors is at:
http://www.conferzone.com/vendor/webconf.html. To locate more web conference solutions, enter the keywords: <online meetings> or <online collaboration> or <web presentation>.

Prices for a 1 ½ hour online web conference range from $50 to $750. Often, pricing is done on a per minute basis per user. Features included vary. They typically provide online training tutorials. Before deciding, test a couple out. They vary in their services, features and ease of use. Before your first web conference, plan in training time and extra setup time. A dry run is also a good idea.

Uses of Web Conferencing

Web conferencing solutions can be used in a variety of innovative ways to allow people to communicate with each other more effectively across any distance at any time. Some common uses of Web conferencing technologies include:

- Employee orientation
- Focus groups
- Sales presentations
- Training
- Meetings
- Educational presentations to small or large groups using PowerPoint
- Support group or therapy sessions

Web conferencing solutions are available to anyone with access to a computer, and an Internet connection. The most obvious benefit from the use of Web conferencing is a decrease in travel expenses. Solutions can promote effective communication between colleagues in separate offices, and can offer a way to communicate with large audiences for relatively low cost.

Determine Your Needs

When searching for a solution that best meets your needs, screen a number of vendors. The number of participants in a web conference can determine the type of technology that is needed; also, which types of materials to be presented: slide presentation, streaming audio, sharing computer program documents (e.g., Word files). Evaluate if special services, like event or project management, are required, and select a vendor based on what it can provide. Remember that some degree of technical support is needed for all web conferencing solutions.

SERVICES OF THE FUTURE

In the not so distant future, we will be electronically communicating with patients to deliver just-in-time care. Patients will give feedback throughout the day on their handheld and home computers. Daily, and even hourly, blood pressure, blood sugars, food records, thought journals, will be stored online for those health professionals treating a patient, to access at any time. Physicians and healthcare providers will be able to set triggers or thresholds for data that will initiate an e-mail to the patient's health care team members. For example, when a patient's blood sugar rises above a specified amount, an e-mail is sent to his or her physician, Registered Dietitian, case worker, and the patient. The e-mail contains the high blood sugar value and a tailored message to the patient on what they should do before the doctor or physician's assistant calls to discuss adjustment of insulin or oral medication.

References

1. Web Trends: E-mail therapy may be effective for eating disorders. Internet Healthcare Strategies; September, 2001.
2. "Information therapy" offer provides a new avenue of patient education, Medicine on the Net; March 2002.
3. Reid B. Rx for the Future: Get an Ix: Washington Post; June 25, 2002.
4. Elias M. Internet therapy clicks for patients. USA Today; May 23, 2001.
5. Bergman M. The Deep Web: Surfacing Hidden Value, BrightPlanet's Website; February 22, 2001, available at: http://www.brightplanet.com/deepcontent/tutorials/DeepWeb/index.asp. Accessed on July 10, 2002.
6. Guernsey L. Mining the 'Deep Web' with Sharper Shovels: NY Times; January 25, 2001.

Chapter 22

Website Basics

Teresa Pangan, RD, PhD and Julie M. Horner
Owners, Puttin' On The Web

Do I Need a Website?

It seems like everyone has a website or is scrambling to get one. It's easy to assume that you have fallen behind the times if you haven't staked out a place of your own on the World Wide Web. This assumption is inappropriate, however. The decision whether or not to create a website should be made only after careful assessment of what you expect that website to accomplish. That is basic business planning and the first step toward designing a website that will meet your needs. This chapter will help you to make that assessment.

WEB APPLICATIONS

First and foremost, a website is a means of communication. Information is made available on-line; responses may or may not be solicited. The variety of website styles is infinite, but virtually all websites communicate at one of three levels.

- The first level is strictly informative and functions much like on-line brochure by listing its goals, activities, personnel, office locations, telephone numbers, etc., while a more elaborate version might furnish detailed information on topics, plus links to other sites dealing with those topics.
- At the second level, websites are interactive by inviting an exchange of information through on-line forums, customer service, discussion groups, reply forms, etc.
- At the third level, websites are designed to "do business" with the user. This category includes e-commerce sites where items are sold, plus renewing memberships, making appointments, interactive continuing education or fund raising.

Level One: On-line Brochure

To assess the value of this communication tool, you have to focus on what you want to communicate. Do you want to attract clients (or customers or members) with a simple brochure-type website that describes your organization, its objectives and addresses and telephone numbers? Would this improve your business' professional image? What about more detailed information, such as press releases, meeting schedules, product descriptions, membership applications, etc.? By posting this information on-line, would you reduce the time and expense involved in providing (and updating) the same information by telephone, mail or other means? Will your clients and potential clients appreciate the convenience of having this information at their fingertips at any hour of the day or night?

Level Two: Interactive Site

What about interactive communications? When someone shows interest in your organization by visiting the website, do you want him to provide an e-mail address, telephone number or other means for follow-up contacts? Would an on-line suggestion box be useful? Do you want a visitor to ask a question when it is convenient for her, while allowing you to answer when it is convenient for you? In some situations, there is no satisfactory substitute for real-time, person-to-person contact. However, for routine inquiries and feedback, on-line messaging can frequently deliver appropriate answers more effectively than letters or telephone calls.

Many companies further reduce demand on staff time by posting Frequently Asked Questions ("FAQs") with stock answers. How about an on-line order form for brochures, books or other materials currently requested by telephone or mail? After mulling over the typical applications mentioned in this paragraph, take the time to focus on your enterprise's day-to-day communications. Ask yourself and others how an interactive website might improve your business or improve your customer service.

Level Three: Business Transaction Site

Interactivity moves to a higher level when the website is designed to conduct some form of business with the client. On-line catalogs immediately come to mind. More and more, people with goods and services to sell are meeting their customers in virtual showrooms. Specialized websites allow you to renew an automobile registration, join a professional organization, enroll in a class, set a tee time for your next round of golf, transfer funds from one bank account to another, donate to your favorite charity or complete any number of other transactions that a very short time ago, simply could not be done from a computer keyboard. What operations can you streamline by letting your clients complete their own "paperwork" on-line? How many customers can you attract or retain by making it easier for them to do business with you?

WHAT'S THE PLAN?

After identifying several web applications that could work for your business, are you ready to hand the project over to a website designer and sit back to wait for the finished product? DON'T DO IT! The next critical step is for you to establish specific purposes for the website and rank those purposes by importance. In other words, you need a plan. You need to tell the website designer what you want the website to do so the designer can build the website to meet your needs. It is certainly helpful to get input from the designer as you flesh out your plan, but you have to design the plan and set the priorities.

Establishing Purposes and Priorities

The purpose of the website is the most important element. Because the typical website may have several purposes, it's necessary to sort through those purposes and set priorities. Website design involves any number of trade-offs. If you do not tell the web designer what is important to you, he or she has to guess. At best, a wrong guess will cost you the expense of more design time. At worst, it could weaken the effectiveness of the site. If you are going to the expense of a custom design, make sure the designer knows your priorities. Several basic website purposes are listed below. Select one (or a variation) as your primary purpose and then list whatever others may apply as secondary purposes. (1)

1. **Improve/ create business or professional image.** This purpose strives to increase credibility in a specific field (e.g., professional organizations, dietetic programs) or increase visibility as an expert in a specialty area (treatment of burns, diabetes, medical nutrition therapy, kitchen design or menu consultation).

2. **Better serve your current clients.** Enhanced customer service is often the primary reason why existing enterprises establish new websites, but it also saves staff time. Examples of this purpose include: interactive customer service of all types; product and service descriptions; placement of orders; "brochure" and company directories; FAQ (Frequently Asked Questions); hours of operation; and program dates.

Down load diet hx form
pt. hx form
ins. form

3. **Attract new clients/customers/members.** For some businesses or organizations, the Internet will be their only advertising medium. Others will opt for multiple forms of advertising. As with any kind of advertising, it is critical that you and your web designer understand the target market. In designing a site for a dietitian who counsels private clients, the designer will "advertise" the site differently than if the dietitian sells products to other health professionals, consults to restaurants, or is a motivational speaker to organizations. (See more on advertising and promotion in Chapter 20.)
4. **Market products.** The marketing of products or services is closely associated with attracting new customers, but they aren't always the same thing. A registered dietitian or DTR who gives food safety demonstrations, for instance, might attract new customers by displaying past projects on the web, expecting that sales will come later. The design of that website will be different from the design of a site meant for on-line, retail sale of educational materials. Shopping malls, corner stores and other physical retail outlets require careful attention to details such as layout and decor. E-stores are no different. Something as simple as listing the steps of placing an order and having the buttons clearly marked can make customers happy, yet many sites don't do it.
5. **Provide educational resources.** This is usually a secondary purpose, unless you sell continuing education. It may be used to attract repeat visits to a site or promote goodwill. Dietetics professionals might include sample diets or information on the basic food groups or an area of expertise like eating disorders or allergies. Organizations might see education as the primary purpose of their websites. One example would be an association that serves as a clearinghouse for information about a rare disease.

HOW MANY "HITS" (VISITS) WILL I GET?

Numbers are important, but they tell only part of the story. In theory, your new website will put you in contact with more people than you could reach with a one-minute Super Bowl advertising slot. In practice, only a tiny percentage of web users will ever visit your site. Even that number is not as significant as it first may seem. The point is that most websites will succeed or fail on their ability to attract "hits" (visits) from people who are already interested in what that website has to offer. Obviously, the mass retailers look for massive numbers of site visits but most websites achieve their success from a special niche. The gross number of site visits is far less significant than what you achieve in new sales or new memberships or whatever else has a direct impact on your success or bottom line. If you will pardon the pun, only the "net" amount is important.

A well designed website will attract customers, members, clients, etc. who are actively looking for what you have to offer. To make this happen, however, you have to identify your target market. Actually, you may have more than one target market, but each will have an identifiable set of characteristics. The site should then be designed to attract visits by web users who share one or more of those characteristics.

WHO WILL DESIGN THE SITE?

Some readers may be thinking of creating their own websites. For those with the time and ability, that may be the way to go. The starting point, however, should be a library or bookstore. You will need working knowledge of site navigation, graphics, hosting options, and numerous other technical factors that will determine how your website will function. Study the guidebooks and be prepared to work and re-work the site as needed to fix the glitches that are bound to crop up. Instructions for a do-it-yourself project are beyond the scope of this chapter. That is probably just as well because site design is a developing art, and the technology and recommended guidelines change frequently.

Choosing a Web Designer

There are numerous individuals and firms who can design your site for a fee. They may be found by looking at sites you admire and asking for the designer's name, through referrals, an Internet search, or from the Yellow Pages. The trick is to find an appropriate designer for your needs and price range. You can obtain a basic website in an off-the-shelf format for a fraction of what custom design services will cost. You should visit sites created in the same format you are considering. Ask an experienced friend to critique a few sites you like. However, the most important test is how the sample sites perform the functions identified in your plan. Can they do what you want done and can they do it effectively?

The choice of a website designer can be difficult because the average web user sees only the result, not the technical decisions that go into producing that result. The user can appreciate a pleasing visual layout, but may not notice details of the functional design. Both elements--style and function--are critical to the effectiveness of a website. The following steps are suggested to help you make an informed choice about a web designer:

- Look at the design firm's portfolio long enough and hard enough to decide whether or not you like their work; (2)
- Obtain references and contact as many customers of the firm as it takes to give you a reasonably consistent rating of the firm's performance;

- Ask the designer to walk you through the design process, step by step, to make sure you will be invited to review and comment at frequent intervals;
- Determine the timetable for the initial design process, but also ask about response time for post-production glitches (There will be some!) for updates, etc;
- Determine the approximate cost (A cost range is usually appropriate because the designer can't foresee how the project will change as the designer learns more about your needs and you learn more about what the website can do for you.);
- Decide whether you like the designer because personal chemistry, especially the element of trust, can help or hinder a project of this magnitude.

The above suggestions hint at a post-production relationship. Unless you plan to part ways with the design firm as soon as the site is up and running, you might ask about additional services such as:

- Maintenance--Does the design firm offer maintenance beyond the initial site set-up?
- Training--Will they train your personnel to maintain your site?
- Hosting--Does the company offer hosting services? You may avoid buck-passing by having a single firm responsible for design, maintenance and hosting.
- E-commerce solutions--Can they develop an e-commerce package? Do they offer a secure server, shopping cart software, on-line credit card acceptance set-up?
- Database setup and management--Do they have the capacity to setup a database driven site for interactivity (for such things as a site search function, on-line shopping, or on-line directories)?
- Mailing list management--Who will update and maintain the e-mail list for newsletters and promotions?

WHAT DO I NEED TO GET STARTED?

You need ready access to an up-to-date computer with reliable Internet access and a color monitor with good resolution. Your site designer should contact you from time to time to ask you to look at the work in progress and to get your reactions. To keep the process moving, you want to be able to respond quickly. Additionally, if you have not addressed this as part of your business plan, you should anticipate changes in your business after the website is open to the public. Will you need more hardware, software, personnel, or computer training?

WILL EVERYBODY KNOW MY NAME?

Domain names

Each website is identified by a specific IP (Internet Protocol) address. An IP address is numerical and looks something like this: 123.000.123.00. (3) Since words are much easier to remember, each IP address is also assigned a domain name.Each URL (www.yoursite.com) or domain name is the distinct name that is associated with one specific IP address. A DNS (Domain Name Server) keeps track of which domain names are assigned to which IP addresses. From this hodgepodge of technicalities comes one simple conclusion: You need a domain name that you can call your own.

Choosing a domain name

Some helpful hints for choosing a name:
- Choose a domain name that closely matches your company's name.
- Keep the domain name short and easy to spell.
- Choose a domain name that is distinctive and easily recalled.

Registering a domain name

Cost of a Domain Name
The cost of a maintaining a domain name varies from one registration service to the next. Current annual rates generally run in the range of $20 to $35.

Trademark Your Domain Name?

There have been disputes over who is entitled to register a domain name. Obviously, Nike, the footwear giant, should be entitled to the name "nike.com," but does "tyco.com" go to Tyco Electronics or Tyco the toy maker, each a giant in its own industry? While you may never get into a legal hassle over your domain name, you should give it as much protection as is reasonably possible. (3) See Chapter 12 and ask your attorney about the necessity of registering your domain name with the U.S. Patent and Trademark Office. This does not guarantee that no one will ever challenge your ownership, but it does strengthen your case if a challenge does develop. (In practice, no one loses much sleep over this issue.)

I HAVE AN ADDRESS, BUT WHERE IS MY HOME?

Perhaps the most difficult concept to grasp is the fact that every website needs a home. More exactly, there has to be a physical device (a "server") that stores-electronically--all the computer code that constitutes any given website. Generally, the physical location of that device is insignificant, so long as the server is connected to the Internet. There are several options (4):

- **You can be your own server.**
You could host your site on your own server with the appropriate hardware and software. The biggest benefit of hosting your own site is that you have complete control over the site. For a small enterprise, however, the cost far outweighs any benefits. For the larger organization, self-hosting may make sense, but it should not be attempted unless you have experienced personnel to set up and maintain the server.

- **"Free" web space from ISP, Cybermalls, E-Commerce Services, etc.**
Some hosting services are "free," but there are some drawbacks: they tend to lack space and features, and most require that you invest in advertising with a banner ad, pop-up ad box or logo. Another disadvantage is that the website can't use its own distinct domain name or URL. Instead, the site must use a URL that is a sub-domain under the host's domain name. (For example, instead of having your own name www.yourname.com you would be a subdomain of the company, www.thehostingcompany.com/your-name.) If you change hosting services in the future, you will have to change your URL as well. The bottom line is that you should care-fully research why the service is "free" before committing to hosting with a free web space provider.

- **Web hosting company**
Without question, this is the recommended option for hosting a serious web site. You or your web designer can contact several, and inquire about available services, options and pricing.

Choosing a Web Hosting Company

There are multitudes of web hosting companies available. Conducting a simple search with the key words "web hosting" will give you an exhaustive list to choose from. Start first with each company's home page. See how the information is organized, and how much information you can get from each web site. The hosting package that you will need depends on what you want to do with your site. If you are planning on a simple informative site, you can get a basic package anywhere around $15 - $20 per month from a reputable web hosting company. If you are planning on building an e-commerce site, or using any interactivity that requires a database, plans will start at $35 - $60 depending on your needs.

WHAT SHOULD MY SITE LOOK LIKE? ─────────────

The overall look and feel of your site should reflect the image you want to portray. If your business has brochures, business cards, etc. that you like, continue with the "look" and tone (colors, wording, style of writing, etc.) of your offline promotional materials. This may entail using slightly different colors and design elements online, but the overall atmosphere is consistent with the offline feel.

A website's tone is a very important design decision. This sets a site's overall atmosphere and mood. The tone information will be used to determine a site's colors, design accents (bullets, horizontal bars, buttons, etc.), font, and layout. Most importantly, the tone should be consistent throughout the site.

Come up with three adjectives to describe the tone you want visitors to your site to feel when browsing your site. What adjectives do you want visitors to use to describe your site to their friends? Business-like? Cutting-edge? Warm and inviting? If you want a warm, inviting site, consider which colors would portray that image. If your business is geared towards children, consider fonts, colors, and graphics would give your site a lively, fun tone.

Design Limitations

Graphics. When using graphics, it is important to remember that the more graphics on a page, the slower the page will appear on the screen to the user. Graphics should enhance a web page. Graphics need to have a purpose or else their purpose is simply to slow the download time of the page. (5,6)

Animation. Animation can be overused or used incorrectly. Any animated feature on a page will draw the viewer's attention to that spot. If you want their attention drawn there, then use it. If you don't have a purpose for drawing attention, then don't use it. (7)

Fonts. There are only a few standard fonts that can be used for text on your site. If you use a non-standard font, you run the risk that most computer browsers will show the font with their standard font, instead of your font.(8) You want to try to keep control of the look of your site and not put it in the hands of other browsers. If you feel the need to use a non-standard font, you can make the font into a graphic instead. This will keep the font consistent from computer to computer. However, as mentioned earlier, you want to limit the amount of graphics because it makes the site harder to update, it makes your pages load slower, and search engines do not recognize the words in graphic designs.

What Should I Put on My Site?

64

Content is the core of the Internet. It's one of the unique advantages of the Internet. What content is included, how it's packaged, and whether it's easy to access determine if a website shines among the rest or is lost on the Web. Take the time to strategically plan the content you will include when your website is launched and over time as it expands.

The content included on your website must be of value to your target market. It must be updated and changed frequently. New and updated content gives your viewers a reason to come back to your site. Adding interaction gives another reason for visitors to come to your site and revisit it.

Adding Interaction

Interaction (two-way communication with visitors) sets the Internet apart from traditional media. It engages visitors. It's very effective at establishing a non-emotional relationship with visitors. Interaction adds value to the viewer. (9,10)

Feedback helps your viewers contribute to your site through suggesting links to your site or filling out feedback or survey forms. Visitors feel a sense of contribution if the questions are worded properly and if their input is taken seriously. This is also a good way to obtain comments from satisfied customers. Typically, demographic questions are included in order to get to know site visitors better. If you have narrowed down your target market, most links submitted by your visitors about specific topics will be useful to others visiting your site.

An e-mail newsletter can be used to announce new services, provide dates and locations of presentations, tips on using products, brief articles and information left out of publications. The newsletter must provide something your target market values. Typically, a newsletter encourages readers to visit your website. By pulling your target market to your site, they will more likely to buy or do what you really want them to do--view a page with advertisers' banners, read a collection of articles you wrote, or schedule a one-on-one chat with you.

Discussion groups or chat rooms are effective methods of interactive communication. You can host a discussion group that focuses on a topic of interest to your target market or set up a chat system for customer service. Another option for chat is where visitors with a question press a button on the screen and it sounds a telephone ring on the computer at the other end to alert whoever is taking calls that someone is online with a question. This is one-to-one chat. Customer service is the most common use for this, but there are many other uses like: Dietitian-on-call, online customized food orders, and tutoring during an educator's office hours. Chat also can be used for two-way discussions at pre-set times with a leader in charge, or a guest speaker where questions are held until after the speaker is done presenting online.

A calculator is a great interactive tool for anyone associated with nutrition. A calculator can be as straightforward as a calorie calculator, or more advanced as an eating disorder risk calculator (score indicates a risk level for development of an eating disorder) or nutrient assessment calculator. Calculators typically require CGI scripts and access to a server that allows CGI scripts. Calculators require a web developer well versed in programming calculators. This may require some investment upfront to hire someone to program the calculator. However, it can be an effective method for drawing in visitors to your site.

This list of ways to add interaction is far from exhaustive. Use your imagination and take advantage of this unique edge interaction on the Internet offers.

Confidentiality

Keep in mind, whenever you are asking for information from visitors you need to prominently display or link to a privacy and confidentiality statement. This statement should tell visitors what data you are collecting, how the site will use collected data, who will have access to the data (third parties need to be identified), how visitors can revise/update their data, and if data will be reported as individuals or as a group. Many sites unfortunately do not post this policy information. In coming years, this will become a very hot issue for sites. Many big health websites have already been publicly criticized for not doing this and have lost large numbers of visitors because of it.

Be certain your system is secure for e-mails as well. Encryption is a possibility. Limit the employees who have access to clients' and patients' e-mails. Be sure all e-mail-handling procedures treat e-mail as confidential. An increasingly popular method of security for e-mail is to go through a website rather than an e-mail box. You receive an e-mail informing you there is a message waiting online. You must then log onto a website to read your waiting messages or print your orders. The message is stored and read in a secure area on the website. The user can compose and send messages while logged onto the website. Users do not need to download the email onto their own hard drive. This is an avenue for providing secure communication.

ELEMENTS EVERY WEB SITE SHOULD HAVE

There are features every website should include for credibility and user friendliness.

1. Home page - The homepage answers the questions "Where am I?" and "What does this site do?"(11) This is accomplished through graphics and text. The graphics include a large logo and company name prominently displayed, and design elements strategically placed to lead a first-time visitor's eyes through it all. Text provides visitors information to help them decide whether they should stay or go. Helpful information includes overview of services, products, and site features. Include at least two sentences of text. Avoid using only graphics on the homepage (11). Search engines can't index words in graphics. When a visitor enters a search phrase at a search engine, the search engine index matches the search phrase to text words found at sites it has visited. A homepage with graphics and no text misses on the opportunity to be indexed properly and thus isn't found at search engines. The homepage example below has both graphics and text that work together to answer the questions "Where am I?" and "What does this site do?"

EXAMPLES

Details what the site is all about, with a balance between graphics and text.

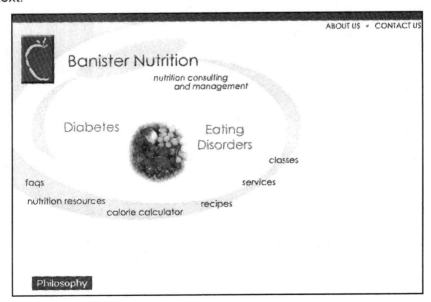

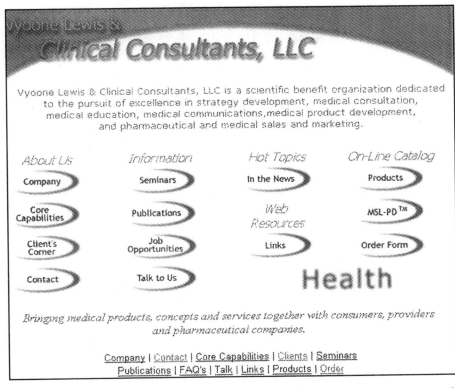

Splash pages have gained popularity recently as homepages. A splash page is a visual introduction page (often with an animated clip) that points the visitor to the main page when the animation is finished. This can be effective if used correctly, with apparent links to an inside section or home page. If used improperly, it can be a way to drive away your viewers, who don't realize there is more to the site behind that page.(12) Also, splash pages often take a long amount of time for visitors with dial-up modems to download; this is a big turnoff for first-time visitors. Search engine optimization experts warn against using splash pages on a site's homepage.

2. About/Bio - Information on the business and owner. It should give some history on the business and the purpose of the website. Include a resume or highlights of professional career and training too.

Information about the author with links to more detailed information

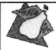

Hope Warshaw Associates

Food • Nutrition • Diabetes

Home
About Hope
Books
Ordering
Services
Faqs
Monthly Recipe
Links
Contact Us

About Hope

Hope S. Warshaw, MMSc, RD, CDE
has nearly 25 years of expertise as a dietitian (RD) and certified diabetes educator (CDE). For the first 10 years of her career she gained expertise as a nutrition and diabetes counselor in a variety of health care settings - from hospitals, to out-patient settings, from inner city to university referral centers.

For the past 15 years, Hope has owned her consulting business, Hope Warshaw Associates. In this business she applies her knowledge of diabetes and passion for people with diabetes. She provides an array of services to an array of clients - from counseling people with diabetes, to

3. Navigation helps - The navigation helps are determined by the size of the site and expectations of visitors. Examples of navigation helps are a navigation bar that remains consistent throughout the

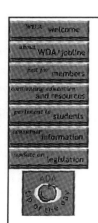

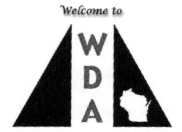

Welcome to

W D A

WISCONSIN DIETETIC ASSOCIATION
Your Link to Nutrition and Health

Our Mission
The Wisconsin Dietetic Association promotes optimal nutrition an people by advocating for its members.

The goals of the Wisconsin Dietetic Association are:

site, site map, site search engine, index page, next page prompts, introductory pages to website areas, and top and bottom prompts. Every web page should have a text navigation bar.

Company | Contact | Core Capabilities | Clients | Seminars
Publications | FAQ's | Talk | Links | Products | Order

4. References - References add credibility to content and the overall website. Provide links directly to references and links to sites for additional information if appropriate. A reference list can be provided for the entire site or for each article. *65*

5. Advertisers/Sponsors - Disclose all sponsors and advertisers and how they are involved in the site. Whether they contribute any content and if so, what content should be clearly indicated. Also, an advertising policy should be described. Several big health websites in the late 1990's received stiff criticism that hurt their credibility when it was disclosed that they were misleading visitors regarding advertisers' contributions to the site.

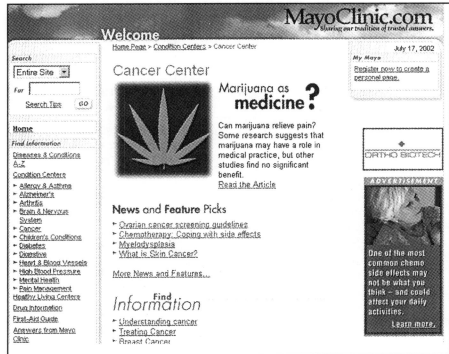

Advertisement policy is given.

6. Privacy/confidentiality--This refers to any information collected at the site. If visitors are required or voluntarily give information, disclose what will be done with the information, who will have access to the information (any third parties), how users can update/modify their personnel information, and if information will be reported as individuals or a group. (16)

An example of a privacy policy

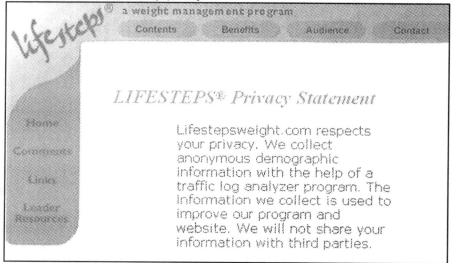

7. Contact information - This should be displayed on every page or link every page to a separate contact page.

Contact information is listed on every page. Also, a link to a contact page is given.

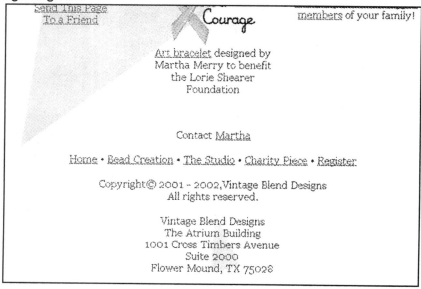

WEBSITE QUESTIONS

Why is stating you meet "high standards" a problem?

You are making a promise on your website and if the reader finds out there are newer research findings, you can be found at fault. It isn't that RD's don't meet high standards, you don't want to set yourself up for legal problems. As a RD, if you made this statement you would need to be very careful about updating content all the time.(This malpractice information is taken from a health lawyer's column in an Internet Health publication.) Now, there is even insurance for spelling and grammatical errors in Internet content. The insurance covers errors that occur in how your advice appears on someone's screen, if they follow your advice and it wasn't what you intended. When your content is out there for the world to see, new issues surface and this is one of them. These are red flags for malpractice problems. (19) It may be in your best interest to rewrite these areas so they provide general information without promises. See page 290.

Why is this a problem if the information is accurate?

The problem isn't the information you are providing, it's more the lack of adequate patient information. There are too many assumptions. The patients may not be revealing everything about their cases, and *very importantly, you probably didn't conduct a thorough assessment, which should be done before ever dispensing treatment advice.* The problem is that the persons reading the information or receiving your response may believe you are treating them. If they do, you can get in hot water since you have not performed an assessment. Every program I have been to on on-line counseling or protecting yourself on-line, advocates getting consent from an on-line 'patient' before starting any type of counseling or MNT relationship. Practitioners must be aware they need to use caution in posting answers to message boards and to questions e-mailed off the website. I am not referring to answers to questions from established patients. Any erroneous advice you provide, perhaps due to incomplete information from the patient, could lead to a malpractice claim. Also, ask yourself if the appropriate course for a patient's question is a face-to-face meeting or phone consultation rather than a "cyber chat." Advise the patient appropriately.   Teresa Pangan

It is important to respect state licensure. If a state outside of yours doesn't have licensure, it's fine to counsel a patient there, but if there is licensure, you need to look deeper into the licensure specifics. Dietetic licensure encompasses a state's scope of practice for dietetics. It is designed to protect the public from fraudulent practice and services being provided by untrained persons. If you work in a state that has licensure and work only with clients who also live in that state, professional liability insurance is sufficient if practicing within ADA's Scope of Practice. (20, 21) Crossing state lines to states without any required dietetics licensure also is covered. The gray areas begin when counseling clients who live in states outside yours that have mandatory dietetics licensure. In these states, avoid establishing a professional-patient relationship with individuals. Counseling patients living in states where you are not licensed is uncharted territory and the best guideline is caution to avoid legal messes down the road.

Additional website areas to consider:
- Testimonials/comments from satisfied clients/users
- FAQ--frequently asked questions, often these are questions that take a significant amount of time to answer regarding business products or services
- Site map/index--especially useful if homepage is starting to get cluttered
- Map to office--at least two versions, "zoom-in" and "zoom-out" should be included. The maps can be password protected if for a home office or if security is a concern.

ARE THERE OTHER ISSUES I NEED TO BE CONCERNED WITH?

Accessibility

Designing for universal accessibility used to be optional for webmasters in designing websites. Not true any longer. The American with Disabilities Act mandates equal access to computer systems for users with disabilities.(13,14) Additionally, the federal government has required that all businesses that contract with them and provide services via their website, must comply with accessibility standards (U.S. Section 508 Guidelines). (13) The term 'disabilities' when referring to the Internet does not refer to disabilities in the traditional sense.

Disabilities on the Internet refer to computer users with special considerations: (24)

- Difficulty with selecting small navigation buttons because of mobility impairments
- Difficulty with making sense of a cluttered screen due to a learning disability
- Difficulty viewing large graphics because of a slow Internet connection
- Difficulty comprehending content with puns because English is not native tongue

The Center for Applied Special Technology has developed a HTML validator program called Bobby that tests a webpage's accessibility.(15) It helps identify changes in a webpage that will help users with disabilities more easily use the page (http://bobby.cast.org). Additionally, there is an international industry consortium called the World Wide Web Consortium with accessibility guidelines to help webmasters and Web developers make Web content accessible to people with Web disabilities (Web Content Accessibility Guidelines 1.0 at: http://www.w3.org/WAI/). (15) The principles in the World Wide Web Consortium's Guidelines are based on (25):

- Provide alternatives to auditory and visual content
- Don't rely on color or graphics alone, words are important too
- Use standard HTML markup language and consistent design across a Web site
- Create tables and new technologies that transform gracefully across all major browsers, older versions too (may require creating alternates for older browser versions)
- Design for device-independence
- Provide clear navigation elements

Security

Security for a web site is both security of your visitor's information, as well as security for your site's information. There are several methods of promoting security. The more methods you employ, the more secure your site will be. You should constantly be updating your security methods and checking for security problems.

The first step to check the security of your site is finding out more about your web hosting company's security methods. You can ask them to provide you a copy of their security policy. It is important to know who has access to your site files within their company as well as what methods of security they employ to prevent hackers from accessing your site files (firewalls, encryption, etc.).

As mentioned earlier, if you are asking viewers for any personal information, you should have a copy of your privacy policy available on your website. The privacy policy should tell them what information you are collecting as well as who has access to that information. Private information should only be collected over a secure server. You can further secure your site's information by protecting your content. Read on to learn more.

Protecting Your Content

Stealing content on the Internet unfortunately is a common practice. There are two ways of stealing online content. First, content can be lifted and posted on another site--so the other site is getting credit for writing the information. Second, content can be linked inside a frame setup so that visitors think they are reading content developed by the site in the address bar, but in reality, the content is from another site. The infringing site can have its own navigation bar, but someone else's content in the main section of the site.

The most basic way to protect your content is to display your copyright notice; the "c" in a circle or the word "Copyright" followed by the date and your name (i.e. Copyright 2000, Mary Jacobs or Your Company Name). You can also protect your content by renaming your pages periodically. If you change your page names, the hyperlinks to your pages will be useless. If another site displays a page of your site, trying to pass it off as their own, their viewers will get a "Cannot find page" error message if you have changed your page name. This protects you from others using your pages as links from their site, and trying to pass them off as their own.

For photographs and graphics, learn to use digital watermarks on your images. A digital watermark is encoded in an image file. If someone copies your image file off of the Internet, the digital watermark stays with the image. When the image is displayed on a website, the copyright information is displayed on the title bar as well. Your images can also be tracked through some digital imaging companies.

Malpractice

Carefully review any statements on your Web site concerning nutrition treatment, "cures," outcomes, and professional qualifications to guard against malpractice. Are you promising cures? Do you claim your care meets the highest standards?

On-line message boards or forums, and questions e-mailed to you from website visitors, not established patients, are potential malpractice landmines. Make sure answers you post do not establish a professional-patient relationship - even if you have never seen the patient. (19)

Many health practitioners offer information based on established standards of care such as those published by the ADA, the American Diabetes Association, and other professional associations. (20) This is done instead of counseling online. The result is avoidance of counseling online and establishing a professional-patient relationship.

When responding to nutrition questions via e-mail, only answer specific questions for established patients. (19) Create policies that designate for what purposes patients can use e-mail.(17) Discourage the submission of revealing questions and information in e-mail. This type of information is best handled over a telephone, office visit, or during a secure web conference.

Posting frequently asked questions often protects against malpractice while still providing desired health information. All informational content and e-mails should include a disclaimer such as:

"Information contained in this Web site (e-mail) is general in nature, and should not be relied on for medical treatment. If you need nutritional advice or services, please contact your physician or a Registered Dietitian in your area."

There are fewer risks in using the Internet for scheduling and administrative functions. For instance, e-mail can be a good way to do appointment reminders and schedule appointments. Post established protocols and turnaround times on your site.

Print copies of all communications with patients and place a copy in patients' records. (22) It's recommended that an autoresponder (an automatic e-mail response setup by your e-mail program) be configured in your e-mail system (17, 23) to acknowledge receipt of all patient messages (consult your e-mail help center). A sample autoresponder message is:

"Nutrition and Associates at contact@nutritioncompany.com has received your e-mail. We will respond to you within 48 business hours. If this requires an immediate response, call our office at 972-321-XXXX. If you have not previously checked, you are encouraged to view our Frequently Asked Questions at http://www.nutritioncompany.com/faqs/ to see if your question has been answered there."

Request patients notify you when they receive your messages. Lastly, perform regular backups of e-mail into long-term storage and keep for the same amount of time as paper records. (17, 23).

The American Medical Association (AMA) developed guidelines for medical and health information websites: Guidelines for Medical and Health Information Sites on the Internet: Principles Governing AMA Web Sites: (http://jama.ama-assn.org/issues/v283n12/ffull/ jsc00054.html) (17).

The AMA developed these principles to guide development and posting of Web site content to ensure site visitors' and patients' rights to privacy and confidentiality. While these guidelines were developed for the AMA Web sites and visitors to these sites, they also are useful to other providers and users of health information on the Web.

(My disclaimer: This information is not comprehensive and is not meant as a substitute for legal counsel. If you have questions or concerns, consult a lawyer specializing in Internet law.)

TESTING AND PROOFING THE SITE

It's essential to test and proof your site before letting visitors have access to it. Since browsers and browser versions can display pages differently, it's important to check all the major browsers. Look at your site with Microsoft Internet Explorer (www.microsoft.com), Netscape Navigator (www.netscape.com), and WebTV browsers (download the viewer at: http://developer.msntv.com/Tools/WebTVwr.asp) (18). Browser updates are released periodically, and each update becomes a new browser version (e.g. Internet Explorer 5.5, Internet Explorer 6.0). You can check the company's website to see what the newest version of the browser is, and then find computers that have that version of the browser, as well as the last two browser versions. Newer browser versions can be updated onto your computer right off of the Internet. Check at least two of the previous versions of each browser. Your check list should include:

- **Visual Appearance**
  Is the site interesting?
  Are the colors appealing?
  Is the site legible in a smaller browser window?
  Is the text easy to read?
  Does the site look too busy or cluttered?
  Does the site give you the feel or tone that you are after?
- **Links**
  Check all links: both internal to the site and any external links to other sites.
- **Forms**
  Run test forms to check functionality.
- **Grammatical and spelling errors**
  Check and double check for grammatical and spelling errors.
- **Print out pages for proofing**
  Printing out the pages may help you catch errors you missed on the screen.

MAINTENANCE AND REPEAT TRAFFIC

In addition to creating value on your site, something must change on your site periodically to bring visitors back and create repeat traffic. Examples for content that might change on your site to draw repeat traffic:

- Useful articles on a topic of value to your target market with new ones added monthly.
- New sweepstakes every month.
- New articles added monthly on how to use a nutrition calculator posted on your site.
- Weekly chat room hosted by different experts.
- A nutrition tip that changes every two weeks.
- Monthly feature of a vegetable and fruit with tips on buying, storing, and how to prepare.
- Foodservice special diet menus that cycle weekly.

The first time visitors browse your site, they may not buy your service or product nor comprehend the information you are providing. It may be on their second, third or fourth visit when this desired behavior occurs. This is why repeat traffic is a key to success.

Related to this is time and money. Time and money must be budgeted for maintenance right at the start of planning a website. One of the biggest mistakes small businesses make in developing a website is not allotting sufficient time to update the site and money to promote it.

Before the website is finished, determine who will be responsible for updating and adding to the website once it is operational. Someone will need to be responsible for coordinating new content, maintaining the graphic and editorial standards, and assuring that the programming and linkages of all pages remain intact and functional. Don't let your site go stale by starving it of resources just as you begin to develop a following of clients.

Webmasters often are the best people for the job. Many have reasonable rates for maintenance. Another option is to contract someone to train you on how to update your site (if you didn't develop it). Allow sufficient budget for training on how to update your site. Some dietitians combine the two. They reserve the simplest monthly/quarterly updates/revisions for themselves to carry out and the more advanced revisions and additions to the site are done by a contracted webmaster.

THE LAST STEP

After planning, developing, evaluating objectives and making changes to your website, the cycle starts again. Think about how you want your business to grow, and begin to plan and outline those changes. Then take action on those plans, collect feedback, evaluate the results, and incorporate what you learn into your site. A website is a work in progress. It constantly evolves to respond to the needs of its visitors. Think of your online business like a garden that thrives with attention, careful watering, and pruning.

REFERENCES

1. Pangan T, Bednar C. Dietitian business Web sites: A survey of their profitability and how can you make yours profitable, JADA, 101(4):399-402, 2001.
2. Kent P. Chapter 6 Designing Your Web Site. In: Poor Richard's Web Site: Geek-Free, Commonsense Advise on Building a Low-Cost Web Site. Lakewood, CO: Top Floor Publishing; 2000.
3. Kent P. Chapter 5 All About Domain Names. In: Poor Richard's Web Site: Geek-Free, Commonsense Advise on Building a Low-Cost Web Site. Lakewood, CO: Top Floor Publishing; 2000.
4. Kent P. Chapter 3 Where to Put Your Web Site. In: Poor Richard's Web Site: Geek-Free, Commonsense Advise on Building a Low-Cost Web Site. Lakewood, CO: Top Floor Publishing; 2000.
5. Nielsen J. Chapter 2 Page Design. In: Designing Web Usability: The Practice of Simplicity. Indianapolis, IN: New Riders Publishing; 2000.
6. Lynch P, Horton S. Chapter 7 Web Graphics. In: Web Style Guide: Basic Design Principles for Creating Web Sites, New Haven, CT: Yale University Press; 1999.
7. Nielsen J. Chapter 3 Content Design. In: Designing Web Usability: The Practice of Simplicity, Indianapolis, IN: New Riders Publishing; 2000.
8. Lynch P, Horton S. Chapter 5 Typography. In: Web Style Guide: Basic Design Principles for Creating Web Sites. New Haven, CT: Yale University Press; 1999.
9. eTRENDS:Making a site "sticky" calls for a diverse menu of tactics, Internet Healthcare, October 2000.
10. Kent P. Chapter 11 Web-Sites Are Two-Way Streets - Adding Interaction. In: Poor Richard's Web Site: Geek-Free, Commonsense Advise on Building a Low-Cost Web Site. , Lakewood, CO: Top Floor Publishing; 2000.
11. Nielsen J, Tahir M. Homepage Guidelines. In: Homepage Usability: 50 Websites Deconstructed, Indianapolis, IN: New Riders Publishing; 2000.
12. Nielsen J. Chapter 4 Site Design. In: Designing Web Usability: The Practice of Simplicity, Indianapolis, IN: New Riders Publishing; 2000.
13. Francis W. Web sites must be made more accessible to the blind. Medicine on the Net, January 2001.
14. Hirsch R. Is your Web site ADA compliant? Internet Healthcare Strategies; February 2001.
15. Jones M. Designing to give everyone access to the Web. Inside Web Design; October 2000.
16. Loch K. How Does Your Website's Privacy Policy Rate? Beyond Computing; September 2000.
17. Guidelines for Medical and Health Information Sites on the Internet. JAMA. 2000;282:12: 1600-1606.
18. Kent P. Chapter 9 Creating an Effective Website. In: Poor Richard's Web Site: Geek-Free, Commonsense Advise on Building a Low-Cost Web Site, Lakewood, CO: Top Floor Publishing; 2000.
19. Johnson L. The Internet and malpractice risk. Medical Economics; November 9, 1998.
20. Grieger L. Working Online: Are Your Covered? Today's Dietitian; November 2001.
21. Horton Eastwood A. Success Online: A Valuable Resource. Ventures, 17(2), Spring 2001.
22. Palumbo C. Using new technology for nutrition counseling. JADA; 99(11): 1363-1364, 1999.

23. eRisk Guidelines for Physician-Patient Online Communications. Medem Website. Available online at: http://www.medem.com/corporate/corporate_erisk.cfm. Accessed June 29, 2002.
24. Burgstahler S. Making Web Pages Universally Accessible. Computer-Mediated Communication Magazine; January 1998, available online at: http://www.december.com/cmc/mag/1998/jan/burg.html. Accessed June 29, 2002.
25. Check your site's accessibility. Medicine on the Net; March 2000.

BIBLIOGRAPHY

Books

Kent, Peter. Poor Richard's Web Site: Geek-Free, Commonsense Advise on Building a Low-Cost Web Site. Lakewood, CO: Top Floor Publishing; 2000.

Lynch, Patrick and Sarah Horton: Web Style Guide: Basic Design Principles for Creating Web Sites. New Haven, CT: Yale University Press;1999.

Nielsen, Jakob: Designing Web Usability: The Practice of Simplicity. Indianapolis, IN: New Riders Publishing; 2000.

Nielsen, Jakob and Tahir, Marie: Homepage Usability: 50 Websites Deconstructed. Indianapolis, IN: New Riders   Publishing; 2001.

Siegel, David: Creating Killer Web Sites, 2nd ed. Indianapolis, IN: Hayden Books; 1997.

Articles

Flory, Joyce. New on the Net: Special Focus: Privacy & Patient Confidentiality. Medicine on the Net; August 2001.

Rourke, Kathleen, Hern, Marcia and Lisa Cicciarello. NetWellness: Utilizing a consumer health information Web site to access nutrition professionals. JADA; 100 (7): 757-759.

Net Resources: Making sites more accessible to the disabled. Medicine on the Net; March 2001.

Techno Web: Getting really small: an ongoing battle with file size. Inside Web Design; February 2000.

Learning to use color on your Web site. Inside Web Design; June 2000.

McCray, Katherine. Designing around the different browser sizes, Inside Web Design; November 2000.

Casey, Carol. Accessibility and the Educational Web Site, Syllabus; September 1999.

Chapter 23

Promoting Your Website

Teresa Pangan, RD, PhD and Julie M. Horner
Owners, Puttin' On The Web

Marketing your website online does not require a large financial investment, but it does require time commitment. Even if you decide to hire a website designer, you need to know what you are hiring the person to do. You need some familiarity with terms and function, so you can evaluate whether the person is doing a good job for you. After you read this chapter, you will know to ask your web developer to see your meta tags or keyword description before you pay a dime, or sit and wait for business to roll in.

From the first draft of your website, plan on budgeting time for online promotions. At the start, a lot of time is spent optimizing a website so search engines will find your site. After a site is optimized, it can be submitted to search engines. When a site's promotion plans unfold, time is directed into multiple activities like reciprocal marketing, posting to listservs or advertising in an e-mail newsletter.

If you are investing in a web site, use Appendix 23A Promotions Worksheet at the end of this chapter to complete as you read along. Before reading on, make a commitment to regularly set aside time to promote your website.

SEARCH ENGINE OPTIMIZATION

More than eight in ten American Internet users go to search engines to find information on the Web.(1) This emphasizes the importance of optimizing a website for the search engines. There are several simple things that can be done to increase your site's position in a search engine's results list.

First, the search engine optimization process starts with determining your critical keyword phrases. Next, the keyword phrases are placed in strategic locations throughout your website. All web pages need to be optimized. Different pages on your site will be indexed for different terms since they cover different topics. You will want to use keyword phrases related to each page's topic in titles, headings, image alt tags, meta tags, text and links, not just on the homepage or a couple of front pages. You will bring in more traffic to a page if it is optimized for a very specific phrase, not a general one. The Internet is better with niches. This results in a high ranking for searches done with your critical keyword phrases. If done properly, search engines will send visitors your way.

Keyword Analysis

Keywords refer to words that describe your site. They are words your target market uses to search for your site in a search engine. It may be helpful to ask members of your target market for words they would use to describe your business.

A common mistake for website developers is to only use keywords they feel are most logical to locate the website they are developing. The words may be different than the target audience would use. An example is the word "dietitian." If the public is your target market, it is best to use additional words like "nutritionist", or "dietician" (spelled with a "c") along with "dietitian" (spelled with a "t") on your website. The words "nutritionist" and "dietician" are more commonly entered on a search engine.

Key Words

To begin, brainstorm 25-50 keywords to describe your site. Then narrow these keywords down to the best 10-15 keywords and keyword phrases (2-3 word phrases). Go with keywords and keyword phrases that (2):

- are simple,
- are not hard to spell,
- include synonyms,
- include 2-3 word phrases, and
- include plurals if your target market enters plurals at the search engines.

Rarely is a single keyword appropriate. A single keyword is misleading. For example "consultant." Does "consultant" refer to a food service consultant, banking consultant, pharmaceutical consultant, or tax consultant? Visitors will be disappointed if they came to your site using the keyword "consultant" and expected tax information. They will press the "back" button immediately. The goal is bringing targeted traffic-buyers interested in what you have to "sell"--- not just traffic.

Power Combinations

Come up with multiple (2-3) keyword combinations that your target market uses in searches that match your site's content and purpose. Additionally, look for keyword combinations that do not have a lot of competitors. Once you find keyword combinations that satisfy these three criteria (content, purpose and few competitors), these are your critical keyword phrases or power combinations.(1)

Complementary and Narrowly Focused

Expand your brainstorming into complementary areas. Often this will lead you to discovering a niche where there isn't a lot of competition. General nutrition keywords include:
- nutrition consultant
- nutritionist
- nutrition therapy
- nutrition educator

Examples of complementary, more narrowly focused nutrition keywords are:
- menu analysis
- wellness nutritionist
- spa nutritionist/ spa dietitian/ spa dietician
- diabetic cooking
- renal dietitian/ renal dietician

Often it is easier to attract your target market to your site for a complementary, narrowly focused nutrition area. Narrowly focused keyword combinations typically have less competition than broader, more general keyword phrases.

Tools to Help Pinpoint Critical Keyword Combinations

There are a handful of software programs to help in identifying the most popular keywords and keyword combinations used at search engines. Industry experts often recommend two programs for this function: Wordtracker (http://www.Wordtracker.com) and WordSpot (www.WordSpot.com).

WordTracker is an online subscription service. It compiles a database with the most popular words people have used at various search engines. It obtains/buys its data from metasearch engines. It uses this data in combination with equations and other data to predict the frequency a keyword combination is used in search engines.

WordSpot (www.WordSpot.com) works very similar to Wordtracker except the database it uses to analyze results is smaller. To find other programs and services enter the keyword phrase <keyword report> at any search engine.

Integrating Keyword Analysis Results into Your Website

After identifying your critical keyword phrases, they need to be sprinkled at strategic locations throughout your site. Search engines will then index your site higher for your intended keyword phrases on a search results list.

Meta tags

Meta tags are HTML code tags (the behind-the-scenes programming code for webpages) that are placed in a Web page's program coding. Browsers know not to display meta tags, simply skip over them. Meta tags are intended as a method for Web developers to communicate information to search engines and other developers. The most talked about meta tags that relate to search engine rankings are:

- keywords
- description

Meta means "information." So meta tags are information about other data. See Figure 23.1 for an example of meta tags. For years, meta tags have been a critical part of improving your search engine positioning. However, due to "spamming" techniques (repeating the same words over and over for pages), and refinement of search engine relevancy equations, the weight given to meta tags by search engines has diminished over recent years.

Figure 23.1

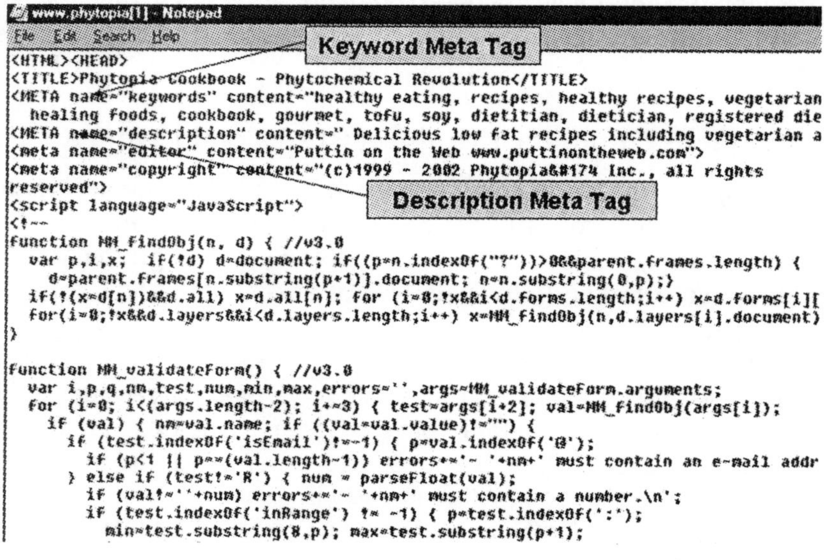


```
<HTML><HEAD>
<TITLE>Phytopia Cookbook - Phytochemical Revolution</TITLE>
<META name="keywords" content="healthy eating, recipes, healthy recipes, vegetarian
  healing foods, cookbook, gourmet, tofu, soy, dietitian, dietician, registered die
<META name="description" content=" Delicious low fat recipes including vegetarian a
<meta name="editor" content="Puttin on the Web www.puttinontheweb.com">
<meta name="copyright" content="(c)1999 - 2002 Phytopia&#174 Inc., all rights
reserved">
<script language="JavaScript">
<!--
function MM_findObj(n, d) { //v3.0
  var p,i,x;  if(!d) d=document; if((p=n.indexOf("?"))>0&&parent.frames.length) {
    d=parent.frames[n.substring(p+1)].document; n=n.substring(0,p);}
  if(!(x=d[n])&&d.all) x=d.all[n]; for (i=0;!x&&i<d.forms.length;i++) x=d.forms[i][
  for(i=0;!x&&d.layers&&i<d.layers.length;i++) x=MM_findObj(n,d.layers[i].document)
}

function MM_validateForm() { //v3.0
  var i,p,q,nm,test,num,min,max,errors='',args=MM_validateForm.arguments;
  for (i=0; i<(args.length-2); i+=3) { test=args[i+2]; val=MM_findObj(args[i]);
    if (val) { nm=val.name; if ((val=val.value)!="") {
      if (test.indexOf('isEmail')!=-1) { p=val.indexOf('@');
        if (p<1 || p==(val.length-1)) errors+='- '+nm+' must contain an e-mail addr
      } else if (test!='R') { num = parseFloat(val);
        if (val!=''+num) errors+='- '+nm+' must contain a number.\n';
        if (test.indexOf('inRange') != -1) { p=test.indexOf(':');
          min=test.substring(8,p); max=test.substring(p+1);
```

Meta tags are still important to develop. However, don't be misled into thinking they will drastically boost your ranking. By following all of the search engine optimization techniques recommended here, your search engine results ranking will increase significantly, but following only one will not do it alone.

Description Meta Tag

This is a brief description of the content of a particular web page or site. It should not be more than 150 characters with spaces since this is the maximum length most search engines will index.(3, 4) Use at least two of your critical keyword phrases in the description.

Think of the description meta tag as a very short billboard ad. Many search engines will use the description meta tag as the description displayed in its results listing. It should reflect accurately and enticingly what the content on that page or site is about.

Keyword Meta Tag

Use your top ten keyword phrases together to create your keyword meta tag. See Figure 23.1 for an example of a keyword meta tag. List them in order of importance with the most important listed first. Repeat them no more than three times. The maximum length is 750 characters with spaces. Typically, you will not come close to using this many characters, but this is the cut off point for most search engines. Also, do not place the same word next to each other. For example, do not insert these keyword phrases together: (3, 4, 5) "sports nutrition," "nutrition education materials." The word "nutrition" is repeated next to each other. Reversing the order would be fine. Also, no word should be repeated more than four times in the entire keyword meta tag. The word "nutrition" often is used in multiple keyword phrases (nutrition educator, nutrition expert, nutrition education materials, nutrition menus, nutrition services) and may result in appearing more than four times. Search engine software programs will leave out your site altogether if they detect a keyword meta tag is repeating a word too often or words are too close together.

Use Keywords in the Body Copy

Make sure keyword phrases appear in the text on each page the description meta tag is inserted. Search engines cross-reference keywords in meta tags with the content of the page. They will not index keywords and phrases that do not appear in the webpage's text as well. Search engines are constantly refining their equations in order to locate webpage's that have higher relevancy for a search phrase. They require that words on a page's titles, alt graphic tags, headings and meta tags must also appear on a page's text for relevancy. If not, they will not index the page for those terms. (Alt tags are "alternative text" programmed into a webpage that is displayed. This text is helpful for the visually impaired or those who choose not to download images on Web pages in order to increase their surfing speed. With most browsers, this text appears when you put your mouse over an image or icon.)

- First 25 words---important area to include critical keyword phrases (3); include at least one, or preferably two.
- Last 25 words---search engines also look here. Search engine owners believe it must be a good descriptive word or phase for that page's content, if a keyword phrase appears in the first and last 25 words. (3)

Keyword weight is the number of times your keyword appears on a page in relation to the total number of words on a page. Search engines keep an eye out for too high a keyword weight. They are screening for spamming. Spammers will repeat a keyword phrase (10 to 100 times) in hopes of improving their ranking. If a search engine detects this, that page will not be indexed and possibly will be put on a black list. Most resources recommend a keyword weight of 3-10 percent (3). We don't recommend calculating your keyword weights, instead read your webpage content out loud. If it sounds choppy, that is your best sign you may have placed a keyword phrase too many times in your content. Go back and take a closer look.

Title

Title refers to the uppermost phrase in your browser window. It appears as a "bookmark title" if you bookmark the page. See Figure 23.2 for an example of a title.

Use descriptive words in your title. The title should tell visitors what to expect on that page, not on the entire site. If possible, start with a keyword. Search engines do index titles, and the more you can pack into it the better. Words like "Welcome, One," or "Best," are poor choices to start a title. They are a waste of prime search engine real estate. (3, 6)

A title length should be 60 characters or less. The first 40 characters should contain at least one critical keyword or keyword phrase. Some search engines index 60, others 40. Examples:

"Nutrition: prevention & chronic disease (41 characters) management services (61 characters)"

"Plant based recipes: easy to make (35 characters) in thirty minutes (52 characters)"

Figure 23.2

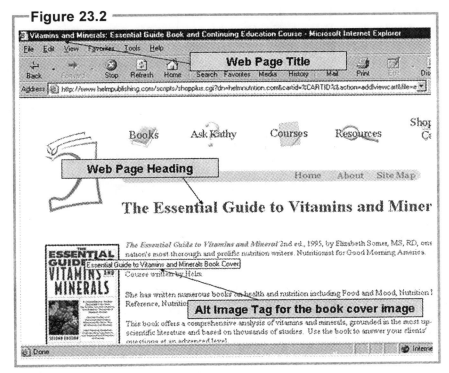

Headings

Headings are commonly called titles and subheadings in books and normal printed text. See Figure 23.2. In HTML coding (the behind-the-scenes coding for websites), there are Headings ranked 1 through 6 with Heading 1 being the most important heading on a page, and Heading 6 is a sub, sub-heading.

When developing a page's format, it is important to label headings as Heading 1 through 6 in the HTML code and not simply enlarge and bold the text until it visually appears like a heading. Search engines read the HTML coding and give a higher weight to words labeled as Headings 1 through 6 than regular content text. This opportunity is lost if headings are only formatted as large, bold text.

Links

Another behinds-the-scene technique that contributes to a higher search engine ranking is words in links. A search engine gives more weight to words highlighted in a link than non-linked content text. Words like "click here" will not help your search engine rankings, but the phrases "diabetes menu planning" and "vegetarian recipes" (words in blue with underlining) linked to the appropriate pages will. A good web page designer will know how to do this.

Links should describe what a visitor expects to find when they follow the link. It is not necessary to link an entire sentence, just the descriptive keywords.

Alt Image tag

This is an optional HTML tag used to label a graphic. Alt image tags are displayed when moving your mouse over an image or icon (called "mousing"), a phrase will appear over the graphic. See Figure 23.2 for an example of an alt image tag. Not all Web designers remember to program this in. Ask your developer to include alt tags for all your graphics. Search engines will index these words. They cannot read words in a graphic or artwork, but they can read words programmed into an alt tag.

It is a mistake to use very generic words in an alt tag. Examples are:
- Concerns
- Fruit
- Man

Descriptive alt tags will generate more keywords for a search engine to index and helps explain the purpose of a graphic. Improved alt tags for the examples given above are:
- Frequently Asked Questions
- Great ideas for a smoothie
- Man with cancer visits with dietitian

SEARCH ENGINE SUBMISSION

Once a site is optimized, it is ready to submit to the search engines. It's important to wait until a site is completely ready to go, before submitting it. The resultant search engine ranking will be higher with a completed site than with a rushed, not quite finished one.

There are two methods for entering a site into search engines and subject directories:
1. free or paid submission service, and
2. entering your website by hand.

The second option is the most time consuming, but it often more effective than the first option. Many experts recommend entering a site by hand into the top search engines and subject directories. (7) When submitted by hand, the submissions can be customized. Submission services, both free and commercial, use software to submit a site. Some customization can be done, but not as much as by hand. Many search engines say they are on the lookout for software programs because it is ten times more likely spamming is present with software programs.

Site Submission Services

If you are tight on time, here is a sampling of services that can enter your website into 25 or more search engines and subject directories.

@Submit	http://www.uswebsites.com/submit/
Register-It	http://register-it.netscape.com/
SubmitIt!	http://www.submit-it.com/
NetMechanic	http://www.netmechanic.com

To find more search engine submission services use keywords: <submission +"search engine">. Fill in the name of each search engine you want to use.

Entering Your Site by Hand

To enter by hand, go to any of the sites below for a list of links to search engines and subject directories.
* Search Engine Guide
  http://www.searchengineguide.com/
* All Search Engines
  http://www.allsearchengines.co.uk/
For more sites with links to search engines use the keywords: < Internet +"search engines" +directories>.

Go to each search engine or subject directory and look for a link labeled something like "Add Link" or "Add URL" or "Recommend a Site." They frequently are located near the bottom of the page in small type. Use your completed Promotions Worksheet for keywords, descriptions, and titles requested in each search engine submission form.

Two to four weeks after submitting your site, check your site's position in all the top search engines and subject directories. This should be done even if you used a submission service. You may need to re-enter your site if it is not listed yet. Many sites never make it into a search engine's index.

In addition to general search engines and subject directories there are some specialized health search engines and subject directories.

Here are some you should consider submitting your site to:

Achoo	http://www.achoo.com
HealthWeb	http://healthweb.org
Medical Matrix	http://www.medmatrix.org/index.asp
MedHunt	http://www.hon.ch/MedHunt/

Fee Based Search Engine and Subject Directory Submissions

The trend in recent years has been for a handful of the top search engines to charge for a submission to their index. Yahoo started charging a hefty $299 annual fee.

Yahoo can be worth the money to be listed for many web businesses (nonprofit organization listings are free) because at this time Yahoo has control over 30 percent of the traffic on all search engines. That means nearly 40 percent of all searches performed on the Internet are at Yahoo.(8,9)

To determine if it's worth the fee for your site, enter your keyword phrases at Yahoo's search query and assess the categories that appear in the results list. How many listings are there in these listed categories? It may not be worth the Yahoo fee if your main category has six pages of sites listed and your business name begins with a "W" (since Yahoo lists companies alphabetically). Be sure when you do submit a description for your listing, it does not go over the word limit. Yahoo editors are known for their discriminating taste and will trim a description for a site if they get wind of any "marketese" language (overblown misrepresentation) in a description. They prefer straight forward descriptive submissions. Look closely at the other descriptions in your main category. Follow their lead.

People in the industry believe many more search engines will follow Yahoo's lead. The key is to look at your competition in the search engine's category you would be listed under. Paying the fee may be worth it, if the search engine covers 15% or more of the search engine traffic and the competition to your business is not overwhelming.

Looksmart currently charges a $49 annual listing fee and requires a minimum investment of $15 a month ($180/year) to pay for 100 impressions. If you receive more than 100 impressions a month, you pay more. Looksmart's search engine gives you access to your account at any time. This allows you to view how quickly your initial investment of 100 impressions is being used and assists in making a decision as to whether you want to increase the number of impressions your site receives on a month-by-month basis. Look carefully at the search engine submission terms and conditions before submitting. Their submission process and fees can change without any notice. Looksmart doesn't attract a large percentage of search engine traffic on its own. You may not have heard of it before. However, it provides directory content for some other big contenders in the search engine field. Looksmart provides directory content for iWon, MSN, Excite, Juno and over 370 ISPs. MSN has around 12% and Excite has 2%. The total is over 15% of search engine traffic. To help split up the initial investment in submission fees, small business sites will submit to Yahoo and then 4 to 6 months later submit to Looksmart. Yahoo submission is done first because it attracts a larger share of the search engine traffic market than Looksmart. (10)

PROMOTION METHODS- MORE TIME BUT LOW COST

E-mail Signature File

A signature file is an Internet business card tacked onto the end of your e-mail messages. It tells people you communicate with on the Internet: who you are, what you do, and how to contact you. There are four basic parts to a signature file: name, contact information, website address (URL), and teaser line.

Name
Give your full professional name with credentials and the name of your company or employer.

Contact Information

This includes e-mail address, telephone number, fax number, and address. Not all this contact information is necessary, but at least one form of contact should be included.

With e-mail addresses, be sure to put "mail to:" before the actual e-mail address. This tells the e-mail software program to pop-up an empty e-mail box with your e-mail address in the "to" box. Example: Lynda@crazy4RDs.com; in a signature file it is:
e-mail: mail to:Lynda@crazy4RDs.com.

Website Address (URL)

Include your (URL) Website/ Webpage address in your signature file, if you have one. Be sure to put "http://" before the Web address. This ensures that the web address is an active link, viewers can click on it and go to your site immediately. Example:
www.hunger.com; in signature file it is: http://www.hunger.com.

Teaser Line

A teaser line provides at least one or two strong reasons to draw people to visit your Website or contact you when they read your signature file. It should convey the benefits of your services, products or content.

A teaser line gives more information on your products or services than saying simply "Nutrition Consultant", "Book Author", "Educator", or "Nutrition Manager." Examples:

- "The roots of education are bitter, but the fruit is sweet." Aristotle
- See our Special Valentine's Day offer, get 20% off all weight loss nutrition videos this week only
- Food trends and news in supermarket products
- Get Free tips for controlling your blood pressure
- Find out how to bring Full Flavor back into your life
- Managing quality nutritional care and people

Teaser lines often are quotes, specials, phrases, enticements with the word "Free," or a condensed mission statement.

Overall, signature files should be no more than 50 words and 5 lines. The idea is to catch the attention of a viewer and entice them to contact you or keep you in mind for future reference.

Most e-mail software programs have an option for creating signature files. Consult the help menu of your e-mail program. This way, every time you send e-mail it will automatically attach your e-mail signature. Two example e-mail signature files are:

Krista Foley, RD, LD
Nutrition Visions   http://www.nutritionvisions.com
"Learn to manage your weight for a lifetime."
e-mail: mail to: Krista@nutritionvisions.com

Tanner Bonneman, MS, RD
Scott County Hospital Nutrition Services
"Food to nourish the soul."
http://www.sch.org
e-mail: mail to: Tanner@sch.org

Use your signature file every time you send out an e-mail message. It's the simplest method to increase visibility and to bring visitors to your site.

Writing for a By-line

An old-fashioned promotion method is to write content for another website-for a fee or simply for the exposure--and always ask to include your by-line with a few words about yourself and a link to your website. Websites are frequently in need of new, fresh content. Find sites where your target market spends time. You should be well-read and up-to-date on the topic. Choose topics your target market may be interested in reading.

First, pitch the article idea to the webmaster or owner of the website. Wait for "the go ahead" to pick up your pen and get the creative juices flowing. The website may turn down your offer, revise the idea, or accept it as presented. Make sure there is an agreement to include your by-line and link with the article.

Discussion Groups

A very effective way to promote a site is by posting comments to online discussion groups. This encompasses giving away information and advice, while including an e-mail signature in the posting. By becoming respected in the discussion group as an expert on a topic, people will come to trust and respect you. When they have a question or need in your area of expertise, they will consult with you. Be forewarned, this promotion method can eat up a lot of time, but it is very effective when done properly for the "right" reasons, like establishing your career as a speaker or author, when running for office (letting others know of your expertise) or for your enjoyment. (11) There are two types of discussion groups: newsgroups and e-mail based groups.

Newsgroups

Newsgroups function like electronic worldwide bulletin boards. In a newsgroup you can post, view messages or reply to someone else's comment. The system on which the newsgroups are posted is called Usenet. Usenet is not part of the World Wide Web.

There are thousands of newsgroups, and the trick is finding a newsgroup where your target market is likely to be in large numbers. Also, which newsgroups and how many someone has access to depends on the person's Internet provider. There also are public access sites that offer a public news server, a service that allows you to read newsgroups your service provider does not subscribe to.

To locate a newsgroup by topic start at: Google http://groups.google.com/ For more sites with newsgroup listings use the keywords: < usenet +"Internet newsgroup"+ "public access">, and <usenet +Internet +"keyword for topic" >. (I would try one keyword first, do another keyword if your results are poor with the first one.)

E-mail Based Groups

When referring to discussion groups, an e-mail based group is a "listserv." Listservs are two-way e-mail based groups. E-mails sent to the mailing list are then forwarded to everyone who subscribes to the group. Only members can post to the group. Members can respond to the individual who sent the posting or respond to the entire group by e-mailing their response to the full mailing list.

Start looking for a discussion group in a topic where you have expertise: Publicly Accessible Mailing Lists http://www.paml.net.
Just like newsgroups, the trick is finding a discussion group where your target market is likely to be in large numbers.

Before posting your own message to the group, get a feel for what is acceptable and always read several group postings. Also, when you join the group, there should be a welcome letter or FAQs (Frequently Asked Questions) document with information on what material is and is not acceptable to post. The ultimate goal is to be known as an expert in a specialty area that falls under the discussion groups' overall topic. Subscribers to the discussion group will come to respect you as a credible expert in that area and call upon your expertise or visit your website when they have a need in that area.

Avoid subscribing to too many lists. A single list may generate 20-50 messages a day. It becomes time-consuming wading through numerous postings. Subscribe to a group for at least two weeks and then decide if the list meets your needs and move on to another if it does not. Try to check your e-mail daily, so your backlog does not become unmanageable. Also, consider adding another e-mail address just to receive communication of this sort.

E-mail a Webpage to a Friend

This is a very inexpensive way to bring targeted traffic to your site-through friends of friends. All that is needed is a program function that forwards e-mail copies of your most interesting web content pages. The program or service allows visitors of those pages to e-mail the page or article to a friend. Typically, there is a form that visitors complete which asks for their e-mail address and their friend's e-mail. The listed friend then receives an e-mail with a link back to the webpage.

E-mailing a webpage to a friend boosts the credibility of your website. Friends are more likely to visit a site recommended to them than a site listed in an e-mail newsletter. Companies that offer this service are:

Recommend It   http://www.recommend-it.com/
Suggest This   http://www.suggestthis.com/
A web programmer can develop a simple program to do this same thing on your site.

If you will be collecting e-mails submitted in the form, be sure to obtain consent and inform visitors of how the data will be used (a confidentiality and privacy statement).

Press Release

A press release can be a very cost effective promotion method especially if you are offering something unique at your website. Press releases are frequently used to announce new websites. However, the only way a media outlet is going to be interested in your story is if you stand out from other websites. You need to find a "hook" when developing your idea for a press release. A press release should focus on benefit to the user.

The maximum length of a press release is two double-spaced, single-sided pages. It is critical that you create a newsworthy press release. Thousands of press releases are generated every day and sent to the various media. Give your reader a reason to set it aside for further research and not throw into the round filing cabinet next to his or her desk. Resources on writing an effective press release are:

PRW	http://www.press-release-writing.com/
eReleases	http://www.ereleases.com/

For more sites with press release writing tips use the keywords: < "press release" + "tips">

There are free and pay services for distributing a press release. It may be effective to pay for help in distribution. Here are some distribution services that are both pay and free.

WebWire	http://www.webwire.com/
URL Wire	http://www.urlwire.com/
Internet Media Fax	http://www.imediafax.com/
Eworldwire	http://www.eworldwire.com/
Xpress Press	http://www.xpresspress.com/
News Bureau	http://www.newsbureau.com/
PRWeb	http://www.prweb.com/

For more sites that distribute press releases use the keywords: < "press release" +services>. So you will understand it more clearly, don't waste your time with this type of marketing unless you have a very unique idea, product or service.

Links   73

Links are typically webpages with a list of links. The links are 10 to 20 websites with similar or complementary services, products or information to your website. Often a reciprocal agreement is established with the linked websites (you post a link to their website and in exchange for a link to your website). This arrangement is only appropriate if the other website has something beneficial to offer your visitors.

Also, only link to credible, well-maintained websites. It does not help your credibility in the eyes of your visitors if you lead them to an unprofessional site. Also, it is not recommended that you list your direct competitors. For example: if you wrote a book to sell on your website, link to sites with tips on publishing and writing. It would not be in your best interest to include links to sites selling similar books.

If you have recipes on your site, link to sites that sell reputable kitchen gadgets and sites with cooking terminology. Link pages are called: "Resources," "Links," "Library," and "For more information."

Some of your best visitors will come from linked websites. Linking your website to high quality websites is equivalent to having "word of mouth referrals" offline. When customers come by referral, there is already a level of trust established, even before they get to your site.(12)

A good method for finding websites that are complementary is to enter your keywords and keyword phrases at several different search engines. Browse the first 30 or so websites. Find some that offer a benefit to your visitors, and are not competitors. E-mail their webmaster with the following information:

- Name of their website, and what you really liked about their website,
- Name and domain of your website,
- Ask to establish a link between the pages,
- How your website will benefit their visitors,
- Contact information, and
- (If they are interested) HTML coding they need to paste a link to your website (Typically you do want to send the HTML coding with your initial e-mail so that if they are going ahead and adding you in as a link, they have what they need to do it and another communication is not needed to send them the HTML.)

Backlink Checking

You also can find possible link pages by backlink checking. This is finding web pages that have links to a specific webpage or website. You can do a backlink check for sites that are linked to a website that came up in the top 30 results for sites that offer complementary content or services. Currently the search engines Google.com and AltaVista.com can perform backlink checking. This is a quick way to find several sites on a topic. If you know <www.foodtolive.com> is a great site that you would like to request a link to your site on, do a backlink search on the URL. It may lead to other good websites to also ask to link to your website.

For AltaVista (www.AltaVista.com) type in URL <foodtolive.com> and in this search engine do not include http://www before URL. For Google (www.Google.com) the format to backlink check is <link:food-

tolive.com>. This is the largest of the search engines that performs backlink checking.

Backlink checking is also an excellent way to keep track of the number of sites linked to your site. Many search engines give a site more weight if they have a large number of sites linked to them. The thinking is the more links a site has the more popular it is, thus the better a website it is. That isn't always the case of course.

Reciprocal Marketing

Reciprocal marketing is the 21st century form of bartering. It's an agreement with another business to link with one another at no cost to either party. The link is placed at the end of the buying process of one site in order to give site visitors incentive to buy from a partner site. It may sound like, but isn't the same as a reciprocal link page. Read on.

Some of the big players doing reciprocal marketing are Barnes&Noble.com with Proflowers.com.(13) Barnes&Noble.com has reciprocal marketing deals with Expedia.com, JCrew.com, LLBean.com, 1-800-Flowers.com, and VitaminShoppe.com. Agreements are setup where Barnes&Noble.com offers a link to each partner site on the post transaction page that appears each time a visitor buys an item from its site. Many of the links offer a discount for visitors who click to their site. A typical discount is a $10 discount coupon or a two-for-one coupon. Additionally, each of the companies involved in an agreement with Barnes&Noble.com offers a similar link to Barnes&Noble.com's site, which also offers a discount if a customer clicks through to their site.

The agreement allows each of the companies partnering with Barnes&Noble.com to put its message in front of a large portion of the bookseller's entire customer base. They are given the opportunity to acquire a whole new base of customers while reducing the cost of acquiring customers overall. Additional benefits are:

- no money is exchanged,
- no third party advertising entity is involved,
- visitor privacy is protected since no customer data is exchanged, and
- customers are ready to buy since they have their credit card in hand.

"Reciprocal marketing programs are a win-win for customers and any participating merchants," says Shel Horowitz, a low-cost marketing consultant and author of *Grassroots Marketing: Getting Noticed in a Noisy World* (13), "You add more value to the customer's purchase, and at the same time, allow the partners in the deal to tap into each other's customer bases."

Web Rings

Web Rings are groups of similar web sites that have banded together to form their sites into linked circles. Their purpose is to allow more visitors to reach them quickly and easily. (12)

Through navigation links found most often at the bottom of Web Ring member pages, people can visit all or any of the sites in a Ring. They can move through a Ring in either direction, go to the next or previous site, jump to a random site in the Ring, or survey all the sites that make up the Ring. In theory all the sites are strung together in a big "circle," so by clicking on the next link over and over, you should be able to travel all the way around and come back to your starting point. Sites participating in a ring use special HTML code that creates the Web Ring navigation links. The largest organization with resources and directories to Web Rings is WebRing at http://www.webring.org/.

There are Web Rings on all different topics. The disadvantage is if your site does not stand out from the other Ring websites and you risk visitors moving immediately to the next site in the Web Ring. Very narrow and unique topics tend to work best with Web Rings.

Other names for Web Ring are loopring and railway. To find Web Rings on a specific topic use the keywords: <"Web Ring"+"keyword for topic">.

PROMOTION METHODS-LOWER COST

Most small businesses do not have large promotion budgets. The following promotion methods require a little investment. However, in the long term, they can pay for themselves by attracting target market visitors to your site.

Before getting deep into low-cost promotion methods, you need to become familiar with the term "cpm." CPM is cost per thousand.(14) The "M" stands for 1,000. Advertising prices generally are stated in terms of cmp, or cost per thousand impressions.

For banners, "impressions" refers to the number of times the banner's webpage is loaded. One thousand impressions does not mean the ad was seen 1,000 times---only the banner. A visitor may choose not to look at the ad even though it is loaded at the top or bottom of the webpage they are reading.

In e-mail advertising, impressions are the number of e-mail messages sent out that contained the ad. Just like for banners, an e-mail impression does not mean the ad was seen. Recipients may delete the message without opening it. E-mail newsletters are often forwarded to colleagues to read which increases the number of people who read the ad.

New Terms:

Click through or clickthru---is when a visitor clicks on a banner ad or clicks on a link in an e-mail ad. (14) This is more accurate but does not always translate into the number of people who saw the banner or e-mail ad because a visitor may cancel before the page completely loads.

Click-through rate--percentage of people viewing your ad that click through. (14)

Banners

Banner ads work for a small group of websites and companies. Much of the hype about banners paints a better picture than usually happens in reality. Banners are best for building awareness but not actually bringing targeted visitors to a site. Awareness building works better for large companies with the larger budgets. It's difficult to justify a banner add for a lower cost item-profits don't easily cover the cost of the banner.

The best places to consider banner advertising are on sites where your target market definitely spends time. Find a page on a site that is complementary to your website. You also might combine two promotional methods together. For example: buy an advertisement in another website's e-mail newsletter to its customers, and while that ad runs, post a banner ad on their website. The hope is that readers of the e-mail newsletter will read your advertisement in the newsletter and see your banner ad on the website, which takes them to your site.

If you want to give banner ads a try, be sure to first calculate what click through rate you will need in order to breakeven on the sale of your product or services. Prices for banner ads vary all over the map starting from a cpm of around $5 to $60 and up. (15) Additionally, not everyone who clicks through to your site is going to buy. Resources to help you get started are:

24/7	http://www.247media.com/
Ad-Up	http://www.ad-up.com/
DoubleClick	http://www.doubleclick.net/
ValueClick	http://www.valueclick.com/

To find more resources on banner promotion services use keywords: <banner +Internet +promotion>. Resources to design an effective banner are:

BannerTips	http://www.bannertips.com
Voytech	http://www.voytech.com
Adbility	http://www.adbility.com

To find more resources on banner design use keywords: <banner +Internet +tips>.

E-mail

E-mail newsletters are an overlooked form of promotion. It also can be the most cost-effective. There are thousands of e-mail newsletters, some operated by websites and others by companies. Many allow advertisers to have a text advertisement for a small fee.

E-mail newsletters vary quite a bit in their content. Some are brief with the purpose of announcing new products, others are content rich and lengthy. Typically, you want to focus on those that are content rich. Lists of e-mail newsletters are at:

Publicly Accessible Mailing Lists   http://www.paml.net
To find e-mail newsletters on a specific topic use the keywords: <"e-mail newsletter" + "keyword for topic">.

Search by keywords to locate newsletters that offer topics your target market is interested in and will likely subscribe to. For example, if you have a website that offers customized menu and recipe writing for the well-to-do, consider advertising in e-mail newsletters on vacations at well-known health spas in the summer and exclusive ski resorts in the winter.

Before handing over some money to advertise in an e-mail newsletter, read at least two past issues. First, check the number of advertisements the newsletter allows. Too many ads turn readers off. Readers program themselves to skip over the long list of ads. The placement of the ads is important too. If the ads are all placed in the same location, readers will also learn to skip them. The ideal is for only a handful of advertisements to be accepted and the ads to be placed randomly throughout the newsletter. (15) Avoid having your advertisement placed at the very beginning or end of the newsletter---these are the least read placements. Research indicates near the middle is better. (15)

Sponsorships

Sponsorships are increasing in popularity on the Internet. A sponsorship is when an advertiser pays to sponsor content, usually a section of Website or an e-mail newsletter. In the case of a site, the sponsorship may include banners or buttons on the site, and possibly a tag line. (16)

The disadvantage is the same as with banner ads: a large initial investment before a financial return. However, sponsorships in recent years have gained popularity over banner ads. Part of the draw is the flexibility of sponsorships. A company can sponsor content with a low-end involvement like a simple tag line: "This section is brought to you by MediNutrition Inc." Or, there could be a more involved sponsorship commitment with banner ads, content in an entire section, an e-mail newsletter tag line, or even a mini-website within the website.

Arrangements vary widely, depending on several factors (17):

- whether sponsorship is exclusive or joint,
- how much of the site is included,
- how involved the sponsor gets, and
- what the sponsor plans to accomplish.

Sponsorships appear at this early date to be effective for building brand awareness in a particular niche market. (16) The secret is to go where your customers are already spending time, and sponsor content they read. Sponsorship pricing varies depending on the popularity of the site, structure of the arrangement, and the sponsor's level of involvement. Often there is a monthly fee with an extra charge when e-mail newsletters are distributed. Unfortunately, there are no resources presently on locating or arranging sponsorships. The best method is to approach sites where you believe your target market is spending time.

Resources

General Web Development
Poor Richard's Web News — http://PoorRichard.com
Webmonkey, — http://hotwired.lycos.com/webmonkey/
Web Developer's Journal — http://WebDevelopersJournal.com

Domain Names
InterNIC web site — http://rs.internic.net
Registration Authority: — http://www.register.com/

Trademarks
Basic Facts About Registering a Trademark, US Patent and Trademark Office, http://www.uspto.gov/web/offices/tafc/doc/basic/

Copyrights
U.S. Copyright Office Web Site — www.lcweb.loc.gov/copyright
The Copyright Website — www.benedict.com

Security Issues
Center for Info Technology, — www.alw.nih.gov/Security/security.htm
WWWeb Security FAQ, — www.w3.org/Security/Faq/www-security-faq.html

Internet Newsletters and Journals
InfoWorld, InfoWorld Media Group Inc., 155 Bovet Rd., Ste. 800, San Mateo, CA 94402.
Inside the Internet, ZD Journals, 500 Canal View Boulevard, Rochester, NY, 14623.
Inside Web Design, ZD Journals, 500 Canal View Boulevard, Rochester, NY, 14623.

Bibliography
McClelland, Deke & Eismann, Katrin: Web Design, Studio Secrets, IDG Books Worldwide, Inc., Foster City, CA, 1998.

References

1. Pew Internet & American Life: US Internet users seek info via search engines, Nua Internet Surveys Website; available online at: http://www.nua.ie/surveys/index.cgi?f=VS&art_id=905358133&rel=true. Accessed on July 10, 2002.
2. Marckini F. Choosing the Right Keywords in the Right Combinations. In: Search Engine Positioning. Plano, TX: Wordware Publishing, Inc.; 2001.
3. Marckini F. META Tabs, Metadata, and Where to Place Keywords. In: Search Engine Positioning. Plano, TX: Wordware Publishing, Inc.; 2001.
4. Bowman JB. Meta Tag Optimization Tutorial. On: Spider-Food.net Website; available online at: http://spider-food.net/meta-tags.html. Accessed on July 10, 2002.
5. Sullivan D. How to Use HTML Meta Tags. On: SearchEngineWatch.com Website; available online at: http://www.searchenginewatch.com/webmasters/meta.html. Accessed July 10, 2002.
6. Kent P, Calishain T. Web Site Checkup: Preparing for Indexing. In: Poor Richard's Internet Marketing and Promotions: How to Promote Yourself, Your Business, Your Ideas Online, Lakewood, CO: Top Floor Publishing; 1999.
7. Marckini F. Submitting Your Site. In: Search Engine Positioning, Plano, TX: Wordware Publishing, Inc.; 2001.
8. Sullivan D. Nielsen/NetRatings Search Engine Ratings. On: SearchEngineWatch.com Website; available online at: http://www.searchenginewatch.com/reports/netratings.html. Accessed July 10, 2002.
9. Sullivan D. Jupiter Media Metrix: Search Engine Ratings. On: April 29, 2002, SearchEngineWatch.com Website; available online at: http://www.searchenginewatch.com/reports/mediametrix.html. Accessed July 10, 2002.
10. Wordtracker Search Engine Traffic Database Results; Wordtracker.com Website, June 2002.
11. Kent P. Calishain T. Promoting in the Newsgroups and Mailing Lists. In: Poor Richard's Internet Marketing and Promotions: How to Promote Yourself, Your Business, Your Ideas Online. Lakewood, CO: Top Floor Publishing; 1999.
12. Kent P, Calishain T. Other Placed to Register Your Site. In: Poor Richard's Internet Marketing and Promotions: How to Promote Yourself, Your Business, Your Ideas Online. Lakewood, CO: Top Floor Publishing; 1999.
13. Campanelli M. Give and Take: Why It Pays to Partner Up on Your Marketing Efforts. Entrepreneur Magazine; March 2001.
14. Marckini F. Buying Advertising on Search Engines. In: Search Engine Positioning. Plano, TX: Wordware Publishing, Inc.; 2001.
15. Kent P, Calishain T. Advertising Your Site. In: Poor Richard's Internet Marketing and Promotions: How to Promote Yourself, Your Business, Your Ideas Online. Lakewood, CO: Top Floor Publishing; 1999
16. Wegert T. Sponsorships: The Pathway to Clicks. ClickZ Website, March 28, 2002; available online at: http://www.clickz.com/article.php/998091. Accessed July 10, 2002.
17. Internet Business Forum: Interview: Richard Keis (Part 1 - 4), ibiz Interviews Website, July 2000; available online at: http://www.ibizinterviews.com/richard1.htm. Accessed July 10, 2002.

Look for these computer chapters (with examples of websites) as online CPE Mini-course after February 2003 at   <www.helmpublishing.com>

Appendix 23 A   Web Promotions Worksheet

Search Engine Optimization

1. Brainstorm 25 - 50 keywords that describe your business/website.

2. Narrow keywords to best 10 - 15 keywords and keyword phrases>

3. Refine keywords to 10 narrowly focused keyword phrases.

4. Description Meta Tag: Describe site in 1 to 3 sentences (150 characters or less) using at least 2 keyword phrases.

5. Keyword Meta Tag: List top 10 critical keyword phrases, do not put same words next to each other or repeat a word more than 4 times in the entire list.

6. Site Title: Use for site submission to search engines (60 characters or less) Try writing in several and count 40 and 60 characters, including spaces.

SEARCH ENGINE SUBMISSION
Date(s) submitted/resubmitted to search engines:

Date(s) checked site in search engines:
PROMOTION METHODS (Choose ones to pursue, give date began, and any details):

___Signature File

___Writing for by-line

___Discussion groups

___E-mail a webpage to friend

___Press Release

___Links

___Reciprocal Marketing

___Web Rings

___Banners

___E-mail ads

___Sponsorships

Additional Ideas:

—— Developing Your —— Professional Practice

Words of Wisdom:

"If you don't invest very much, then defeat doesn't hurt very much and winning is not very exciting."
Dick Vermeil

"Never, Never, Never Quit."
Winston Churchill

Chapter 24

Jobs With Physicians and Other Accounts

Becky McCully Varner, M.S., R.D.

Presenting a professional image is imperative if an entrepreneur is to work successfully with other professionals. This includes a positive attitude, the ability to communicate without distracting gestures or habits, a neat and updated appearance and dress, consideration, cooperation, and tact. Showing respect for another professional's expertise and expecting others to respect yours is important.

MAKING CONTACTS

Making contacts to find work or to network with professionals can be accomplished in many ways. Remember to keep visible and audible. Be seen in public frequently. Be careful not to limit opportunities. Be broad-minded in thinking, and explore all possibilities as future contacts. Develop a filing system or use your computer to record all contacts. Include names of individuals, what was discussed, the reaction of the person contacted, telephone number, address, date, and a recommended follow-up procedure. Add personal information about the individual, such as children, or an upcoming trip, or a remark, to trigger your memory the next time you contact the person. This helps the person feel you are taking a personal interest in them.

When making personal contact, always have business cards available. Anything else with your name and phone number, such as handouts, fliers, brochures, and so on, would be helpful to leave. Remember to keep visible!

Who Should Be Contacted?

The number and type of contacts you choose to make are essentially unlimited. Below is a list of potential organizations and people to approach, but the list should be individualized according to your interests.

- Professional health organizations, such as American Heart Association, American Diabetes Association, American Lung Association, Arthritis Foundation, etc.
- County and State Medical Associations
- Education centers (vocational-tech schools, community colleges, nursing schools, etc.)
- Clinics and hospitals
- Women's and men's groups (business and professional organizations, etc.)
- Fitness centers and spas
- Sports facilities and teams
- Individual physicians
- Newspapers, television stations and magazine editors
- Church groups
- Civic organizations (Lions Club, American Legion, VFW, and so on)

How to Make Contacts

There are three ways to make an initial contact--an introductory letter, a telephone call, or a personal conversation--and each can be appropriate for different situations.

Introductory letters. Although a letter is not as personal as a conversation, it is an effective way to introduce yourself and what you have to offer. It allows you time to preplan and edit the message. The letter should vary according to the particular needs of the person being addressed. Keep the letter simple, clear and concise. Additional information about you, such as a resume, brochure or letter of reference, could be included. Brochures are also available from the Nutrition Entrepreneurs Dietetic Practice Group of the American Dietetic Association, which explain the services provided by a nutritionist.

Telephone contacts. Whether networking or marketing your business, decide what needs to be said and outline the points to be emphasized before making the call. It may not be possible to talk directly to the individual in charge. Be concise and yet give enough information so the person will want to schedule an appointment for you. Be flexible in offering times to meet. Offer to go to the physician's or owner's office, or suggest a luncheon meeting at your expense. If the individual is interested, an appointment time will be arranged. If not, neither of you has invested much time. Be conscious of voice tone on the telephone. Voice sound and the spoken message are the only tools for making a first impression. Speak clearly and slowly.

Personal interviews or conversations. Whenever possible, personal contact is a "must" to build a business. People refer jobs and patients to other people they feel they know and respect. You are seen, heard and have the opportunity to leave printed material. Plan and organize the entire presentation. Dress appropriately. When contacting a physician or business owner, a business suit would be appropriate. Even if the meeting is with an individual at a sports or fitness center, your dress should still present a professional image. Dress to feel comfortable for the specific interview.

Body language speaks loudly. Practice role playing and, if possible, have a friend film it. This allows you to observe your mannerisms, gestures and body movements. Constant movement, such as swinging a foot, shifting weight, wringing hands, and so on, are distracting and will take away from the presentation.

It's a good idea to take impressive marketing materials that can be left behind for the person to review. For example, if contacting a physician, include:

- a business card,
- diet prescription blanks,
- a sample of a patient's progress report that would be mailed to a referring physician,
- a newsletter or published article you have written, and
- types of services you can provide.

If the physician specializes, it would be helpful to include articles on nutrition intervention related to the specialization.

When approaching an owner of a fitness center or clinic director about providing group services, present a brief overview of the particular program. For example, if you are offering a weight reduction class:

- show in a 3-ring binder presentation, but do not leave,
- a schedule of class topics,
- a brief summary of information to be presented in each class, and
- sample handouts.

OPTIONS FOR WORKING WITH PHYSICIANS

There are many options for working with one or a group of physicians. A creative arrangement with a physician allows you to get a taste of what private practice is all about, without the risk of opening a free standing practice initially.

Besides individual consultation on diets for medical nutrition therapy, normal and sports nutrition diets, suggested programs could include weight control groups, diabetes education programs, seminars on specific diseases, such as cardiovascular disease and hypertension, wellness and prevention programs, cooking classes for various types of diets such as low calorie, low sodium, and diabetic.

Development of handouts, information sheets, newsletters, and articles is also a part of a well-designed nutrition program. Although these may or may not directly produce income, they are effective educational and advertising tools. Such creative tools are enriching to a program. Be sure to include your name, address and telephone number on all printed materials. They will become very inexpensive advertising.

My attorney strongly suggests that in cases where long-term association with a physician or clinic is envisioned, the nutritionist consult an attorney for preparation of a formal contract. The investment in a more detailed contract may pay for itself many times over if there is a problem.

An Employed Position

If the physician strongly desires your services in his practice, it's possible he or she will take more financial risk than if there are questions regarding the importance of nutritional services. The physician may work out an arrangement to hire you as an employee. Although this is different from opening a practice, it can be advantageous. There is little risk to the nutritionist, and it gives the opportunity to try consulting with patients and develop programs for patients before opening a practice.

If the physician hires you as an employee, benefits such as health insurance, malpractice insurance, paid vacation, use of office space, equipment, office supplies, and receptionist are usually included, as well. The patients are financially responsible to the physician and the physician pays the nutritionist a salary while billing patients' insurance companies. Although this type of working relationship may be beneficial in gaining experience, it has limitations.

You are dependent upon the physician to refer enough patients to use you efficiently without large open blocks of time. (Other physicians are not apt to refer their patients to a nutritionist who is employed by a physician.) With this arrangement, the nutritionist may be expected to see patients when they come to see the physician and, consequently, will not have much control over the daily schedule. The physician may or may not have specific nutrition guidelines he or she wants the nutritionist to use. The nutritionist may have to compromise personal philosophies to work for the physician.

Independent Contracting with a Physician

It's common for practitioners to work as independent contractors in a physician's office. This arrangement gives much greater flexibility of time and scheduling and more opportunity to control your business. It also will involve more financial risk and investment of personal capital.

Practitioners contract with physicians in a variety of ways:

- A contract may be for a predetermined number of hours per week, or it may vary with the patient load.
- Another option is to have a percentage of the nutritionist's fee paid for the use of the office space.
- Finally, the nutritionist may pay the physician a flat rental fee for the use of the office facilities. The physician refers patients to the nutritionist, but incurs no financial responsibility if the patient does not show.

Working with a Group of Physicians

It is also possible to work as an employee or independent contractor with a group of physicians in a medical complex. This option offers more variety and sometimes more professional challenge as one works with the different philosophies of physicians. Be sure the physicians specialize in areas of medicine compatible with your interests. Generally speaking, family physicians, cardiologists, internists, endocrinologists, renal, diabetes specialists, obstetricians, and allergists use the services of a nutritionist more often than specialists such as surgeons, urologists and dermatologists. Sports orthopedic specialists, Functional Medicine practitioners and chiropractors are growing markets also.

WORKING WITH REGISTERED NURSES

Numerous types of programs benefit from the combined efforts of various health professionals. Consider combining the consultation services of a registered dietitian with a registered nurse. One example would be a diabetes education program. The expertise of each specialist can mesh beautifully to form a well-rounded program.

A diabetes program could be designed in a variety of ways, including a two or three hour class, a weekend seminar, a series of classes meeting daily for a week, or a weekly class meeting for a specified number of weeks. This program could be presented in a clinic, hospital, community center, or on a college campus. The nurse could cover information about the disease itself, mechanisms of oral hypoglycemic agents and insulin, insulin injections, and complications of diabetes. The dietitian could present the principles of the diabetic diet, recipe conversion, eating out, traveling, and shopping. A cooking demonstration and grocery store tour would be helpful.

Another program could be a hypertension control program. This could be offered through a clinic or hospital, or to individual patients. Suggested topics for the nurse include the disease process of hypertension, medications and how they work, complications of uncontrolled hypertension, and how to take blood pressure readings. The nutritionist could present various aspects of nutrition intervention, including sodium restriction and calorie control. Videos, actual foods, pamphlets, and dietary flash cards are good tools for teaching specific principles. Discussions on seasoning foods without the addition of salt, cutting calories and eating in restaurants are all applicable.

In prenatal/postnatal programs, the nurse could present information on pregnancy, delivery and caring for an infant. The nutritionist could discuss nutritional needs during pregnancy and lactation, as well as infant nutrition. An exercise specialist could plan individualized exercise programs for each woman.

OTHER GROUPS

There are numerous opportunities to develop nutrition programs with well people. Examples include directors of fitness centers, schools, libraries, and recreation centers. Managers and chefs who work for grocery stores and restaurants are also potential clients.

Working With Fitness

YWCA/YMCAs, fitness centers, school athletic departments, corporate fitness, and senior community groups contract with nutritionists. Programs for weight control, sports, eating disorders, and wellness are all possibilities. Contact the person responsible for coordinating all programs to determine the primary age groups and the various needs of people who use the facility. Get feedback about the types of programs they feel are most appropriate.

Cooking School Directors

A director of a cooking school may be interested in offering a variety of health-oriented cooking classes. These classes could include cooking for a healthy heart, low calorie cooking, diabetic or vegetarian cooking, healthy snacks, and so on.

When setting your fee, consider the mechanics of the class. Will you only be teaching and cooking, or will you be doing the grocery shopping, pre-preparation of the dishes, and clean up also? Will you help advertise the class, or will the cooking school absorb this cost? These factors must be considered before quoting a price for conducting the class.

If you are doing a series of classes, design a creative logo and a style of writing recipes. This helps to establish your identity. Again, be sure your name, address and telephone number are on each original recipe. Obtain permission to use copyrighted recipes and always add the permissions line, i.e. "Used by permission. Copyright 2003 Jane Parker."

Libraries and Book Stores

Frequently, libraries offer classes to patrons on various subjects. Consider doing book reviews for a book store or library on diet books, having discussion groups on various nutrition topics, conducting weight control classes, diabetic classes, and so on. These classes may not prove to be financially lucrative, but your name will be exposed to the public, and this may be a good referral source. Remember to keep visible!

Grocery Stores

Many grocery stores now make nutrition information and some-times foods classes available to customers. This may be in the form of grocery store tours, healthy cooking classes, a series of nutrition book-lets, healthy recipes using ingredients sold at the store, or creative advertising of new products for special diets.

As a corporate dietitian, you could coordinate consumer education, store food campaigns, answer online questions from customers, work with the media, and so on.

Other Dietitians and Dietetic Technicians

Involvement is important with the local and state dietetic associations and Dietetic Practice Groups like Nutrition Entrepreneurs, Sports and Cardiovascular, Nutrition in Complementary Care, and Dietitians in Business and Communication, or Dietetic Technician DPG. Group members provide support and involvement keeps you visible, as well as up-to-date with what other practitioners are doing.

Corporate Wellness

Many employers are interested in providing employees with fun, health-oriented programs as mentioned above, as well as individual medical nutrition therapy, to improve job performance and cut health care costs (see Chapter 30 for more information on this topic). Consider a wide variety of companies, especially those in prosperous industries that are self-insured and those with progressive employee programs.

Chapter 25

Consulting in Long-term Care

Becky Dorner, R.D.
Owner, Becky Dorner and Associates

By the year 2030, the population over 65 years old in the U.S. will double to an estimated 70 million (from today's current 35 million). The population over 85 years old will also double, to almost 9 million.(1) For the first time in our nation's history, one in five Americans will be in the over 65 years category. The Institute of Medicine report, Informing the Future: Critical Issues in Health, indicates that more than 85 percent of this population "has hypertension, diabetes, or blood lipid disorders due to chronic disease."(1)

Statistics like these indicate there are opportunities available for those who enjoy working with older adults in nursing facilities, assisted living facilities, retirement centers, residential care centers, home care, and congregate feeding, or Meals on Wheels. This chapter will discuss the entrepreneurial opportunities to work as a consultant dietitian (RD) to those agencies or facilities that provide care and services to the older adult population, and to other population groups.

Regulatory Environment

The nursing home industry is one of the most highly regulated industries in the U.S. In its quest to protect the public and Medicare/Medicaid funding, the government has developed very precise regulations governing these licensed facilities. Because those regulations require a qualified dietitian to perform certain duties, and because so many nursing home residents are malnourished (studies estimate 35-85 percent [2]), opportunities have been created for dietitians in the long-term care industry.

Many smaller facilities have 100 beds or less, and do not require a full time dietitian. They prefer to use a consultant, as it is more cost effective than hiring a full time person. Most of these facilities employ a certified dietary manager (CDM) to run their food service departments, allowing for a dietitian to oversee the clinical duties of the facility. The RD may also assist in guiding the CDM to provide high quality food service to assure safe food, provision of special diets, and meeting the many diverse needs of today's nursing facility population.

CONSULTING IN LONG-TERM CARE

If you are looking for diversity and challenge in your career, long-term care may be a great choice for you. The skilled nursing facilities of today provide highly skilled care to residents who would have been in hospitals 10-15 years ago. Higher acuity levels translate into the need for more nutritional intervention due to complications such as weight loss, dehydration, pressure ulcers, and malnutrition.

Clinical challenges to the RD include:
- therapeutic diets for chronic disease states, dialysis, ventilator patients;
- enteral and parenteral feedings;
- providing nutrient dense foods and fluids for those who cannot consume enough food to maintain nutritional status;
- providing appropriate consistencies of foods and fluids for dysphagia patients (studies indicate the prevalence of dysphagia in nursing facility residents is as high as 53-74%); (3)
- caring for end-of-life nutrition and hydration needs.

The greatest challenge may be to assure a quality experience at mealtime. To provide safe, wholesome and high quality foods that meet the needs of each individual; promote a dining environment that is conducive to a pleasant and dignified social experience; promote independence with eating; provide feeding assistance for those who need it, and assure adequate intake to meet nutritional needs.

The demands of clinical documentation are great in nursing facilities, as regulations specify the need for assessment in the first 5 days, re-assessment at 14 days, 30 days and a minimum of every 90 days thereafter. Regulations are very specific as to parameters for nutrition care, weight loss, pressure ulcers, hydration, enteral feedings, and dining issues.

Dietitian consultants in long-term care are expected to have an excellent working knowledge of the following:
- federal and state regulations for nursing homes,
- the survey process,
- nutritional assessment and care planning,
- nutrition interventions for the older adult,
- food service and sanitation,
- cost control,
- therapeutic diets, and more.

334

Because the RD is acting as a consultant, the expectation is that his or her knowledge level is above the level of an employee. In addition, because most consultants work with multiple facilities, information sharing between facilities is important, but one must be careful not to share any confidential information.

Standards of Practice in Long-term Care

At this time, the climate in long-term care is extremely litigious. Facility professionals, including RDs, are being named in lawsuits related to malnutrition, weight loss and pressure ulcers. Because of all the intense regulations in long-term care, and because of the current litigious environment, it is imperative for RDs practicing in this area to be sure they are up-to-date on critical information. It is also important to carry malpractice insurance.

The Consultant Dietitians in Health Care Facilities (CD-HCF), a dietetic practice group of the American Dietetic Association, provides members a great deal of information and resources on the practice of dietetics in long-term care. It is a great resource for anyone new (or experienced) to the field. There are also state CD-HCF organizations, and even some local chapters. CD-HCF publishes "Standards of Practice for Consultant Dietitians in Health Care Facilities", a helpful guideline of the expectations of excellent practice in the long-term care setting. The standards of practice include six standards: (4)

1) Provision of Services: Provides quality service based on clients' expectations and needs;
2) Application of Research: Effectively applies, supports and participates in dietetics research to enhance practice;
3) Communication and Application of Knowledge: Applies food, human nutrition and management knowledge and communicates with others;
4) Utilization and Management of Resources: Uses resources effectively and efficiently in practice;
5) Quality in Practice: Systematically evaluates the quality of effectiveness of practice, and revises practice as needed to incorporate the results of evaluation;
6) Continued Competence and Professional Accountability: Engages in lifelong, self-development to improve knowledge and enhance professional competence.

Changes Affecting Long-term Care

There are major changes occurring in long-term health care. Facilities are experiencing staffing shortages. Changes in the survey process are promoting increased scrutiny in the areas of nutrition and hydration. Changes in reimbursement for Medicare and Medicaid encourage the consultant to concentrate on more cost effective health care interventions. Increased consumer pressure (from advocacy groups, residents and families) demands improvement in quality of care, customer service and hospitality. Unfortunately, a lack of improvement in these areas leads to increased occurrence of litigation cases. Changes in the use of technology in facilities eventually may result in better efficiencies and improved quality of care.

Employer's Expectations

As a result of the above changes, consultant dietitians need to have more knowledge and learn to keep up with the rapid pace of change. Even though clinical documentation consumes the majority of a consultant's time, just keeping up with documentation is not enough. Employers expect consultants to identify potential problems, bring viable solutions and implement systems that work. They want consultants to keep them informed about pertinent happenings in their buildings, and bring them new information from outside sources (on nutrition, recent surveys, regulation changes, etc.). Employers expect consultants to ask them what their needs are--what's important to them as customers--and then fulfill those needs. They want more than just a documenter. Employers want consultants to address quality issues, cost control issues and to give them new solutions for old problems

Employers want consultants who have entrepreneurial skills:
- to think for themselves,
- make good decisions,
- work independently,
- have good management skills, and
- take calculated risks.

Consultants must be able to sell themselves and the benefits of their services to the employer. Good communication skills (speaking/writing skills) are necessary to communicate messages clearly.

In addition, the consultant must be financially savvy and learn:
- how to read profit and loss statements,
- how to develop and follow a budget, and
- how to advise the facility on cost controls.

Consultants must know their worth--how their work saves money, decreases costs, decreases patients' health complications, increases customer satisfaction, quality of care and quality of life, and improves the image of the facility. A consultant also must have time management and organizational skills to be able to prioritize and get all of these things done in the limited amount of time available.

Other Opportunities in LTC

There are many other opportunities available for consulting work in the long-term care area. Assisted Living Facilities (ALF) have varying needs for RDs. Each state has different state regulations (there are currently no federal regulations for ALF). So it is best to check the regulations in your state. Generally speaking, most states will promote the use of pre-written menus, proper sanitation and food safety. Most ALFs do not want to be considered institutions and will fight the institutional mindset. Their focus is on hospitality service. Fine dining and restaurant style service is common. Some ALFs will want RDs to be involved with providing in-services to the kitchen staff on a regular basis to assure proper knowledge of food safety, sanitation, preparation, and special diets. Some will want to purchase menus or menu services, or have a RD do a sanitation inspection on a regular basis. And some will want the RD's involvement to assist with prevention or intervention for weight loss and other nutritional issues. Realize that the work is not as steady in this area, as most ALFs will only use an RD on a very limited basis (once per quarter or once per month).

Retirement villages and independent living facilities may use a consultant RD if they have a nursing facility or ALF associated with them. Otherwise, the involvement of a RD is usually limited, although some may hire RDs to provide preventative care services, such as presentations on proper diet or one-on-one counseling for residents.

Mentally retarded/developmentally disabled (MRDD) facilities also need the assistance of consultant RDs. These are usually smaller group home settings with 8-10 residents. They may be adults or adolescents. There are also larger facilities, but most of the care of MRDD residents is moving into the community setting with a goal of assimilating residents into society. RDs are needed for consultation on menus, special diets, food preparation, safety, and service.

Home health care is an area where RDs are needed but, unfortunately, there is not much funding available through Medicare/Medicaid to pay for RD services. This work is often sporadic, and difficult to schedule. The assigned home visits may come few and far between, and may necessitate a lot of driving time. Remember to negotiate a fee that will cover your visit plus preparation time, travel, reviewing charts, documentation, and a percentage of development time for educational materials.

Correctional institutions are also a growing area of dietetic practice. Correctional facilities need RDs to consult on menus, special diets, food preparation, and sanitation. This area is also highly regulated, so it is important to understand the state and federal regulations for correctional food service. The main difference for the consultant in this area is the issue of personal safety when visiting a facility.

STARTING A BUSINESS IN LTC CONSULTING ―――――

To get started in long-term care, a RD must have knowledge of the field. CD-HCF is a good resource of information on all of the above settings. To be a consultant, one must really have some experience working as an employee in LTC, have knowledge of the state and federal regulations and the survey process, have skills in clinical documentation and care of the older adult, and have a clear under- standing of food preparation (including food safety), and meal service.

For those just starting, a sole proprietorship is the most reasonable form of business, however, be sure to have proper liability coverage. As you grow, if you plan to subcontract to other RDs, DTRs or CDMs, it is best to incorporate in the form of an S Corporation, LLC or C Corporation for protection of your assets. Realize when setting your fees that consulting may require quite a bit of driving time, depending on your geographic location in relationship to your contract accounts.

As with any other business, a good bookkeeping system is essential. Many long-term care accounts prefer to pay every 45-60 days after the invoice is received. The initial wait may be long, but it is good, steady income. Consider running credit checks on individual facilities before accepting them, to help assure payment for your services. Most consultants work 30 days before billing, and then wait another 45-60 days before collecting on the invoice. (This means you won't be paid for your work until up to 3 months after the work is completed.) If you can negotiate a better payment term, do so. For a sample contract, see Appendix 25 A at the end of this chapter.(4)

Determining a Reasonable Amount of Time to Consult

The amount of time it will take to complete your work is totally dependent on what is expected. A great resource for calculating the amount of time needed to consult to a facility is the CD-HCF "Adequacy of Consultant Hours Worksheet".(4) (See Figure 25.1.) When interviewing for a position as a consultant dietitian, ask the following questions:
• What is the RD's role?
• What dietary concerns do you have? Any concerns on the past 3 surveys? What are your quality indicators for unintentional weight loss, pressure ulcers, dehydration? What kinds of systems do you have in place?
• Do you need assistance with your dining program? With sanitation/food safety? In-services?
• Are there any staffing concerns that might inhibit nutrition care?
• Can I do a mock survey on first visit?
• Are there clearly defined roles and responsibilities agreed upon by both parties?

- What is the time allowed for monthly consulting work? (Be sure it is reasonable time for the work expected--ask for more time if expectations are too high for time allotted.)

Figure 25-1

Adequacy of Consultant Hours Worksheet

These are averages. You need to add or subtract any duties that are different from what is listed.

TASK	Estimated Time	Number Min.	Total
Clinical			
Nutrition Screen - deduct 15 min/res if someone else screens resident	15 min/res		
Nutritional Assessment for moderate to high risk	45/60 min/res		
On-going at risk documentation, wt. loss, pressure sores, tube feeding	20 min/res		
Care Plan Conferences	1 hr/week		
Summary Conferences - with Administrator, DNS and DM	60 min/month		
Weekly Communication with nursing - nursing to give you wt. changes, skin and TF info	30 min per visit minimum		
Travel time between resident and where you chart			
Management			
Sanitation Inspection	60 min/month		
Writing 4 week cycle menu	20 hrs/cycle		
Additional modified diet writing	90 min/diet		
Gathering Outcome Data	60 min/month		
Communication with dietary manager or tech	30 min/visit		
Education			
In-service	30-60 min/month		
Discharge Instruction	30 min/res		
Weekly nutrition team meetings	30-60 min		
Total			

Reprinted from the CD-HCF strategy paper "Adequacy of RD Hours" by Jody Vogelzang, RD MS LD FADA and Pam Womack RD   Consultant Dietitians in Health Care Facilities (CD-HCF) 2000

SUMMARY

To be successful in long-term care consulting, it takes the following magic ingredients:

- a desire to achieve your dreams,
- the ability to focus your time and talents on your goals,
- the drive to overcome all obstacles,
- the ability to value mistakes and learn from them, and a commitment to constant improvement.

Resources:

Consultant Dietitians in Health Care Facilities (CD-HCF)   www.cdhcf.org
American Health Care Association.   www.ahca.org   800-321-0343
   (The Long-term Care Survey Book~$28.00)
Am. Assoc. of Homes & Serv. for the Aging www.aahsa.org
National Institute on Aging   www.nih.gov/nia
Nutrition Screening Initiative   202-625-1662
National Pressure Ulcer Advisory Panel   www.NPUAP.org
Web MD   www.webmd.com
Dietetics Online (LTC/ALF site - many links) www.dietetics.com
Administration on Aging   www.aoa.dhhs.gov
Am. Assoc. of Retired Persons (AARP)   www.aarp.org
Merck Manual of Geriatrics   www.merck.com/pubs/mm_geriatrics/
Food Code 2001   www.vm.cfsan.fda.gov/~dms/fc99-toc.html
Gateway to Government Food Safety Info. www.foodsafety.gov/
The National Food Safety Database   www.foodsafety.org
USDA Food Safety & Inspection Service   www.FSIS.usda.gov/
ASPEN   www.clinnutr.org
American Heart Association   www.americanheart.org
American Diabetes Organization   www.diabetes.org
National Kidney Foundation   www.kidney.org
Becky Dorner & Associates   www.BeckyDorner.com
      1-800-342-0285
"Everything you need to get started in business in long-term care consulting"

References

1. Informing the Future: Critical Issues in Health. Washington, DC: Institute of Medicine, National Academy of Sciences; 2001.
2. Greene-Burger S, Kayser-Jones J, Prince-Bell J. Malnutrition and Dehydration in Nursing Homes: Key Issues in Prevention and Treatment. National Citizen's Coalition for Nursing Home Reform; June 2000.
3. Disease State Management: Dysphagia; Proceedings of the Furth Annual Ross Medical Nutrition and Device Roundtable, Charleston, SC; April 1999. Vol. 14, No. 5, Supplement to Nutrition in Clinical Practice. ASPEN.
4. Consultant Dietitians in Health Care Facilities (CD-HCF), a dietetic practice group of the American Dietetic Association. www.cdhcf.org

Appendix 25 A Sample Contract

(Copyright CD-HCF, Used by permission. To order contact CD-HCF.)

SUBCONTRACT FOR DIETARY SERVICES

THIS SUBCONTRACT entered this _____ day of _____, 1993, by and between David Dietitian of 1111 East Second, Evansville, Indiana 47714 ("David") and

_____ of _____

_____ ("_____").

WITNESSETH:

WHEREAS, David's business of providing dietary consulting and related services is expanding and David desired to subcontract portions of such services to the Subcontractor; and

WHEREAS, the Subcontractor desires to subcontract such work from David according to the terms and conditions set forth herein below.

NOW, THEREFORE, in consideration of the mutual ter~ ~ons and covenants set forth herein below, the parties hereby agree as follows:

1. Subcontractor Service D~~~ ~id, the Subcontractor shall provide one or all of the following services for ~ ~e facility or other health or educational institution (collectively "Insτ

a. evaluation of Ins ~artment with
   recommendations . ~eet recognized standards of service;

b. review of existing menus and/or alteration of the Institution's existing menus;

c. the Institution's planning for and personal evaluation and/or revision of medically prescribed diets

d. observation of the Institution's meal service and preparation with
   recommendations for improvement to meet recognized service standards;

e. correlation and integration of the Institution's special diet, aspects of care,
   with documentation in resident's medical records;

f. development and presentation of Institution's inservice education for
   personnel, with documentation made of each presentation;

g. assistance in developing the Institution's managerial and supervisory skills of
   its director of nutrition services through on-the-job education and/or correspondence courses;

h. advising the Institution on the development of appropriate policies and
   procedures relating to its food service and dietary functions;

i. consultation with the Institution's administration following each visit to
   include findings and recommendations, progress, and evaluation of goals; and

j. assistance to the Institution with an y group purchasing program that might be in place or recommended.

2. Service Area. The Subcontractor shall be ready and able to provide upon reasonable notice the service above-described in the following described geographic area
   ("Service Area"):

341

Chapter 26

Talking and Writing About Food

Mary Abbott Hess, LHD, MS, RD, LD, FADA, and Jane Grant Tougas

Dietary guidelines, food pyramids and nutrition labels pack a lot of information, but when it comes right down to it, eating is believing. Survey after survey confirms that people want food that tastes great, as well as being easy to prepare and economical. For dietetics professionals, excellent ways to promote healthful eating are to give food demonstrations, develop recipes and menus and write cookbooks that are as flavorful and convenient as they are nutritious.

Traditionally, food skills were considered important primarily for dietitians in foodservice and food management. Today, practitioners in all areas of dietetics need food-related knowledge and skills. Counselors must be prepared to teach clients how to select and prepare foods, especially those clients on modified diets. Community dietitians must be ready to inform caretakers how to cook for all ages of family members. In addition, more and more dietitians are active in the food industry and the media. There is a growing demand for dietitians with excellent food communication skills.

To strengthen the positioning of dietitians as food and nutrition experts, the Food & Culinary Professionals dietetic practice group of The American Dietetic Association has proposed a comprehensive set of competencies for entry-level practitioners. These competencies include:

- Sensory perception and evaluation skills
- Basic cooking skills
- Menu and menu planning
- Ingredient selection
- Recipe development and modification
- Communicating about food

In this chapter, we will review some of the basic food demonstration skills, recipe development, menu planning skills, and cookbook writing that can enhance your impact as a food and nutrition communicator.

COOKING DEMONSTRATIONS

Trend spotter Faith Popcorn calls it "homemaking voyeurism", watching other people cook. The popularity of the Food Network, Home & Garden TV and PBS food programming is testimony to this phenomenon. Food demonstrations also have become part of the regular line-up on morning television. Appearing on these shows, and in their own series, has made personalities such as Julia Child, Martha Stewart, Emeril Lagasse and Jacques Pépin contemporary legends.

Across the nation, chefs (the famous and the not-so-famous) are teaching in their restaurants, community colleges and community centers. Culinary schools are doing a booming business, offering both basic and advanced cooking classes. Even grocery stores offer food demonstrations and classes. National organizations, such as the American Institute of Wine & Food and the American Culinary Federation, sponsor programs all over the country showcasing the work of food experts. The Culinary Institute of America in Hyde Park, New York, offers an excellent series of instructional videos, and the food sections of many newspapers list local cooking classes and demonstrations. The exhibition Bon Appetit! Julia Child's Kitchen at the Smithsonian at the Museum of American History in Washington, DC showcases the kitchen that Julia Child used in filming many of the classic cooking shows. Many Americans learned to cook by watching Julia on public television.

Food demonstrations offer great show-and-tell opportunities for dietitians. Cooking classes allow exploration of new ingredients, flavors and procedures in an environment that is conducive to experimentation and discovery. Learning is enhanced when people are able to smell, touch and taste healthful food, as well as watch it being prepared.

One of the best ways to master a new skill is by observation and practice. This is as true for learning how to cook as it is for learning how to present food demonstrations. Start by watching a variety of television food shows and taking some notes. You will notice significant differences in skill, technique, content, organization, sanitation, and. personal style. Some really good cooks simply can't explain clearly what they are doing and why. Others excel at succinctly describing and demonstrating proper technique, while also entertaining and sharing insights on topics such as nutrition and food history.

After you have done some basic research, plan a food demonstration, and practice setting up and presenting the demonstration in a limited amount of time. Have an imaginary audience or, if it is comfortable for you, invite friends or neighbors to observe. When you are confident of your skills, try offering classes at your worksite or in a community setting. After additional practice, consider approaching the media, including local cable stations that may be are looking for programming.

If you are not particularly comfortable handling food, find a local chef with which to partner. Work out each of your roles. Many chefs have great cooking skills but are uncomfortable explaining them. A team approach, if there is good rapport, can be interesting and fun. Many chefs, particularly those educated by dietitians involved in the American Culinary Federation certification, welcome the opportunity to work with dietitians.

Almost all demonstrations conclude with construction of a finished presentation plate. You might have seen Graham Kerr's television series on healthy cooking, in which he analyzed his plate presentations with colorful architectural-style renderings to demonstrate the importance of food placement and color. The ultimate goal is to create a plate that makes observers say "Wow!" and you to think, "I can do that!"

HOW TO BE AN EFFECTIVE FOOD DEMONSTRATOR

At the 1997 American Dietetic Association annual meeting in Boston, Chef Michael Moskwa and Suzanne Vieira, MS, RD, both on the faculty of Johnson and Wales University, presented a session titled "Marketing Your Message with Food: Culinary Demonstrations." Chef Moskwa, who for several years hosted a weekly television show, provided ten tips for effective food demonstrations:

1. Use clear, unadorned equipment. Glass bowls and plain equipment are best to show ingredients and amounts.
2. Use sensory words to describe food. Words such as "juicy", "crunch" and "spicy" engage the viewers' senses.
3. Use household measurements, not metric. Americans do not relate to grams and liters.
4. Make sanitation obvious, but not rigid. Keep work areas clean and neat. Keep tasting spoons handy.
5. Choose colorful ingredients. Bright colors create visual impact and pizzazz.

6. Focus on the food. Don't confuse a food demonstration with a nutrition lecture. Mention a nutrient or two and a nutrient benefit, but concentrate on the food.
7. Be entertaining and informative. When you are on television, remember your viewers have their clickers handy!
8. Wear plain clothing. Your clothes should not be distracting. Neutral clothing keeps the focus on the food and your message.
9. Be aware of taste bias. Respect individual preferences and offer alternatives for different palates.
10. Always be prepared. Identify your most important message or technique. Bring everything you need. Be prepared to show and tell in less time than you expect to have. If you are using an overhead mirror, adjust it properly so the audience can see.

RECIPE DEVELOPMENT AND TESTING

From the food technologist's point of view, a recipe is a chemical formula. From the chef's point of view, a recipe is a magic formula. It's up to the dietitian to blend the science and the art into a seamless whole your customers will experience as great-tasting, health-promoting food. No matter where you practice dietetics, communicating about food and nutrition through recipes and menus will significantly enhance your ability to promote nutritional health.

Recipes are a form of communication, they must be targeted to an audience. For example, the lifestyle, health concerns and available time for cooking by a young mother with children are quite different from those of retired empty-nesters. Likewise, a person with diabetes will have nutritional needs that differ from someone in cardiac rehabilitation. Economic conditions, literacy level, family traditions, ethnicity, and cultural/religious heritage are additional considerations. Depending upon the audience to be reached, your recipes can appear in newspapers, magazines, books, calendars, or on posters, bookmarks, websites or client materials.

Cooking Terms

One easy-to-overlook variable is cooking skill. Many recipes and books by chefs and very experienced cooks assume that recipe-users know basic cooking terminology and methods. For example, their instructions may say: "Blanch beans." Blanching entails briefly cooking vegetables in boiling water and then "shocking" them in ice water to retain their bright colors. Inexperienced cooks need to know that to blanch beans one must:

1. Bring a large pot of salted water to a boil.
2. Fill a large mixing bowl with cold water; add about 20 ice cubes.
3. Put trimmed beans in boiling water for 1 minute only.
4. Drain beans and plunge them into ice water to quick chill. Drain well.

When you explain each cooking method and technique in detail, however, the result can be a long recipe that appears complex and time consuming. Complexity and time commitment not only scare inexperienced cooks, but also turn off people who know how to cook, but are too busy to enjoy it. The trick is to be as brief as possible, while still being very clear. Some famous cookbook authors, such as Maida Heatter, are known for their very specific directions. Although Heatter's recipes do tend to be long, the cook who follows each step knows what to expect and can be confident the recipe will work, taste wonderful and look beautiful. Books such as Julia Child's, The Way to Cook, use photos to enhance instruction and understanding, but most recipes and cookbooks do not have the budget to cover expensive food photography.

Is the Recipe Fail-Proof?

Everyone has a story about "the recipe that didn't work."? Make sure that story is never about one of your recipes! Those who spend the time and money to use your recipes deserve to have success when they exactly follow the recipe. Test and test again. Here are some points to remember as you are establishing your recipe testing procedures:

- Set up your laboratory—your kitchen. Use an oven thermometer to check the accuracy of your oven. Make sure you have all the basic measuring utensils (good quality measuring cups and spoons, a food scale, a timer, meat and candy thermometers, etc.).
- Use only the kitchen appliances, tools and gadgets you would expect to find in your readers' kitchens. Avoid unusual ingredients (unless you are developing an ethnic recipe, in which such ingredients are essential).
- Plan ahead, so you can prepare a detailed grocery list. If you are going to be testing a lot of recipes, group them according to common ingredients.
- Think about what you are going to do with all that prepared food! Serve it to family and friends; freeze it to eat later; make arrangements to donate it to a local shelter; or deliver it to a homebound or elderly person you know.

When testing a recipe, remember these tips:
- Develop a worksheet so you can keep track of the ingredients and methods you try and what you finally use (see Figure 26.1).
- Measure ingredients very carefully. Measure liquids in glass or clear plastic measuring cups intended for liquids; measure dry or solid ingredients in metal or plastic cups. Measure dry ingredients in dry measuring cups that can be leveled off with a straight edge, such as a knife. If the recipe specifies sifted flour, sift before measuring. Disregard that some flour comes pre-sifted, and sift it again.
- Use whole purchase units when possible. For example, using 1 (15-ounce) can of tomato sauce, rather than 2 cups of tomato sauce, makes shopping easier and avoids leftovers.
- Use large eggs in recipes. Do not substitute other sizes, unless there is a specific reason to do so.
- Specify pan sizes, especially for baked goods. Measure skillets and baking pans across the top, not the bottom. Remember that thickness influences cooking time and texture.
- Keep track of how long it should take an average cook to make the recipe. Also note how long it takes to complete steps such as reducing the liquid or cooking the vegetables. You might want to add this information to the recipe. Inexperienced cooks don't know what consistency or degree of doneness is correct, so time estimates help.
- Taste test. Get some second opinions. For example, if the dish is meant for children, enlist the help of a taste-testing youngster or two.
- Recipes with reduced salt or fat may require several taste tests with varying levels of additional herbs, flavoring agents or different cooking techniques. Recipes suitable for modified diets should be flavorful enough for anyone to enjoy.
- If you are planning to make adjustments/substitutions to create a healthier dish, you might want to make the original recipe first to see what it looks, smells and tastes like-these are the baseline expectations. Make any adjustments/ substitutions you want to try, and prepare the dish again.
- The finished product must look and smell appetizing. If you have made adjustments/substitutions, the revised recipe does not have to taste exactly like the original, but the flavor should be balanced and the texture should be appropriate for the dish. If you want to try some changes in types or amounts of ingredients, method of preparation, cooking time, etc., retest the recipe until you are happy with the final product. If your recipes don't taste wonderful, they will disappoint the people who use them and destroy your credibility.

Figure 26.1

RECIPE TESTING FORM

Recipe Working Title: Date Tested:
Project: Recipe Source:
Test #: Number of Servings:
Total Yield: Size of Servings:
Pan(s)/Equipment Required: Pan Prep:

Cooking Temp: Preheat: ___Yes ___No Total Cooking Time:

Ingredients & Quantities
Adjustments/Substitutions

Method (Steps of Preparation)
1.
2.
3.
4.
5.
6.
7.
8.

Notes for Nutrient Calculation (deduction for waste, discarded ingredients and weight):

Garnish: Serving Suggestions:

Secondary Recipes Required:

Comments/Taste/Evaluation:

- Keep in mind that a recipe is a chemical formula. Because chemicals react in different ways under various conditions, you may not be able to halve or double a recipe and expect it to turn out the same as the original "formula." When testing a recipe, prepare the entire recipe. You need to know the final yield (volume) to determine the appropriate number of portions.
- Many recipe testers take a photo of the final dish as a reference. When testing a lot of recipes, it is useful to have written descriptions to refer to at a later time.
- Know when to give up. Some of your ideas that look great on paper, may not work—ever!

When modifying recipes to meet a specific nutritional need, review the recipe and determine if it is appropriate to modify. Certain recipes can be prepared with substitute ingredients, if adjustments are made to assure pleasing texture and flavor. Other recipes, however, will never be successful without particular ingredients. Sometimes it is wiser to substitute another recipe entirely, rather than create a poor imitation of the real thing. For example, there is no such thing as a low-fat croissant!

Adapting Recipes to Meet Medical Needs

Low Fat

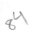

When adjusting recipes to meet nutritional needs, the most common modification is in the type or amount of fat. There are thousands of low-fat and "healthy" cookbooks available that describe how to modify fat content. Dietitians write more and more of these books. Some are successful; some are not. Similarly, some low-fat recipes are wonderful, while others disappoint. For example, although it is a commonly suggested modification, simply substituting fat-free yogurt for sour cream or substituting skim milk for cream usually does not work. Such substitutions can be made, however, if other ingredients and seasonings are adjusted appropriately and if the recipes are tested and evaluated. Even substituting low-fat or fat-free salad dressings for full-fat dressings requires taste-testing. Simply expecting a recipe to taste good is not enough. Only taste-testing will tell.

Low Sugar

Lowering sugar content is another common recipe modification. Remember that sugar adds more than sweetness to many recipes.

For example, it enhances browning and adds crispness to baked goods. Sometimes simply using less sugar is satisfactory. Sugar substitutes or alternative sweeteners can be used to add more sweetness with fewer grams of carbohydrates. Although individuals with diabetes or hypoglycemia need to count the carbohydrates in their foods, they are less likely to be on the "sugar-free" diets of the past.

Low Salt

When salt must be restricted, other flavoring ingredients, such as fresh herbs, garlic, pepper, lemon juice or citrus zest, should be used to perk up flavor. Often, sodium can be reduced significantly by reducing the amount of salt used in the early stages of cooking and adding some salt just before serving. Course-grain Kosher salt has less sodium per teaspoon than regular fine-grain salt. Small amounts of monosodium glutamate (MSG) can be used to intensify and blend flavors and replace salt in some recipes. MSG is a potent flavor enhancer with one-third the sodium of salt.

Increased Nutrients

Recipes also can be adjusted by adding ingredients that boost nutritional value. Vegetables, fruits, legumes, and grains rich in fiber and phytochemicals will improve the nutrient profile of many recipes. Artfully using fruits and vegetables as edible garnishes can also make plate presentation more attractive.

Many foods used as ingredients in recipes are fortified or enriched to boost their nutrient contribution. Flour and many pastas now have added folate, as well as B vitamins and iron; fruit juices are available with added calcium and/or vitamin C; fortified rice and soy beverages can be used as milk substitutes in preparing foods for those with lactose intolerance. Dietitians can help their clients meet specific medical needs with great-tasting and beautiful foods.

TECHNIQUES TO REDUCE FAT CONTENT

- Use cooking techniques that require little or no fat, such as grilling, broiling, roasting, poaching, steaming, stewing, or baking.
- Use nonstick pans or pan spray to reduce the amount of fat used to control "sticking."

- To enhance mouth-feel and "gloss," add a small amount (1 tablespoon) of butter or margarine to a sauce immediately before serving, rather than using fat earlier in preparation.
- For "creamy" soups, use pureed vegetables thinned with broth or skim or evaporated skim milk. Add the appropriate seasonings.
- Meringue cookies and tart shells are easy to make and fat-free. Use them with fresh fruit or sorbet for a luxurious low-fat dessert. Some stores and bakeries sell ready-made baked meringue shells.
- Reconsider what portion sizes are adequate and appropriate. Use different pan sizes, or reduce portions. For example, make smaller muffins or bake brownies in a larger pan to create a "thinner" product. Smaller means less calories and fat per serving.
- Use low-fat salad dressing as a meat or poultry marinade and drain it before cooking. Before doing a nutrient analysis of the recipe, deduct the discarded marinade.
- When using fat, choose the optimal type and use only the amount needed to create a delicious product. Olive, safflower, sesame, and canola oils are considered more "heart healthy" than other oils. Various olive oils have different flavors; canola is bland and neutral. A small amount of chicken fat (also monounsaturated) adds a lot of flavor to sautéed onions. Intense flavors help minimize the amount of fats needed. For example, nut oils and seasoned oils (lemon or garlic oil) can be brushed over cooked vegetables just before serving. Butter has a distinct flavor and should be used where appropriate.
- Toast nuts to intensify their flavor, and use half the amount called for in recipes.
- A mixture of nonfat yogurt and ricotta cheese can fill in for cream cheese in desserts and dips. Fat-free buttermilk can be seasoned to use in delicious low-fat salad dressings and to make low-fat mashed potatoes and some sauces.
- When possible, shift the balance in a recipe to increase the amount of vegetables, grains and fruit, and while reducing the amount of meat and/or sauces. This adjustment will reduce total fat, while boosting essential nutrients.
- Cut leftover bread into small cubes, dip in stock to infuse flavor, and then bake until crisp. A non-fried, crunchy alternative, these tiny croutons add texture to salads and can be use as a topping for soups and casseroles.
- Use fruit salsas and chutney (fat-free), instead of sauces with hot or cold meats, and to mix with poultry or seafood for high-protein salads.

- Thinly slice steak and other meats. "Fan" the slices on a plate to make 3 or 4 ounces look like a much larger portion of meat.
- When vegetables are being used as ingredients, roast, grill, or "sweat" them, rather than sautéing them in fat.

RECIPE WRITING

Whether you are writing recipes for publication or to use as presentation handouts, the most important thing to remember is consistency. Choose a recipe format and develop an alphabetical style sheet to keep track of your decisions on matters such as capitalization, spelling and word choice. (See list of resources at the end of this chapter for books that discuss various recipe-formats.)

If you are writing for a magazine or newspaper, study the publication's recipe style and follow it as closely as you can. If you are writing a cookbook, review other cookbooks you enjoy using, select a recipe style you like and stick with it. Basic cooking techniques are explained particularly well in The Culinary Institute of America's Techniques of Healthy Cooking, and in Julia Child's The Way to Cook. Techniques for low-fat baking are explained in Alice Medrich's book, Chocolate and the Art of Low-Fat Desserts.

Eventually, a copy editor will edit your recipes into the proper style for a particular publication. This task will be much easier if you have been consistent in the recipes you submit. Below are some general guidelines for recipe writing.

A Recipe for Your Recipes

Ideally, the person who is using one of your recipes will read it through once before beginning to cook. Less methodical cooks, however, will dive right in. For these people, especially, it is important to be a clear as you can and to anticipate any areas in which you think confusion might occur.

Title

Baked Alaska and Better than Robert Redford Cake aside, make your recipe titles fairly simple and descriptive of the dish. If you are preparing recipes for a book that will be indexed, straightforward titles will make it easier for readers to find what they are seeking.

Headnotes

In this introductory blurb, you can include an acknowledgment, a historical fact, serving ideas, tips on seasonal ingredients, a personal recommendation, or even a fond memory associated with the dish. Be creative. Remember that some people enjoy reading recipes more than they enjoy cooking them! (Not every recipe has a headnote, but this information can give a recipe some extra pizzazz.)

Ingredients

List ingredients in the order they will be used. When order doesn't matter or when several ingredients are added at the same time, list the dry ingredients in descending order according to volume followed by the liquid ingredients, also in descending order by volume. Only list water in the ingredient listing, if it must be heated or chilled before use. Avoid using brand names unless, of course, you are developing a recipe for a food manufacturer. Use standard kitchen measurements and avoid abbreviations (exception: F for Fahrenheit). A "dash" or a "pinch" can be used for less than 1/8 teaspoon of dried herbs.

Be as clear as possible about amounts, sizes, weights, and dried/canned/ packaged vs. fresh. For example, if you say, "1 can of tomato sauce," the reader might interpret this to mean an 8-ounce, 15-ounce or a 29-ounce can. The amount of tomato sauce used would dramatically alter the success and character of the recipe. Different types of food have different standard size cans and packages. Check the weight and list it.

When possible, give measurements in both units and weight, such as:
- 1 (8-ounce) can tomato sauce
- 1 (16-ounce) package angel hair pasta
- 6 medium potatoes (about 2 pounds)
- 4 ounces of cheddar cheese, shredded (about 1 cup)
- 1 medium pork chop (about 5 ounces)
- 1 (10-ounce) package frozen leaf spinach
- 3 cups fresh spinach leaves, packed tightly
- 1 teaspoon dried oregano
- 1 tablespoon chopped fresh oregano

Because you learned it in school and see it on measuring cups, you might assume that 1 cup (volume) equals 8 ounces (weight). Don't convert weights to measures based on this 8 ounces = 1 cup assumption. While it is true of water, foods have widely varying weights per volume measure. For example, a cup of un-sifted, all-purpose flour weighs about 4 ounces (115 grams); 1 cup of rice weighs 5 1/2 ounces (150 grams); and 1 cup of honey weighs a whopping 13 ounces. For baking, it is especially important to list both weights and measures. Check ingredient amounts by weight and measure when testing recipes.

Include preparation procedures, such as peeling, chopping, slicing, separating, thawing, bringing to room temperature, and precooking in the ingredient list. For example:

- 1 large baking potato, peeled, cooked, chilled, and sliced
- 2 (15.8-ounce) cans kidney beans, drained, liquid reserved

Be aware of the impact one misplaced word can have. For example, measuring before or after chopping or processing can make a significant difference, as in:

- ½ cup chopped walnuts versus ½ cup walnuts, chopped
- ½ cup whipping cream versus ½ cup cream, whipped

If an ingredient is used more than once, you can take one of two approaches:

- List the total amount needed the first time the item is used, and add the word "divided," as in "2 cups of flour, divided." The cook then knows the total amount of flour needed. In the recipe method, you will instruct the cook how much flour to use at different points in the recipe.
- List the ingredient twice in the appropriate amounts as it occurs in the recipe. This option takes up slightly more space, but may prevent errors.

Method

Write the recipe instructions in a concise, logical efficient order. Begin sentences with a verb followed by equipment, treatment, time, and doneness check. For example:

"Place onion slices in a 12-inch nonstick skillet over medium heat. Stir about 3 minutes until onion is limp and transparent."

Either number the recipe steps or divide them into short paragraphs.
- If appropriate, begin by stating oven temperature for preheating in degrees Fahrenheit (F), and identify any pots or pans that must prepared.
- Explain what type and size bowls, utensils and appliances to use and how to combine ingredients.

- Explain what type and size cooking vessels to use and how to cook ingredients. Use standard pan sizes. When testing a recipe, check that pan sizes are appropriate.
- When needed, specify a test for doneness: for roasted meats, a temperature using a meat thermometer; for cakes, until top is firm and inserted toothpick comes out clean; for cookies, until they are slightly brown around edges.
- Make garnishing, serving and menu suggestions.

When referring to a mixture of ingredients, identify it by its primary ingredient. For example, say the "egg mixture" or the "flour mixture." When conveying cooking information, describe the method, time and give some visual clues about how the food should look. For example, "Sauté chopped shallots until transparent, about 3 minutes." The method section can end with food storage information, food safety tips, how to vary recipes, or make substitutions.

Yield

Note how many portions the recipe yields. In your notes, you will want to weigh or measure the total yield--for example, "2 quarts" of soup. In some cases, it will be helpful to note the portion size as well, for example, "8 (1 cup) servings." Many recipes featured in the newspaper give an unrealistically large or small number of portions. Indicate a portion that is adequate, but not excessive. Recipes for people with diabetes or on calorie-controlled diets should provide "standard" exchange portions.

Nutrient Analysis of Recipes

A basic per serving nutrient analysis includes calories, carbohydrate, protein, and fat. For some audiences, it may be appropriate to include cholesterol, sodium and fiber, to break fat into saturated, polyunsaturated and monounsaturated; or to note if the recipe is a good source of certain vitamins or minerals.

Because of variations in ingredients and measurements from cook to cook, all calculated or computed values must be only approximations. The  nutrient analysis usually does not include optional ingredients, herb garnishes; the fat used to grease pans, nor suggested accompaniments, unless specific amounts are given.

When a range of servings is indicated, the larger number is typically used for the nutrient analysis. If there is a range in the amount of an ingredient, the smaller amount is typically used. Some analysts, however, prefer to calculate the midpoint of a range. When a recipe lists a choice of ingredients, the first ingredient is the one used in the calculation. Salt is figured only if the recipe calls for a specific amount. Salt added to cooking water is usually not calculated because the cooking water is discarded and so little salt is absorbed.

Subsidiary Recipes

When a recipe includes a number of components, for example, a layer cake with frosting and filling, or poultry with stuffing and gravy, break it down into subsidiary or secondary recipes and label them clearly, so the reader can follow the process easily. If some secondary recipes are used in more than one main recipe, consider having a special section on basic recipes, and refer the reader to that section as needed.

May I Use Your Recipe?

Like a formula, a recipe can't be copyrighted (the cookbook can be), but that doesn't make it acceptable to claim other people's work as your own. Ethically, plagiarism is plagiarism. Recipe writing can be a gray area, one in which the Golden Rule definitely applies.

If you plan to use someone else's recipe in a presentation, ask permission first, and be sure to give that person or book the appropriate credit. If you intend to publish someone else's recipe in an article or book, you must obtain permission either directly from the author of the recipe, or in the case of a recipe in a book, from the publisher. Even if you change the title or make minor adjustments in the ingredients or method, if the recipe is essentially the work of someone else, you should seek permission for its use.

On the other hand, if you are inspired by someone else's recipe, but with substantive changes make it your own, you need not seek reprint permission. In addition, some recipes are considered "standards," for example, basic pastry dough or cake batters don't require permission to use. Likewise, recipes from manufacturers and food advisory groups, such as the Produce Marketing Association or the Lamb Council, generally can be used without prior permission, although a credit line is appreciated.

Send a permission form to request use of a recipe (see Chapter 12). Include the recipe you want to use and its source. Explain how and where you would like to use it. In addition, note exactly how you intend to credit the author/publication, for example, at the end of the recipe or in a list of acknowledgments. Create a check-off area at the bottom of your letter for the recipe author/publisher to respond with YES or NO, and include directions for returning the form to you. Keep in mind that some authors and publishers will charge you a reprint fee, which can be based on how many copies of the recipe will be printed (as in a book, newspaper or magazine) and/or how a book containing the recipe will be priced for sale. If the fee is unacceptable, use another recipe.

RECIPE WRITER'S CHECKLIST

___Does the title give the reader an idea of what this recipe is all about?
___Does the headnote add some interesting or useful information?
___Are the ingredients correct and in the proper order of use?
___Are all the measurements correct? (One typo can lead to disaster!)
___Is the method explained clearly and in a logical progression?
___Are there any simple preparation steps that could be moved to the ingredient list?
___Are all the ingredients in the method on the ingredient list?
___Are all the divided and reserved ingredients used?
___Are the pots and pans measurements standard and correct?
___Are the cooking temperatures and times correct?
___Is the recipe yield indicated?
___Is the specified portion adequate and appropriate?

NUTRITION ANALYSES

More than ever before, consumers want to know what is in the food they eat. Because nutrition labels on supermarket food list calories and grams of key nutrients per serving, many consumers want comparable data on the recipes they prepare at home.

Running the Numbers

In nutritional analysis, you can't believe everything you read. For example, the analyses printed with recipes in some newspapers, magazines and cookbooks quite often are incorrect or misleading. One common cause of error is using the ingredient list as input data without adjusting for losses, such as unused pan drippings from poultry or discarded marinade.

Nutrient values should be accurate, but not unrealistically specific. The rounding rules used for food labels offer sensible guidelines:

- Round 0-50 calories to the nearest 5-calorie increment; 50 or more calories to the nearest 10 calorie increment.
- Round grams of carbohydrate, protein, fat, and fiber to the nearest gram.
- Round cholesterol to the nearest 5 milligrams.
- Round milligrams of sodium to the nearest 5 milligrams, if less than 140 milligrams and to the nearest 10 milligrams, if over 140 milligrams.

Inappropriate specificity, such as 13.628 grams of fat, is also misleading.The calculated value should be rounded to 14 grams. Remember that even excellent databases are based on averaged values of many food samples, and home cooks don't measure with gram scales.

While nutrient analysis and computer printouts will be very specific, the dietitian should translate these numbers to consumer-friendly data. Before analyzing a recipe, review it to determine if all ingredients should be included in the calculation. Your recipe testing notes should indicate if pan drippings, fat from the top of soup or gravy were discarded. If so, delete the gram weight of discarded fat before the analysis is done. To do this, weigh the pan drippings in a small bowl or blot the pan drippings on paper toweling, and weigh it. Subtract the weight of the empty bowl or the clean paper toweling.

Chicken is a common ingredient that presents calculation challenges. The amount of fat gained or lost in cooking depends on the cooking method, length of cooking time, cooking temperature, and the addition of other ingredients. If poultry skin is removed before eating, the skin must be removed, and its weight subtracted.

Proper nutrient analysis is far more than just entering the ingredients into a computer program. A database includes many similar items (for example, types of canned tomatoes or grades of ground beef), and the correct item must be entered. Many dietitians prefer to buy nutrient analysis computer programs and do their own data entry. Others use the services of companies that specialize in nutrient analysis. The decision is often based on variables, such as volume of recipes to be analyzed, cost of purchased analysis versus the cost of software, and the time availability and computer skills of the dietitian doing the work. Even when the recipe is sent out for analysis, you must check the computed values carefully for accuracy. As the author and recipe developer, you are responsible for printed nutrient values.

The format for nutrition analysis on recipes varies, according to the audience and how the information will be used. In some cases, you may use a sentence listing calories and grams of fat. Other times, a food label format or food exchanges may be appropriate. Think about what your audience wants to know, and avoid providing more information than they want or need. Most nutrient analysis software programs provide more information than you will share with readers, but keep records of all your calculations, in case you receive questions from readers or your editor.

Selecting Analysis Software

Many nutrient analysis computer software programs are available. Microcomputer Software Collection, produced by the Food and Nutrition Information Center (FNIC) of the U.S. Department of Agriculture (USDA), offers a comprehensive listing. In addition, the Journal of the American Dietetic Association carries classified ads placed by software companies. Some are reviewed in the "New in Review" section. Software companies also exhibit at the Association's annual meeting each year. Almost all of these companies offer demonstration diskettes or a preview of some type.

Do your homework before you invest! Ask colleagues which programs they use and if they are satisfied. Because software is designed for many uses (foodservice and planning management, inventory and cost control, nutrition labeling, recipe or meal analysis, menu planning, etc.), you must be sure the program you purchase matches your needs.

Before purchasing a program, you will want to understand the quality and quantity of the database. How many items are listed? Does it include the specific nutrients you need? What is the basic cost? How often it is updated? What is the fee for obtaining database updates and enhancements? Is there a toll-free number for assistance? When is the assistance available?

In addition to knowing how many foods are in the database, you also may want to know some of the actual foods. For example, if you are working with ethnic foods, you will want to know if the database includes them. In addition, you will want to know how difficult it is to add foods to the existing database. Imported and ethnic foods now carry nutrition labels, but are not in some databases.

If you're going to use the program primarily for recipe analysis, make sure the process is simple. Are food items easy to access or must you use a code? What information prints out in the report? Can all the analysis information be viewed on the computer screen prior to printing? Can the program convert the data to a label format? Bowes & Church's Food Values of Portions Commonly Used and many databases have "holes" in their micronutrient and macronutrient information, because some information had not yet been collected when Handbook 8 was compiled. Current database information includes some old Handbook 8 data.

You will want to know if a database uses a zero for both missing information and absence of a nutrient or does it specifically identify missing information? You may have to estimate a value from a similar ingredient, rather than use zeros for unknown amounts. For example, if the database you use does not have fiber values for a particular legume (adzuki beans), you should enter the fiber value of a similar legume (kidney beans or small red beans) to calculate an estimated value. An educated guess is better than a zero for a missing value, and all calculations should be checked for missing data. As you can tell, you might be missing a lot if you only look at the bottom line of nutrient totals.

Finally, newer software packages often do not work on older hardware. Determine whether your computer meets the software company's minimum requirements. You will need to know what operating system your computer runs on (MAC, DOS, Windows, UNIX) and the minimum memory (RAM) and hard disk space requirements for the software. The more inclusive databases require larger memory, as do programs that provide graphics and extensive statistics.

CREATING MENUS

While some of us love to cook and take great pleasure in preparing food to share with family and friends, others (perhaps the majority), seek the quickest and easiest way to get food on the table. For people who prefer assembling food, rather than cooking, the food industry provides a full range of convenience and takeout options. And Americans aren't shy about using these options. As editor Christopher Kimball reported in the September/October 1998 issue of Cook's Illustrated magazine, of meals eaten at home, 41% are fast food, 21% are restaurant takeout and 22% are supermarket "home meal replacements", that is, takeout. Only 16% of the meals we consume at home are (presumably) home-cooked, Kimball noted.

Home-cooking allows more control of ingredients and nutrients and it's usually more economical. However, lack of food knowledge and cooking skills in the majority of American homes presents a huge obstacle to cooking from scratch. A survey reported in The New York Times, also cited by Christopher Kimball, found that 75% of people polled did not know how to cook broccoli; 50% couldn't prepare gravy and 45% did not know how many teaspoons are in a tablespoon. And, it doesn't appear that the situation will improve anytime soon: 75% of American children do not know how to cook. (Do yours?)

By suggesting meals and menus, home-cooked or otherwise, dietitians can translate nutrient needs into food choices that complement each other, delight the senses, provide essential nutrients, and preserve the budget. As in any type of communication, "Knowing your audience is rule No.1." Things to consider include:

- How much time does your audience generally have to prepare meals?
- What skill level can you expect?
- What cooking equipment can you assume people have at home?
- Do you need to accommodate any medical nutritional needs?
- Are there any age-related considerations?
- Does your audience have ethnic or cultural food preferences or food traditions?
- Is food budget a consideration?

In an individual counseling situation, you will have access to this type of information from dietary assessments and medical records. In family situations, however, household members can differ dramatically in nutrient needs and food preferences. Among larger groups of people, needs vary even among members of the same group. For example, teen athletes are different from sedentary teens. And within both groups, women's needs differ from men's.

One thing everyone has in common, however, is an appreciation for taste. And because we eat with our eyes as well as our taste-buds, suggesting foods and combinations that are exciting and beautiful can make food messages even more appealing. Borrow good ideas from chefs and other food experts. Scan food magazines, cookbooks and newspaper food pages for menu combinations and ideas. Go to the library or bookstore and peruse award-winning cookbooks. Evaluate what is appealing to you and why. When you go to restaurants, look at plate presentations.

COOKBOOKS

Cookbook writing is an ancient art. One of the earliest cookbook authors was the Greek scientist Epicurious, whom we recall in the term "epicurean". Through the late 18th century, upper-class men who could afford fine ingredients wrote most cookbooks. When women began to write cookbooks, like other women writers of the time, they often published their work anonymously. With titles such as The Frugal Housewife, Cookery Recipes and The Young Housekeeper's Friend, these cookbooks were meant for everyday use and included family health tips, as well as recipes.

Today, anyone can publish a cookbook–and they do! Contemporary cookbooks are often more than a collection of recipes. They preserve ethnic and religious traditions, create adventure, promote health, poke fun, celebrate the seasons, and simply revel in sensual pleasures of food. No wonder so many people enjoy reading cookbooks.

If you have been tossing around an idea for a cookbook, here are some tips on how to start to bring that idea to fruition:

- Think about exactly what you want your cookbook to be. What is your theme? Who is your audience? Write a very brief description. Don't worry about your writing style. This description is for your eyes only, to help keep you centered on your idea as you do some research.
- Conduct market research. Check the Internet. Go to a few bookstores and to the library, and examine cookbooks similar to what you want to do. Are there already a lot of cookbooks using your idea? How could you make your cookbook different? If there are very few cookbooks using your idea, ask yourself why? Is the audience for your concept too small to support profitable sales? Is your idea so new that not many books have been written about it?
- While at the bookstore or library, make a list of publishers who have released books similar to what you have in mind. Make notes on recipe styles that appeal to you. Also pay attention to the number of recipes, different book formats, size of the book, and photography and illustration.
- You can also check Books in Print at your library. This publication, which will be available in printed form and/or on-line, lists all cookbooks currently in print. Literary Marketplace and Writer's Market, both available at the library, list publishers according to subject matter, including cookbooks.
- Using what you have learned in market research, refine your original description, and expand it to include some information on format, length and overall style. Give your book a working title.

Getting your book to market means you either sell your idea to a publishing house or self-publish. The list of resources at the end of this section includes books that tell you how to write a query letter to a publisher, how to prepare a book proposal, and when and how to work with a literary agent. (See Chapter 27.)

If you self-publish, you will act as the "general contractor" for your cookbook. It will be up to you to conceptualize your book, identify your market; decide how many books to print; set a selling price and manage sales. You will have more control, but more responsibility and financial risk. You will need a team of subcontractors: a copy editor, perhaps an indexer, a book designer and production person, perhaps a photographer and a food stylist (plus all the food and props they will need), maybe an illustrator, a printer, a distributor and, possibly, a promotion or public relations professional. Most of all, you will need money!

PUBLISHING OPTIONS

- A publishing house usually offers an author an advance against sales and royalties (percentage of sales price) and other sales, such as paperback rights. If you are using a literary agent, he or she will take a percentage of your advance and royalties. Some publishing houses will simply buy your book outright with no royalty agreement.
- A cookbook packager purchases a manuscript from the author for a flat fee. The packager then designs, edits and sells a complete book, sometimes already printed, to a publisher, who then distributes the book.
- Food and equipment manufacturers and food advisory boards occasionally commission sponsored cookbooks to showcase their products or to offer as premiums to customers. The author is paid a flat fee for this work.
- A subsidy publisher will produce an author's book at the expense of the author. Generally, "vanity publishing", as this approach is called, is looked upon with some disdain.
- In self-publishing, the author assumes complete responsibility, including costs, from writing through distribution and promotion. The self-publisher puts together a team of experts to do what he or she is not able to accomplish alone. Some printers will offer self-publishers design, production and printing services in one package. But this is a very viable option, with e-books published on the Internet or short run publishers who can print one book at a time or a 100, instead of thousands. Self-publishing can be a stepping stone toward being recognized by a national publishing house.

KEY RESOURCES FOR COOKBOOK

Bowes & Church's Food Values of Portions Commonly Used, 17th edition. Jean Pennington. Philadelphia: Lippincott; 1998.
Chocolate and the Art of Low-Fat Desserts. Alice Medrich. New York: Warner Books; 1995.

CookWise. Shirley Corriher. New York: William Morrow and Company; 1997.

Dictionary of Healthful Food Terms. Bev Bennett and Virginia Van Vynckt. Haupparge, NY: Baron's Educational Services; 1997.

Food Writer, bimonthly newsletter, P.O. Box 156, Spring City, PA 19475: Phone (610) 948-6031. Fax (610) 948-6081.

Food Writing Guidelines. Food Writers and Editors Committee of the International Association of Culinary Professionals, 304 West Liberty St., Suite 201, Louisville, KY 40202; 1994.

Handbook of Food Preparation. Food and Nutrition section of the American Home Economics Association, 9th edition. Dubuque, Iowa: Kendall/Hunt; 1993.

Larousse Gastronomique. edited by Jenifer Harvey Lang. New York: Crown; 1988.

Maida Heatter's Brand-New Book of Great Cookies, Maida Heatter. New York Random House; 1995.

Microcomputer Software Collection, produced by Food and Nutrition Information Center, U.S. Department of Agriculture Library, 10301 Baltimore Ave., Room 304, Beltsville, MD, 20705-2351. Phone (301) 504-5719. Fax (301) 505-5719.

On Cooking: Techniques from Expert Chefs, 2nd edition. Sarah R. Labensky, Alan M. Hause and Steven Labensky. Upper Saddle River, N.J.: Prentice-Hall; 1998.

Recipes into Type. Joan Whitman and Dolores Simon. New York: HarperCollins; 1993.

The International Menu Speller. Kenneth N. Anderson and Lois E. Anderson. New York: John Wiley & Sons; 1993.

The Professional Chef's Techniques of Healthy Cooking, 2nd edition. The Culinary Institute of America, New York: John Wiley & Sons; 2000.

The Oxford Companion to Food. Alan Davidson. Oxford: Oxford University Press; 1999.

The Recipe Writer's Handbook. Barbara Gibbs Ostmann and Jane L. Baker. New York: John Wiley & Sons, Inc.; 2001.

The Way to Cook. Julia Child. New York: Alfred A. Knopf; 1989.

Webster's New World Dictionary of Culinary Arts, 2nd edition. Steven Labensky, Gaye G. Ingram and Sarah R. Labensky. Upper Saddle River, NJ: Prentice Hall; 2001.

Mary Abbott Hess, LHD. MS, RD, LD FADA, is president of Hess & Hunt, Inc., a nutrition communications firm in Chicago, Illinois. She is Chairman of the National Board of Directors of The America Institute of Wine & Food, a past president of The American Dietetic Association and founding chair of the Food & Culinary Professionals Dietetic Practice Group. She has written eight books, including award-winning cookbooks. Jane Grant Tougas is a writer specializing in food, nutrition and health. Her company, JGT Ideas, is located near Cincinnati, Ohio.

Chapter 27

The "Write" Way to Get Pubished

Susan Tornetta Magrann, MS, RD, updated by Kathy King, RD

Don't skip this chapter because you think you don't have the skills to be writer. Writing talent is not something you are born with like curly hair or brown eyes. Learning how to write is like mastering any new skill, whether it is skiing or developing healthy eating habits. It is the mark of a truly educated person, a necessary communication tool for the professional practitioner. You need motivation guidance, and practice, practice, practice.

WHY WRITE?

The abundance of inaccurate nutrition articles and books written by pseudo-nutritionists should motivate dietitians to pick up their pencils or learn to use word processing by computer. Complaining about nutrition misinformation will not solve the problem. Even instructing patients in a one-to-one situation won't have a tremendous impact on the public. But dietitians writing interesting articles and books about sensible nutrition will. Just think how many people you can reach with one article---probably more people than you could counsel in a lifetime.

A second motivational factor is the self-satisfaction you experience when you see your name and work in print. It is what will spur you on to write additional pieces.

Writing gives you a chance to be creative. It is like painting a beautiful picture or sewing a gorgeous outfit. You start out with a few basics--paper, pen and an idea---and you can create a masterpiece.

Publishing can give you credibility with your readers and peers. People who write books or articles don't necessarily know more than their peers, but everyone thinks they do. Being published opens doors to speaking, media interviews, top-level committee appointments, tenure for educators, and it makes it easier to become published in the future.

And you can't overlook the financial rewards, but don't spend the money yet. The publications most likely to print your first articles probably will pay poorly. But they do provide the opportunity to get established and perfect your writing skill. Besides, many of these initial contacts can serve as a network to meet the right people from bigger---and better paying---publications.

Having had the experience of writing for a variety of publications helped me convince a large supermarket chain that I was the person best qualified to write a monthly nutrition newsletter for their approximately 200 stores.

There also are other financial gains from getting published. Most publishers, especially those that don't pay well, are willing to print a brief statement about your background and the location of your private practice. This can attract potential clients; also include information about how your book can be purchased. Bartering services like this is how one dietitian is marketing her self-published book.

THE RIGHT START

Ready to dust off the old keyboard? Good. But before you begin, you should polish your writing skills. Attend a publishing workshop, hire a tutor, or take a writing course at a local college. Or, at least check out library books on the topic such as Writing with Precision by Jefferson Bates or On Writing Well by William Zinsser. Two major national writer's magazines---The Writer and Writer's Digest---also offer invaluable writing tips.

Reading newspapers, magazines and books can advance your writing education. Scrutinize what you read. Take a close look at the lead and the format of the article. Analyze what techniques the writer uses to capture your interest. If you spot a poorly written article, think about how you could improve it.

A writer whose style is worth particular study---is Barbara Gibbons. Check if your newspaper carries her syndicated column the Slim Gourmet.

WHAT TO WRITE ABOUT

Now that your fingers are itching to write, you must focus on an idea. It is easy to come up with good ideas if you keep your eyes and ears open. Nutrition is an "in" topic. Listen to what people are talking about. Read a variety of newspapers, magazines and books. Watch the news.

Once you have an idea, you must make it uniquely yours by giving it a different slant. Editors want articles that are timely, and your slant can help update any nutrition subject. For example, more career women are waiting to become mothers. Why not slant your piece toward nutrition during pregnancy for the woman over thirty?

Major national or local news stories can make a nutrition topic timely. Obesity in America is a "hot" topic, but it needs a niche like how heavy people also have fat pets. President Bush's dislike for broccoli opened the door for many articles on vegetables and on children who don't eat well. A recession makes food budgeting especially pertinent to the consumer.

Use your calendar to help inspire timely ideas. Waistline survival tips for holiday partying would be perfect for the December issue of a magazine. But you'd better think about Christmas in July, since editors plan months in advance.

In developing your idea, keep in mind who your readers will be and what would interest them. For example, most senior citizens do not care about basic nutrition for infants. But they may enjoy a story on healthy snacks for visiting grandchildren.

You should be able to state your idea in one sentence. Make it specific. General ideas don't sell. You are more likely to spark an editor's interest with "Ten Tips for Looking Great in a Swimsuit" than a general article covering weight reduction principles.

People love to clip recipes and editors know it. So consider developing recipes to sell your message. Don't just write about the need to use less salt, but include recipes that show how to make delicious low sodium dishes.

Make sure you choose a topic that is of personal interest to you. This will keep you motivated to do the research and survive numerous revisions.

THE COMPUTER AND WRITING

With the growth in popularity of the personal computer, a discussion on writing would not be complete without mentioning how one can be used. Software such as Microsoft Word or Word Perfect can allow you to use the computer as a word processor. This gives you the capability to compose directly onto the computer screen, correct or reword the manuscript as necessary and then print it when you are happy with it. The manuscript can be checked for spelling and grammar with the right software. It can be stored on software, later recalled on the screen and revised by the word, sentence, or paragraph.

Time-consuming handwritten or typed manuscripts are problems of the past. Scanners can read typed manuscripts and record them on software so you can easily revise them. Through voice-recognition software, you don't have to spend hours typing the manuscript.

A modem device and your telephone line can allow your computer to access stored information in larger computer databases. This would allow you to conduct literature, newspaper or scientific journal searches for the most current information and could greatly reduce the amount of time needed for research. For practitioners who do not live close to a good medical or research library, this capability for accessing information is especially invaluable.

It is possible to have an editor, or graphic artist doing layout, check and revise your manuscript on their computer and send it back to your computer---all without anyone leaving their home or office.

FINDING A MAGAZINE/NEWSPAPER PUBLISHER

After your idea is clearly defined, your next step is to find a publisher. You can start by referring to a writer's directory book that should be available in your local library. Writer's Market, Writer's Yearbook and Literary Market Place are the best-known books. (See Recommended Readings at the end of the chapter.) They are updated yearly and contain the names of thousands of newspapers, magazines and book publishers.

In addition, there are market listings in Writer's Digest and The Writer. You also can write directly to a magazine and ask if it accepts material from freelance writers; also ask them to send "spec sheets" or Writer's Guidelines.

The following is a sample of the information listed in the directories for magazines and newspapers.
1. **Name and address of the magazine or newspaper and the editor's name.**
2. **Type of magazine.** If your idea is about nutrition during pregnancy, you would focus on a magazine geared to women in their twenties and thirties. Obviously magazines aimed at senior citizens or men won't be interested.
3. **Date established.** Recently established magazines are more likely to accept your material, since they have not built up a list of regular contributors. At the same time, they are more likely to fold before you ever receive payment.
4. **Circulation.** Generally, the higher the circulation, the higher the pay rate, but this will also mean more competition.

5. **Pay rates and preferred length of articles.** Editors work with a fairly set budget, so there is not much room for negotiating fees unless you're well known or have a really "hot" story.

6. **Terms of payment.** "Payment on acceptance" means that the magazine will pay you as soon as the editors agree to buy your article. "Payment on publication" means they will pay you when your article appears in the magazine. This could be several months after you submit the article. "Kill fee" is a portion of the agreed-on price for an article that was assigned, but the editor decided not to use. You are still free to sell your article to another magazine.

7. **Rights purchased.** When you sell your article, you are selling the publisher the rights to reprint these words, "First serial rights." First serial rights mean the newspaper or magazine has the right to publish your article for the first time in their periodical. "Second serial rights" gives a newspaper or magazine the right to print your article after it has already appeared in some other newspaper or magazine. This term also refers to the sale of part of a published book to a newspaper or magazine. "All rights" means the writer forfeits the right to use his material again in its present form. This is also true for "work-for-hire" agreements because the writer has signed away all rights to the company making the assignment.

8. **By-line.** This means your name will appear on your article.

9. **SASE (Self-Addressed Stamped Envelope).** If you do not include one, and most request it, the editor will probably not reply to your letter.

10. **Lead-time.** Many editors request that seasonal material be submitted a specific number of months in advance. Editors have a lead-time of several months so they don't want to see ideas for a Christmas holiday article in October.

SELLING YOUR IDEA

Now that you have pinpointed which publishers are most likely to be interested in your work, you must sell them your idea.

A Query Letter

Before you write your article, you should send the editor a query letter (see Figure 27.1). Most editors prefer that you do not telephone or send the complete article. The query letter is your sales tool. Since editors will formulate their impressions of you from this letter, it is wise to use quality 8 1/2" x 11" stationery and to make sure your typewriter or computer is printing well.

A query letter should contain these basic components:
1. Description of your idea, why it is timely and your slant. Include an abstract of how you plan to develop your idea and a suggested length and deadline.
2. An explanation of why the editor's readers would want to read the article.
3. Why you are qualified to write the article and resource people you plan to interview. Include a statement about your professional background, as well as one or two samples of published works. If you haven't been published, you need not mention this fact.

The ideal query runs one to two single-spaced pages--just enough to develop your idea but short enough to be read quickly. Enclose a SASE (self-addressed stamped envelope) and your phone number.

Figure 27.1 Sample Query Letter

Susan Magrann, M.S., R.D.
CONSULTING NUTRITIONIST
5252 LINCOLN AVENUE, CYPRESS. CA 90630
PHONE: (714)

Date

John Smith, Editor
Today's Family
1410 First Street
Morristown, NJ 07960

Dear Mr. Smith:

Are your readers buying what they think they are buying when they go to the supermarket? Shopping today is fraught with mysterious codes and language.

Do fruit drinks or fruit-flavored drinks contain more fruit juice? Does the term "lite" mean low in calories? Is Instant Breakfast a nutritious meal? Does white bread contain any nutrients? The answers are all there on the products' labels.

I would like to take the mystery out of label reading by writing a 1000-word article covering the following points:

1. HOW TO INTERPRET A PRODUCT'S NAME. Included would be a chart of the legal meaning for various terms. For example:

If the Label Says:	It Means:
Fruit juice	100% real fruit juice
Juice drink	35 to 69% real juice
Fruit drink	10 to 34% juice
Fruit-flavored drink	less than 10% juice

Your readers will probably be surprised to learn that the term "lite" can refer to   other properties of the food besides calories. "Lite" corn chips aren't lower in   calories; they're thinner.

2. INGREDIENT LISTING. You can learn a great deal about the product's composition, since ingredients are listed in descending order by weight. Included will be a description of hidden sources of sugar, salt and saturated fats. If your readers check the ingredients for Instant Breakfast, they will find that in addition to sugar, corn syrup solids, another form of sugar, is also listed.

3. NUTRITION LABELING. The article will have a detailed explanation of what every line means on the nutrition label and will define the term "RDI."

As for white bread, the nutrition label shows that it does contain some nutrients, although less than what is found in whole wheat bread.

I hope I will have the opportunity to help your readers become better-informed consumers.

Besides being a registered dietitian, my nutrition articles have appeared in several publications including The Jogger. I also write a monthly nutrition newsletter for a large supermarket chain on the West Coast. Enclosed are two samples of my work plus my curriculum vitae.

Sincerely,

Susan Magrann, MS, RD

A Book Proposal

If you're interested in having a book published, the Literary Market Place listings will tell you what types of books a company publishes, how they want the material submitted, and what terms to expect if you're offered a book contract. The author's payment is called a royalty and is usually calculated as a percentage of the retail price of copies sold. For hardbacks, 10 percent is the usual base rate and 7 to 8 percent for paperbacks. Generally, the percentage increases if your book sells well.

You also can find a potential publisher by going to a bookstore or your own library and looking at books that cover a topic similar to the one you intend to write about. Check in the front of the book for the name of the publishing house. Because of the interest in nutrition today, there are publishers who are looking for dietitians with writing or recipe-development talents or someone with a "new" twist on diet and foods.

Karen Mangum, RD, of Boise, Idaho was contacted by Pacific Press, because of her public speaking and good reputation. Pacific Press had decided it wanted to publish a vegetarian cookbook, and she was chosen as its author. The publisher paid for 80 colorful photographs in the book (sometimes the author must share the cost or pay for photos), and the publisher footed the bill for an eight-city media tour.

If you're working on a book or want to be, start by sending the prospective publisher(s) a proposal. The proposal should be about five to ten single-spaced pages and contain all the elements of a good query letter, as well as a synopsis or outline of the chapters. Most publishers would also like at least two good sample chapters or some other published material that shows your writing ability. Send the proposal, along with a large return envelope with postage, so that it can be returned to you if they are not interested. For additional tips, refer to How To Write "How-to" Books and Articles as well as the Writer's Handbook.

Since your proposal can remain under consideration for many months, it is reasonable to send it to two to three editors at the same time. However, you must inform them that others are reviewing the same material by saying "simultaneous submission" or some other similar wording.

Don't get discouraged when selling your book idea. Published dietitians tell stories about the numerous proposals they submitted before a publisher showed an interest. Lack of interest may indicate that the idea needs to be reworked, but it could mean the "right" person had not seen it yet. Try to get as much feedback as possible from anyone who rejects it.

It is curious how some opportunities come so easily and others are hard to find. At an ADA Annual Meeting in the early 1980's, Kathy King, RD, and Olga Satterwhite, RD, were setting up their exhibit in the Consulting Nutritionist's booth when Earl Shepard, an editor for Harper & Row, walked over and asked, "How would you two women like to write me a book?" Kathy looked at his name tag and said, "When do you need it and what do you want it on?" This book is the result of that chance meeting. Kathy states that none of her other book proposals have had such an easy beginning. Earl said later that he had been an editor for twenty years and made the offer because of a gut feeling.

Using A Literary Agent

You don't have to have a literary agent in order to sell your book. Many dietitians have sold their book ideas directly to a publisher.

Dietitians and other authors who have used agents state they do it for several reasons: First, the agent is often able to negotiate a much larger up front advance on your book; second, the agent represents your interests during the contract negotiations to make sure you make all you should on foreign rights and future printings, as well as assure the publisher performs as promised with cover design, promotional support and maybe even media tours. Dietitians can negotiate this for themselves or with a lawyer, but often first time authors don't know what to ask for and where problems arise.

Some agents help their clients get exposure in the media and make the right contacts in the industry. Some agents have writing skill and a knack for helping writers refine their book concepts before a publisher sees them. Many publishers will not look at manuscripts that are not submitted through agents they know and trust. Agents perform the important function of screening many of the thousands of manuscripts that are written each year and bringing only the best ones to publishers.

On the down side, some agents are very popular and thus very busy; they may keep your work a year or more without giving you much feedback. Some agents show initial enthusiasm for an author's work but stop returning phone calls after awhile, leaving the author in a quandary. Unless you're an established writer or have a very good book concept, it will be difficult to attract an agent. Since agents' fees are usually about ten to fifteen percent of your royalties plus some expenses, they want to feel certain you will earn enough money to be worth their time and effort.

Some agents work only on verbal agreements while others have written contracts. In either case, if you feel the agent is not working well for you, you should have an understanding that you can take your manuscript and go elsewhere.

If you decide to pursue getting a literary agent, you can start by asking for suggestions from writers you know. The Literary Market Place contains a comprehensive listing of literary agencies.

Self-Publishing

If you or your agent cannot find an interested publisher, you can always publish the book yourself. Of course, you have to invest your own money. But if you don't have confidence that your book will sell, why should a publisher?

Ellen Coleman, a dietitian from California, originally self-published her book, Eating For Endurance. She decided to self-publish because editors felt the topic did not have a wide appeal and wanted her to dilute the material. Today, she has her book with Bull Publishing because of its wider marketing channels.

It is extremely important before you take this step that you accurately estimate your costs and determine how you are going to market the book. It may look attractive to sell 2,500 books at $20.00 each, but look at the items below to get an idea of the costs involved in publishing your own book, consider the following:

- $1,500+ for computer, desktop publishing and word processing software and laser printer
- $250-500 or more for a graphic artist to prepare the book cover (art professors and students will do it for the best price)
- $50-250 each for copyrighted cartoons, graphs, photographs, and illustrations. An artist or photographer may want his or her money up front, or some will take a percentage of the book royalty.
- $6,500-8,500 to print 1,000 copies of a 300-page book, or $12,000 for 2,500 copies, or $16,000+ for 5,000 copies (this includes page layout for printing, book cover in four colors, binding, and so on). Some printers will let you pay for it over several months, and others will want their payment when the inventory is delivered. Before choosing a printer, see samples of his work, and confirm your time-lines. Although a printer at a distant location may give you a better price than a local one, consider the added costs of delivering the inventory and long distance calls, FAX and overnight mail to check last minute details. The best book printer to use is one who does it for a living, not a printer who will have to make an "exception" for your project and "find" a binder in the area.
- $520 or more per 1,000 people for a direct mail promotion you send out (approximately $.52 per person using a brochure and first class postage with a purchased label; $.42 each if sent bulk mail); a JADA classified ad costs about $120 per month; and state and dietetic practice group newsletters charge $50-150 to run one ad.
- Consider selling your books through NCES or NASCO catalogs for dietitians and other health professionals, and Tuft's University Diet & Nutrition Letter in Boston and CSPI in Washington, DC offer products and books in their newsletters. If they feel your book is a good fit for them, you usually sell your books to them at a discount similar to that given to bookstores.
- $450 plus all your travel and lodging expenses to exhibit in the Product Market Place at ADA's annual meeting for one day;

$1,700-3,500 for a large commercial booth for three days at ADA. For other conventions like Home Economists, Nursing, or Restaurant costs vary, but it takes many book sales to cover expenses. There is the possibility you could share the booth with one or more entrepreneurs or publishers.

- According to Linda Hatchfeld, RD, author of *Cooking A la Heart* and founder of Appletree Press, Inc., if your book is for the public, there are three distribution channels you could use:

  1. **Wholesalers,** who warehouse the book for you and fill orders from bookstores, but do not promote it; you pay them 50-55 percent of the retail price for that service and they sell to stores at a 40-43 percent discount--they make 10-15 percent for warehousing your book.

  2. **A distributor** will market your book to retail stores through their catalog and sales staff on consignment--they don't buy the books, they usually sell them for 42 percent off the retail price. Then they split the remaining 58%, 30/70%, with you getting the 70 percent to cover printing-paper-binding (PPB) and your profit.On a book which retails for $10, that would mean $4.06 to you for expenses and profit.

  3. **A retail bookstore** will ask for a 40-43 percent discount from the retail price and perhaps the right to return any unsold copies.

  If your book is over forty-nine pages and you plan to sell the book in stores or through Amazon.com, you should get an "ISBN" number (International Standardized Book Number) to print on your back book cover (as well as on software, videos, audio tapes with voice, and some calendars). This number makes it easier for bookstores to order your book or other items, and it puts your book in the Books In Print book and database available at all libraries and bookstores. The cost is $300 for a fifteen to twenty-day turnaround to get your listing of numbers and more if you need seventy-two-hour response. To get a number and more information, call R.R. Bowker at (800) 521-8110 or go online at www.bowker.com.

You can easily see in this example it could take almost 1,000 copies of a book just to cover your initial expenses involved in publishing and marketing the book. That is why most people who self-publish try to print as many as they think will sell over a year or two in order to save on printing. After the initial costs are paid for, any remaining inventory is profit except for on-going marketing and storage costs. Even though the cost-per-book drops as you order more, be realistic about how many books you might

REALLY sell-after every relative and friend has a copy.

If your book is for the public and you want to sell it in B. Dalton, Amazon.com or wherever, it's important that the book sells well to remain on the shelves. Mary Hess, RD, author of *The Art of Cooking for the Diabetic,* whose first edition sold more than 350,000 copies, and *Pickles and Ice Cream,* written along with Anne Hunt, reports that her publisher said a trade book has about ninety days to "make it" in the large bookstores. After that, the copies are sent back to the publisher and a new book is ready to fill the space. To have a book that really sells well is the exception, not the rule. Knowing this, you can see why initial marketing is so important!

Is There An E-Book in Your Future?

Since about 1998 a new form of publishing has peaked writers' interest-e-books. First, authors and publishers promoted traditional books with banners and web sites. Then some adventuresome writers skipped the paper and pen, query letters, and begging publishers to take their novels and went directly to the public on the Internet. Web sites were formed to sell the books-sometimes a chapter at a time.

A variety of software and hardware came to market to facilitate reading a book from PalmPilots, Rocket e-book, desktop, or laptop computer. Now, of course, there are e-publishers who make the process even easier. One e-publisher, iUniverse, published over 15,000 new works in 2000.(1) A competitor, Fatbrain, reported that 5,500 authors signed on to write books in just four months. (1)

Self-published authors pay all the bills and make all the profits. They share a larger percentage of the selling price if they use an e-publisher (40-70%) versus 10% from a traditional publisher. Most book prices are very reasonable, typically $3 to $10. (1) Some sites will require that you have Acrobat reader software, which is available for free download from:

www.adobe.com/products/acrobat/readstep.html.(2)

Helpful Resources

- EBookNet (www.ebooknet.com) carries articles about e-book publishing and reading technology.
- The Glassbook Reader helps you read books on your computer; it has a free download at www.glassbook.com.
- Sites to check out: www.hardshell.com, www.sofbook.com, www.diskus.com, www.iuniverse.com, www.fatbrain.com, www.booklocker.com

Illustrations

Don't overlook the value of good illustrations in your book to increase sales. Unless you are talented, your best bet is to find a free-lance professional artist and/or photographer. Contact other writers who have used local illustrators and get their recommendations. Or look in the Yellow Pages under "Artists--Commercial" and "Photographers-Commercial." There may be good, young talent at local universities and art schools.

WRITING YOUR MASTERPIECE

Congratulations! You sold your idea. Now you only have a deadline to worry about. This can cause panic---and an illness called "writer's block." Don't worry--it need not be terminal. There are measures to overcome the condition.

First, find a location--either at home, work, or at the library--where you can work without interruptions. If the phone is a problem, consider investing in an answering machine or unplug the phone for several hours and put your cell phone on mute.

Second, select the best time for you to write and force yourself to stick to it. Most people have a specific time of the day they feel most creative. You will be more productive by spending whatever amount of time you can spare every day at your "peak creative time" than trying to cram the assignment into a couple of 8-hour days.

Third, break your writing into small parts. This will keep you from feeling overwhelmed by the project.

Outline

Maybe the first day will be spent on your outline. It is essential to have some type of outline, since it makes the next step--research--much easier. An outline helps you gather and organize all the pertinent information you need. While doing your research, you may decide to revise your outline.

Research

Begin your research by reviewing materials you have at home or work. Then, you'll want to expand your information by going to a local library and/or medical library or by a computer search.

Interview dietitians and other professionals who are experts in the topic you're writing about. In addition to providing valuable information, they can direct you to reference books and articles.

Don't let the term interview scare you. It's just a fancy name for talking to someone. Most people will be flattered that you value their opinion. To avoid wasting the expert's time, prepare a list of questions before contacting him.

Writing

After research comes the hardest step for most people---writing. Some would-be authors are guilty of research overkill to delay the inevitable. It sometimes helps to scan the collected research the evening before you want to finally sit down to write. The information is fresh in your mind and the best ideas often rise to the top overnight.

It is easier to write your first draft if you don't worry about it being perfect at this point. Just sit at your desk and put your thoughts on paper. Don't stop for any corrections or even crossing out words. Once you force yourself to do the first draft, your work will become easier.

Next, revise and fine-tune your piece. The first revision will probably be the most extensive. Keep in mind you want your work to be clear, concise, accurate, and interesting. Check that your lead sentence is a grabber. Unless you capture the audience's attention, they won't continue to read on. It can take a good deal of time to develop your lead, but it's definitely worth the effort.

Next, take a close look at each word. Specific and short words crowd more meaning into a small space. Cross out unnecessary words and check for spelling.

Avoid overusing a particular word especially within the same paragraph.This is when a thesaurus or a dictionary of synonyms and antonyms is valuable.

Now you're ready to study sentences. Do they flow smoothly? Are the lengths of your sentences varied? Generally, shorter sentences are easier for the reader to understand.

After sentences come paragraphs. Each paragraph should contain a main idea. Avoid paragraphs that are too long. You can even slip in some single sentence paragraphs for a change of pace.

Look for a snappy ending. The reader will then leave the story with a favorable impression.

After your first revision, put your work away for a few days so you will be able to take a fresh look at it. Now you're ready to do your second, third, or however many additional revisions it takes to make it perfect.

Editing

If you lack confidence about your writing, but feel it is near perfect, pay a professional writer to edit it. You can find someone by asking business associates whom they recommend or by contacting a college with a journalism program. There may be an instructor or a senior student who could help.

Depending on your subject, you also may want an expert in that area to check your work for accuracy.

Final Copy

The end is almost near. You are ready to type your final copy, or let your printer do it, if you are using a computer. Don't forget to follow the guide the publisher sent you. After you've cleaned up all those typos, you're ready to mail off your masterpiece. Today, everyone wants the manuscript on disk, as well as a sample on hardcopy. Even if you self-publish a book, the printer will want the final book on disk to make the film---and it's cheaper for you than having the film made from hardcopy.

Since you've invested so much time and energy creating this literary work, you don't want someone to steal your material. If you're not familiar with copyright laws, refer to Chapter 12 on protecting your ideas.

The last step: Relax. You'll need to gather strength before you start your next writing project.

One final piece of advice--resist spending your entire writer's fee buying copies of your work for friends and relatives. On second thought, why not? You should be proud of your accomplishment. And you thought you couldn't be a writer!!!

REFERENCES

1. Kuchinskas S. Publish Thyself. *TIME*. January 24, 2000: B7.
2. Folkers R. Get your book published-electronically. *USA Weekend*. May 5, 2000.

RECOMMENDED READINGS

Magazines
The Writer. Published Monthly by The Writer, Inc.
Writer's Digest. Published Monthly by Writer's Digest.

Books
Marketing Information
Literary Market Place. Bowker, Annual.
Writer's Market. Writer's Digest, Cincinnati, OH, Annual.
Writer's Yearbook. Writer's Digest, Cincinnati, OH, Annual.

Writing and Publishing
Appelbaum Judith: How To Get Happily Published. Harper & Row; 1998.
Hull Raymond. How to Write "How-To" Books and Articles. NY: Writer's Digest Books; 1981.
Day Robert. How to Write and Publish a Scientific Paper. 2nd ed. Philadelphia: ISI Press; 1998.
Graham Betsy P. Magazine Article Writing. New York: Holt, Rinehart Winston; 1980.
Zinsser William. On Writing Well. New York: Harper & Row; 1988.
Henderson Bill, ed. The Publish-it-Yourself Handbook. Pushcart Press; 1998.
Burak Sylvia K, ed. The Writer's Handbook. The Writer; 2001.
Meyer Carol. The Writer's Survival Manual. New York: Crown Publishers; 1984.

Chapter 28
Media Savvy

The unfamiliar world of radio and television can unnerve health professionals who are old pros with one-on-one counseling and public speaking. Interviews with the print media are usually more relaxed, but you seldom have control over what is quoted. Why,then, become involved in something so challenging or risky? Usually, it's because you want to communicate with a great number of people. How else can you discuss nutrition with a million people for five minutes or warn your entire city about a new diet fad? What better way is there to quickly establish your credibility as you open a new business? Once your business is thriving, the media can take your career to new levels.

First chances, much less second chances, aren't always easy to get in any media avenues. Because so many people recognize the value of media exposure, there is stiff competition to become a guest, especially on national programming. Local media and some cable stations are not so difficult.

Jack Hilton, author of On Television!, states, "The electronic media have replaced print as the basic source of information in this country, and the ordinary person is severely limited in the ability to get before a microphone and camera. In fact, even the extraordinary person has found it difficult to reach an electronic forum with regularity." (1)

Even considering all of the benefits, media work is not for everyone. Radio and television seek out people with original personalities; those with something new to say and, of course, the ability to say it. The pace is usually quick and then it's over.

Sometimes the station or newspaper never again has time for another interview, and you never know why. They have time for the chef, the fortune-teller, the gardener, and the police officer, but not the dietitian. At least not you. Was it something you said? Were you too boring? What could you have done differently?

PRACTICE MAKES PERFECT

Experts usually suggest you plan, practice, and seek training if you are really serious about pursuing the media on anything but an occasional, small-time basis. It also helps to have experience. But how can you get it, if no one will give you a chance to start?

Practitioners have trained by first going to small local radio stations and newspapers to learn the ropes and the style that sells. If writing style is a problem, hire an editor to review your work or follow the other suggestions in Chapter 27. If speaking off the cuff is not comfortable, take communication courses, pay a tutor, or practice with another person using a tape or video recorder. It is also beneficial to watch, listen to, or read the media. Train yourself to begin thinking of angles that will make your project (or you) more newsworthy. Review the media topics below:

Food demonstrations on
    Vegetarianism
    Natural food sources of vitamins
    Increasing the healthy omega-3s and why
Discussion on
    Can foods prevention cancer?
    Obesity in children and adults
    The aging gut--eating after 60 years old
    Sports nutrition for the everyday athlete

To prepare for call-in talk shows read back issues of newsletters such as Nutrition and the M.D. and Tuft's University Diet and Nutrition Letter. Read lay publications, such as "Good Housekeeping," "Prevention," and newspapers, to get a better idea what your audience is reading.

Jack Hilton offers some good suggestions to consider before joining the talk show circuit, even on the smallest scale. He states, "Watch every talk show you can. Get a feeling for the rhythm, and for how much can be said. Note how questions tend to be repeated from show to show. Make up a set of questions and answer them in the microphone of a tape recorder. Listen to your voice. If you hear a continuing series of crutch words or sounds (ah, well, I don't know, sure, maybe, and so on), practice talking without them." (1)

It's usually less stressful to be interviewed by a newspaper writer, but answering with concise, clear statements is just as important. An interview should not be interpreted as an invitation to ramble or become too familiar. Don't make statements you hope stays "off the record." Ask to see the quotes the newspaper plans to use from you-often they will be read to you over the phone before the article goes to press. Many times you can make last minute changes, especially if you have a working relationship with the reporter. Radio and TV morning shows are less intense than television news because there is more time to be conversational.

LEGALITIES, LIABILITIES AND CONTROVERSIES

When you appear on the media on the subject of nutrition, you are representing yourself as an expert and as a member of your profession.Obviously, the better you do, the more credible everyone appears. However, there are legal and liability implications involved that you must be aware of:

1. As a nutrition expert, you have the right (and perhaps civic responsibility) to state the facts on an issue as you know them and as your peers would, given thorough research. If someone sues you for what you say, they have to prove that you intended malice toward them.
2. If you are introduced as an officer or representative of your local, state or national dietetic practice group or professional organization, you are speaking not only for yourself, but also for that organization. It is therefore very important, especially when you want to take a very controversial stand, that you think it out ahead of time. Then either only represent yourself by not implying otherwise or make sure the organization is in total agreement with your statement before you make it.
3. Consider carrying media malpractice insurance (call ADA at 800-877-1600 ext. 5000 Member Services to get information).

To help avoid problems with controversial subjects, research the subject thoroughly and then state both sides of the controversy in a fair manner. Quote higher sources to defend your statements. Afterward, you can either state your opinion with your reasons or quote a higher source and give their reasons.

A personal experience by the author helps illustrate the viewers' interest that can be generated by controversy:

After years of doing media work in Denver on subjects that I thought were interesting and sometimes controversial, I learned a valuable lesson. One week Judy Mazel, the author of the Beverly Hills Diet, was a guest on NoonDay, the NBC TV program where I was a weekly nutrition authority. She appeared about 15 minutes before my segment and was lively, vivacious and a "media event". After her segment, the hostess asked if I could quickly look over the book and critique it for my segment instead of talking about what I had planned. I told her I needed more time to do an adequate job, but suggested we give a "promo" for next week's segment where I would give a critique. At least people might wait a week before they bought the book.

That next week I spent three times more preparation time than normal in developing my critique of Ms. Mazel's book. I called several PhDs to get their comments on some of the erroneous statements made on physiology and digestion. The show went very well, but the viewer response to the station was much greater than I expected.

A physician friend, whose opinion I respected, said it was the best show I had ever done, and he gave me a quick review. He stated that the hostess and I first got everyone's attention because we issued a warning about the book. Then my arguments began to crescendo, as each became stronger than the preceding one. At the moment when I had everyone's attention, I quoted a higher source that lent greater credibility, and the hostess and I made light of the author's poor knowledge of the subject.

I hadn't realized what had transpired, but I was glad it was pointed out to me so that I could use it again. My reviewer also told me that I should stop covering such "milk toast" subjects and go after the "hot" controversial ones.

I took my friend's advice and immediately went after the Nestle issue, Dr. Adkins, stagnant schools of thought in nutrition, and the Cambridge Diet Plan (our station received its first threatening phone call for my segment on that one). To prepare for the subjects, I called national headquarters' offices to talk to people, requested printed materials, and read other professionals' reviews. I even had a personal interview with the president of Cambridge International at my home the evening before the televised program on the diet. Phone calls and letters increased to the station and to me, and the station loved it.

BY-LINES AND PROMOTION

We miss many good opportunities to market ourselves in the media because of our hesitation to ask for, and contractually negotiate, by-lines and promotional credits. A by-line is a written acknowledgement in a newspaper, magazine or other printed article that you were the author or at least a contributor. There have been times when dietitians have written magazine articles, assuming they would be given credit, only to find that someone at the magazine was listed as the author. The magazine edited the article to make it appear the dietitian was merely interviewed. The fee was paid, but the by-line credit was worth far more.

A promotion on radio or television usually consists of a short on-air statement about how to contact you directly. It may be simply, "Look for Jane Jones under 'Dietitians' in the Yellow Pages," or "Jane Jones may be reached at 333-421-1234." Do not assume this will be offered to you automatically. The media person can refuse your request, but at least ask. To help establish on-going relationships with media professionals, it helps if you accept the fact they will not always quote you each time they call for feedback or a quote. But if you write an article or column, that is a different matter.

DEVELOPING YOUR SALES STRATEGY

There may be many motives for wanting to pursue the media: Personal challenge or promotion, business exposure, consumer crusading, or all of the above. Whatever the reason, you must demonstrate that your cause is of interest or benefit to many people. But a worthy cause is not enough in itself. Unfortunately, the importance of your cause may be less important than the style in which you sell it.

You must have something new to say about the subject, something you have discovered yourself, engineered yourself, or dramatized in a newsworthy fashion. (1) Appearing each March to say this is National Nutrition Month wouldn't generate much attention if it weren't for the creative dietitians willing to appear on the media, or the school children's colorful projects, or the "new" nutrition facts used to catch the audiences' attention. Television stations and newspapers love human-interest stories with visual content. It doesn't have to be spectacular, just interesting or dramatic.

Becoming involved in "causes" to get media exposure (along with other personal and professional benefits) is a tactic long used by individuals in the know. (2) In many businesses, notoriety or popularity often equates with power or clout. Sometimes doors open to us first because of our popularity or the draw of our name, before our great expertise in nutrition is even considered!

Some suggestions to help develop a sales presentation include: (1)

1. Is there a way to demonstrate a perceived benefit to many people? Could you orchestrate an effort to help the local food pantry? Is there a local fruit or vegetable that everyone grows that is in season and high in nutrients? Is your local water contaminated? Have there been several outbreaks of food poisoning at church picnics? Have you been able to convince several restaurants to offer "petite" portions as a way to satisfy smaller appetites and stop the growing obesity trend?

2. Is there a way to package your cause to make it seem new, even if it's old? Is there new research to prove your point? Selling points

consist of a good strong headline, plus a specific example or anecdote that supports the headline. It's not enough to talk about nutrition, you must add the information that falls in the "I never knew that before" category. (3) For example, "Our nutrition consulting business specializes in working with adolescent obesity. Did you know that if both parents of a child are overweight, the child AND the dog have an 80% chance of being obese too? We are very concerned about that fact and want to teach kids and families how to break that cycle."

3. Is there a dramatic way to illustrate your cause (before and after pictures, charts, films, slides or testimonials)?
4. Can you demonstrate a particular expertise in talking about a subject of continuing public interest? (This is a favorite tactic of professionals who do not advertise widely, but who use broadcast exposure as a way to build a practice.) (2)

How to Get in the Media

You can always call up and ask if you can be on a show or talk to a reporter. By first doing your homework and observing the media, you should know whom to contact, what kind of programming they offer and what topics are current.

In radio and television, first contact the program host.(1) If that person is unavailable, or won't talk to you, speak to the producer. At a newspaper, ask to speak with the editor of the section most likely to be interested in what you have to say.

If the show or paper prefers to have requests made in writing, write a good one-page cover letter, plus a sample newspaper column or the proposed interview topics, and attach your bio or resume to support your credibility. Follow that up with a phone call. Try to call at least an hour or more before any show so the person will have time to speak with you.

You will need to let them know your ideas, what you have to offer and why the audience would be interested. Make sure you have several news "hooks" (unique features about your story) that will draw their interest. Remain flexible in case the reporters or station people have a new twist or approach they like better that still includes you. If the person doesn't like the idea at all, ask why. Offer to rethink the concept and offer a new proposal. Do not, however, ask for recommendations to other media contacts or new approaches for you to try. (1) The information may be offered, but it is not their responsibility to be your public relations consultant.

Gail Levey, RD, was consulting at the New York City YMCA and Heart Association. A reporter from WCBS-TV called to ask if she would do a news segment, and she reluctantly agreed. The interview went so well, she became a "regular" on CBS News, the McNeil/Lehrer Report, quoted in the New York Times, and a regular contributing author to four national magazines.

"Gentle persistence is the key" to finally getting in the media, according to Jeffrey Lant, author of *The Unabashed Self-promoter's Guide: What Every Man, Woman, Child and Organization in America Needs To Know About Getting Ahead by Exploiting the Media* (2). No one should be discouraged if turned down; just keep persisting until someone is interested or the idea finally proves that it isn't right for you.

Before Arriving for the Media Interview

When you work with the media you are selling yourself and your ideas. Be comfortable, prepared, rehearsed, and confident about your appearance. You will not be able to read a prepared speech, so reference material, notes, props, or whatever else you plan to refer to should be accessible, easy to read, and familiar to you. Go prepared! Or don't go.

Many media consultants encourage interviewees to choose only three major points they plan to emphasize. For television, all props, notes, charts, and so on should revolve around those points. All artwork and lettering should look professionally prepared, not homemade. The possibility of "freezing" or getting off the subject is much smaller when you simplify the interview. The audience will remember what is important if it is clear, simple, and restated several times in different ways. After you make the main points, feel comfortable in discussing whatever the interviewer brings up. Plan to close with a summary of your three points.

Wardrobe is important since first appearances are crucial in all forms of the media. Don't wear anything so flashy that your clothes draw attention away from you. Don't overdress or under dress for the occasion. Clothing you would expect to see on a bank vice president or TV newscaster will be good at any hour (1).

On television the color and print of an outfit are important. Try to avoid stark white or black. Instead, use colors like gray, royal blue, purple, red, yellow, and beige. Patterned items, if you wear them, should be quiet, very small, and only one at a time. Avoid wearing herringbone, bright flowers and too busy clothing.

Jewelry can be a problem on television because it can reflect into the camera or keep hitting a lapel microphone. Wedding rings and watches are usually fine, but large reflective bracelets, pins, necklaces, or chains may have to be taken off. Eyeglasses, especially with metal frames, can reflect the light. However, if you can't see without them and you don't wear contacts, don't take them off---the interviewer may ask you questions about the slide showing on the monitor or a cameraperson may try to signal to you.

The Interview

When an interviewer meets a knowledgeable guest, the guest usually gets more freedom to carry the conversation. But this is not always the case, especially when the interviewer feels loss of control. So be aware and flexible concerning others' agendas.

Try to be relaxed and don't forget to smile. Hold something in your hands if you like, but don't play with it or mutilate it. Before an interview on radio or television begins, it's usually possible to take a few minutes with the host to mention the items you feel are most important to discuss. Usually, the details on showing props, slides, charts, or whatever are worked out ahead of time with the host or an assistant, but be sure the host is aware of them and when they are to be used. It is also appropriate to ask if the host is familiar with the topic on which you plan to speak. If he or she is not, offer several key human-interest anecdotes or mention a new study that might be of interest.

Be careful not to explain everything ahead of time, because the host may unintentionally make your points in his or her introduction and cause you to panic. (This happened to the author in Little Rock while on her initial spokesperson tour for Butter Buds. Before my segment, as I spread out my props, I told the hostess, a former Miss America, my three points. On the air she introduced me, and then she gave my three points while she pointed to my props, smiled and turned to me. I was sick. I'm seldom at a loss for words, but that time taught me a lesson about disclosing too much.)

There are interviewers in all the media who enjoy controversy and antagonizing guests, but this is not usually the case. The best way to handle this type of person is to be well prepared and to remain calm. In radio and television the audience will usually side with the person they like and respect the most. When you take telephone calls over the air from the public, there is risk involved, but remaining calm is the best defense, along with a sense of humor and being well prepared. (I always liked answering a caller with, "That's a great question! I will look it up and answer it on next week's show." You can only do that once or twice, however, before viewers want to know what you do know.)

At a newspaper, writers will write whatever they want anyway. So, keep the discussion lively, but keep to the facts as you know them. Try not to be drawn into emotional controversies that have no satisfactory answers. Don't be afraid to have an opinion, however. Sometimes the best answer is to briefly discuss what the research shows and to say there is no proven or agreed upon answer to the problem.

Media Tour

On media spokesperson tours just about anything can and does happen. If you decide to go into this line of work, keep a sense of humor. There will be times the interviewer tells you on the air that your product may be healthy but leaves a lot to be desired in the taste category, or only rich yuppie athletes will buy it, or whatever. They want to get a rise out of you. That is why it's so important to carefully choose which products you represent...because you may have to defend them, and your credibility and reputation are closely associated with the products.

Interviews are cut or lengthened while you are on the air or two seconds before you start. You may be told you have thirty seconds instead of the scheduled two minutes in which you must entertain the audience, introduce your product, and yet not be commercial. You are trying to please the audience, the station, the client, the public relations firm, your professional peers and yourself---the pressure is intense at times. That is why the client trains you to give the key public service messages that position your product in a good light or as the answer to a problem. For example, "A new study shows Americans eat 50% of their daily fat in snacks", and you have a low fat cheese and other ideas for snacks. Or, "Caffeine can make people nervous and have sleepless nights", and you discuss herb teas without caffeine, along with other caffeine-free beverages.

Handling the Session

Be very aware of time limitations. Make your answers interesting and to the point. Unless it is the only appropriate answer, don't just answer with a yes or no. Use examples to make your selling point. And, it's very important that you listen to questions and conversation instead of just thinking about your next statement, because you may be caught off guard with a simple, "What do you think about that, Ms. Jones?"

93 Bridging is a conversation tool used by anyone who wants to change the direction of questioning. The best guests don't evade the difficult questions---they restructure them. Before answering a question you don't like or that doesn't fit your needs, volunteer additional or different information introduced by a lead-in clause, such as: "Let us consider the larger issue here ...", or "We are all upset about that, but you should be aware of...", or "Another issue the public is even more upset about is..." (1)

Trained guests volunteer much more than the required information when they like a question. No question is sacred, and none need be answered slavishly. It is possible, through bridging, to bring up more interesting issues than the interviewer asked. (1)

The A or B Dilemma is where the interviewer asks a question and only gives two answers to choose from, both of which put you on the spot. An example would be, "Why do dietitians have such unrealistic ideas about what people eat? Is it because of poor training or aren't they observant?" What would you say? Probably, the best answer would be to disagree with the original statement or avoid the trap by offering an alternative not given by the interviewer.

Don't echo any negative words like "rip-off" or "cancer-alley."(3) Don't restate hostile questions used by the interviewer.

Whenever you are on the premises of a media interview, be cautious of things you might say or do. When in a radio or television studio, always be aware that a "live" microphone or panning camera may be picking you up. On the premises is not the time to mention in idle conversation to a colleague or friend the hospital kitchen was just closed by the Health Department or a patient is suing you or your client for malpractice.

After the Interview

Obviously, after an interview take a moment to thank interviewers for their time and express a desire to do it again sometime. If no offer is forthcoming, offer to be a resource person, leave your card, and plan to call again in a month or two.

REFERENCES

1. Hilton J. On Television! A Survival Guide For Media Interviews. New York: Amacom; 1981.
2. Lant J. The Unabashed Self-promoters Guide What Every Man, Woman, Child and Organization in America Needs to Know About Getting Ahead by Exploiting the Media. JLA Publications; 1983.
3. Berg K, Rosenau N. CommCore Media Skills Workshop manual. New York; 1990.

HERMAN

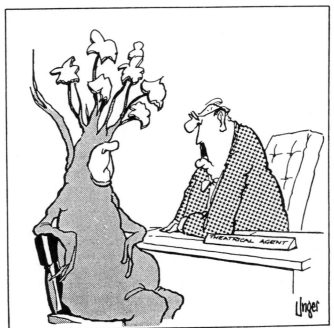

"I know you want to play Hamlet, but for this one television commercial you're a stick of celery."

Chapter 29

Sports and Cardiovascular Nutrition

Marilyn Schorin, PhD, RD, Karen Reznick Dolins, MS, RD,
Updated by Kathy King, RD

These are exciting times to be a sports or cardiovascular nutritionist. Opportunities for dietitians in these areas abound and continue to grow. Dietitians find positions at sports and fitness centers, wellness programs, cardiovascular clinics, spas, and as consultants to sports teams and athletes at all levels and abilities. They are hired as consultants to food manufacturers and as media spokespersons for health or fitness-related products or services.

Crowds in health clubs, spas and wellness programs, and the number of bikers and runners on the streets show the public's awareness of healthy living. Clients' ages and levels of physical conditioning, as well as their motivations, vary, posing a bold challenge to a dietitian's professional capabilities. Young athletes are interested in maximizing performance with foods and timing of meals. Adult clients seek ways to become fit, prevent disease and control their weight.

These two specialties are discussed as one in this chapter, because both have a strong exercise physiology component and deal closely with cardiac output. In practice, many places of employment offer both sports and cardiovascular rehabilitation services, making it necessary for the dietitian to know in-depth information about both. Dietitians' growing interest in this area of practice is mirrored by the growth in membership in the Sports and Cardiovascular Nutritionists (SCAN) Dietetic Practice Group of The American Dietetic Association. SCAN is now ADA's second largest practice group.

WHAT KNOWLEDGE AND TRAINING IS NECESSARY?

We are acutely sensitive to marginally trained lay people or health care professionals (with no background in nutrition) advertising their expertise in our field. It follows, that we must have appropriate training. The dietitian who is an expert in sports and cardiovascular nutrition must have at least a basic knowledge of each of the areas listed below.

Baseline subjects for sports and cardiovascular specialists include:
- Nutritional science
- Biochemistry
- Physiology, especially exercise physiology
- Cardiovascular disease etiology and treatment
- Sports rules, training, common injuries, ergogenic aids, verbiage
- Counseling skills
- Communication skills

There is no degree or certificate necessary to call oneself a sports or cardiovascular nutritionist. However, most practitioners have had special training (in a fitness or cardiac disease, CPR, or sports injury class), or additional degrees in exercise physiology, athletic training, aerobic dance, or nutrition with a sports nutrition emphasis.

Nutrition Science

First and foremost, of course, is a working knowledge of nutrition science and food composition. Sports and cardiovascular dietitians must know general information about foods, as well as such facts as which cuts of beef offer the lowest saturated fat content and which types of fish are the best sources of omega-3 fatty acids. They must know the nutrient composition of specific brand names. For example, which brand of cereal can be recommended for its high soluble fiber content, as well as being low in sugar and sodium? Which fast foods provide a high school athlete with the most amount of carbohydrate, with the least amount of fat?

Always be up on the latest. For example, recommendations regarding optimal carbohydrate concentration in sports drinks have changed in recent years. The sports nutritionist should be familiar with ergogenic aids, and their contents, being promoted to athletes. He or she should know the carbohydrate content and sources (sucrose, fructose, glucose polymers) of the various sports drinks on the market and the practical differences between them.

The mass media picks up on research published in credible medical journals and turns it into news. Articles frequently appear in the newspaper the day after a study has been published, and the implications of such studies are often exaggerated. Physicians and clients alike may ask your opinion on a story-relating intake of oat bran or garlic to blood cholesterol levels. You will gain their respect if you are ready with a knowledgeable answer.

Biochemistry

Sports and cardiovascular dietitians need a working knowledge of the metabolism of macronutrients and the interrelationships among energy-providing fuels. A sports nutritionist should know which substrate is being used for fuel at a particular intensity of exercise. If they have not kept up with lipid metabolism, some advanced training, education or assiduous review of the literature is critical. The biochemistry of exercise is a fascinating, but complex subject, yet it is essential to grasp its intricacies in order to explain it in terms appropriate to each client. It is difficult to advise very learned athletes and fitness enthusiasts on their nutritional requirements without a comprehensive understanding of the biochemistry and physiology involved.

Physiology

A clear understanding of muscle morphology is necessary when talking to athletes, coaches and trainers. The specialist in this field must know terminology like red and white muscle fibers and fast-twitch and slow-twitch fibers when conversing with medical and exercise specialists. Cardiovascular nutritionists will be familiar, of course, with digestion from a background in dietetics, but they need more advanced knowledge of cardiovascular and respiratory physiology, as well as hormones.

Cardiovascular Disease

Cardiovascular dietitians require greater proficiency in the treatment of heart disease. The various drugs used to treat angina, cardiac arrhythmias and hypertension should be recognized. Special emphasis should be made to know the common nutrient interactions caused by these pharmacological agents. The dietitian's effectiveness is increased by knowing other modalities of treatment for heart patients, like techniques for stress reduction, smoking cessation, and exercise prescription.

Sports Knowledge

The best way to become successful as a sports nutritionist is by knowing the sport and the people in sports. You can have all the nutrition knowledge in the world, but if you can't make it apply to the sport you are targeting, you are of no use to an athlete, trainer or team.

Make sure you know the rules of the sport. For example, some sports have weight requirements to limit weight, and other sports want increased weight. Learn about training schedules. Do athletes train throughout the year, or is there a season? How many hours per day do they train? What is their training regimen? Do they cross train? What types of injuries are they prone to? Is nutrition considered an important adjunct in recuperation from injury? When dealing with professional athletes, this point is crucial.

Know the commonly accepted guidelines for body weight and body fat in an athlete's sport. Know that it may be different for various positions on the team. The sports nutritionist can be valuable to a sports team by measuring body composition to determine appropriate body weight based on percent body fat. Keep up on the latest research in the area of sports drinks. Be able to discuss the benefits of different beverages, including water. Know which sports are prone to problems with dehydration.

Advertisements for nutritional supplements are attractive to athletes interested in enhancing their performance and gaining the "competitive edge". The sports nutritionist must be able to discuss this issue with the athlete without appearing judgmental. Remember that placebos often work! Visit the local health food store at regular intervals to keep in touch with the latest in ergogenics.

Know the energy requirements of the sport and which energy systems are used. Power lifters are not going to deplete their glycogen stores, so advice in this area is less valuable to them than to a basketball or soccer player. Baseball players and sprinters do not rely on endurance to win. When addressing them, hydration issues, or possibly weight control for the player, will be a more relevant topic.

Counseling

The dietitian who concentrates on sports and cardiovascular nutrition needs to have well-honed counseling skills. Like all aspects of dietetics, counseling achieves its greatest impact when these three factors prevail: 1) the client is highly motivated, 2) a relationship is established between the counselor and client, and 3) the nutritionist helps the client achieve small, manageable steps. Male and female athletes are motivated by improvements in performance; they constantly seek the competitive edge. Nutrition has been touted to them as a type of snake oil in which anything from carbo-loading to bee pollen may provide that edge. Their motivation is, fortunately, not usually a problem.

On the other hand, the high-risk client for cardiovascular disease may feel "fine" and therefore, resist making any dietary changes. A skilled counselor can dispel resistance, increase motivation, build confidence in client's ability to make dietary changes, and promote maintenance of positive salutary changes.

Communication

Through a concerted effort to expand one's audience, the sports and cardiovascular dietitian can reach many people via other methods. When the message is relayed through an indirect medium, expertise in writing and public speaking is demanded. Some other effective modes of communication with clients include:

- Individualized counseling
- Classes on specific topics
- Lectures
- Articles written in lay publications
- Radio and television appearances
- Web page, sports column on another website
- Online counseling

Commonly used approaches include seminars, supermarket tours or food demonstrations. Classes may be offered through hospitals, adult education programs, junior colleges, or health clubs. More corporations welcome the opportunity to provide on-site instruction for their employees as part of corporate wellness programs.

Should the nutrition specialist prefer to avoid the constraints of regularly scheduled meetings, lectures offer an alternative avenue for educating the public. Finding an audience for lecturing is usually easy. Examples include business and professional clubs, religious and community groups, and self-help groups for topics related to nutrition and the heart. The YMCA/YWCAs, fitness clubs, coach conferences, school groups, and amateur sports groups want speakers on sports nutrition. Some lectures may be given for free, to help market you, and to get to know local athletes and their coaches. At other times a fee may be paid by the sponsoring organization.

WHO IS THE CLIENTELE?

Sports and cardiovascular nutritionists have limitless opportunities. This section will be directed at four specific groups of people who provide excellent targets for our services. These are:

- Professional athletes
- Recreational athletes
- School age athletes
- Patients with high risk of cardiovascular disease

Professional Athletes

The glamour certainly lies with the big names. Who wouldn't want to play a role in the success of such superstars as Michael Jordan, Joan Benoit Samuelson or Tiger Woods? Although such opportunities are not out of the question, there are of course very few of these superstars to go around. Also, there are many other health professionals, coaches and trainers who want the chance to work with the big name athletes and are willing to do it for free or a greatly reduced price. So, competition is sometimes stiff to get your foot in the door. Dietitians with professional football, basketball, hockey, and baseball teams are usually paid good hourly fees, however, there are no full time positions and often only sporadic hours at the beginning of a season and as-needed thereafter. It's not unusual to be "paid" with a T-shirt, season tickets, or a gate pass when the teams or athletes can't afford any other compensation.

Recreational Athletes

Most of us will have a better chance earning a livelihood by focusing on the legions of athletes outside the realm of the top pros. Recreational athletes are overflowing our biking and running clubs, walking trails and pools. Communities abound with health-oriented adults determined to live longer and healthier. Sports and health clubs provide a source of motivated clientele who may wonder why pounds aren't dropping off as they drip buckets of sweat while working out on the Stairmaster or exercise bicycle. Other clients work out on their own and just want to know how to lose body fat and stay motivated on a diet.

Practice settings and financial arrangements vary. Some nutritionists find it helpful to set up shop within a fitness facility or sports medicine clinic, while others set up a referral system and counseling in their own

How Do You Create a Successful Business in a Fitness Center?
Diana Burge, RD

What are the keys to your success for working in a fitness center environment?

My office was located in the reputable sports medical center inside the health club. I heavily marketed my business to the club's personal trainers and membership directors. I tracked who referred the most clients and at the end of each month I gave a gift to the best referral agent. I provided quarterly education workshops for the trainers and the members of the club. Each client's physician received a progress report. I advertised in the local newspaper and Yellow Pages. This opened doors to speaking for groups and becoming known by the local pro sports teams.

How important was support from the club or other referral sources?

I did not receive many referrals from the fitness staff for the first one to two years; it improved after I became established and better known. My main referral sources were physicians and word of mouth. It's important to have multiple sources though because many physicians moved over the years or hired their own RDs.

What kind of arrangement for space do you recommend to other dietitians?

I recommend having your own space-not shared space in a Manager's office or employee lounge. In regards to payment, I recommend starting by paying a percentage of your income with a 40% cap, but hopefully lower. After a year, pay a flat rent per square foot. Don't expect the fitness center to provide for you. You need to be a self-starter and want to work more as a sub-contractor not employee.

offices. Practitioners may choose to work in a facility in a salaried position, at an hourly rate, or set their own rates and pay a percentage to the facility to help cover any overhead. Group lectures can be a practitioner's main source of income, or it can be a marketing vehicle offered for free or at a reduced cost to introduce large numbers of people to the practitioner's services. Working with the recreational athlete can be stimulating and financially rewarding work.

CASE STUDY

When Nancy Clark, MS, RD, was beginning her practice, she wanted the credibility that comes with being part of a large medical practice. Therefore, she contacted Dr. William Southmayd, the medical director of Sports Medicine Brookline, one of the largest athletic injury clinics in the country. He welcomed this opportunity to include a nutritionist on the medical team, and they were able to agree to terms.

Nancy set up shop in the clinic and quickly realized that despite the high traffic flow, she would have to do more than simply put out her shingle and wait for physician referrals. She embarked on a promotional campaign to the patients through brochures in the waiting room explaining the benefits of sports nutrition counseling. She coached her professional colleagues to look for possible nutrition related conditions like anemia, stress fractures and slow-to-heal injuries.

She increased her national visibility through speaking, writing sports nutrition columns for several lay magazines and authoring three books, *The Athlete's Kitchen*, *Nancy Clark's Sports Nutrition Book*, and *Nancy Clark's New York Marathon Nutrition Book.*

Nancy finds it valuable to remain visible to her target markets by being a member of a local bike and a running club in order to be athletic herself. She encourages everyone who wants to become a sports nutritionist to be patient. It takes time to build a client base.

School Aged Athletes

Young athletes provide a wide open market for sound nutritional advice. In the fall an athlete may be using protein powders to bulk up for football, while the winter months may find him eating less than one meal per day trying to make weight for wrestling. Young girls in gymnastics and ballet often skip meals in order to reduce their weight. However, before practice many may succumb to vending machine sweets for a quick "pick-me-up," while after practice there is fast food. A balanced dinner at home may only be picked at.

These students need help, not just in deciding what and how much to eat, but also when. Salient suggestions the nutritionist can offer regarding food choices and timing of meals can make a difference in both their athletic and academic performance. These budding sportsmen and sportswomen must be shown that focusing on weight without regard to body fat or adequate nourishment is an ineffective way to achieve an athletic body.

Nutrition services are not typically included in school budgets. Funding for services may come from a parent, a Booster Club, or the PTA, if there is funding. When money is tight, group talks are the most efficient vehicle for getting the message to the greatest number of people. It also gives an opportunity for nutrition misinformation to be aired. Many sports nutritionists give their time to schools without pay or with only modest payment because of the fun and satisfaction of working with the kids. It's also a good place to hone skills before trying to work with the top athletes, and it may lead to more paying clients or job referrals.

CASE STUDY

Karen Reznick Dolins: I began my private practice while working at a major medical center as a clinical dietitian. A physician with the affiliated medical school was opening a hyperlipidemia clinic and needed a registered dietitian. I made the contact, and I was off and running. When the medical school opened a cardiac rehabilitation facility, I was offered the opportunity to open a private practice in nutrition counseling.

I cut my hours back at the medical center, but my private practice soon took up so many hours, I resigned as clinical dietitian. I maintained my contacts with the dietary department and the hospital physicians, both of whom continue to refer patients.

Once I made the move to private practice, I broadened my referral network by writing to all area cardiologists. Each letter was followed up with a phone call, and invaluable contacts were made. One medical group of six physicians preferred to have an in-house nutritionist. As this large practice provided great opportunities, I agreed to spend one day a week at their office on a fee-for-service basis.

Physicians continue to be a major referral source for me. I see a number of physicians as clients, and they in turn become referral sources. When the NCEP guidelines were published, I took advantage of them by sending a copy to all the physicians I work with, highlighting the areas about the value of the RD. Now that I am well established in my community many clients are referred by former clients. My practice has grown over the years to include a variety of corporate clients, athletes and a teaching position at a local university.

I tried advertising in local papers early on, but found it to be unproductive. I found that word-of -mouth advertising was my best promotion. To enhance my skills, I took advantage of a nutrition-counseling workshop offered by the local chapter of the American Heart Association. In addition to making me more proficient in this area, the workshop gave me the opportunity to network with other RDs involved in this type of counseling. My advice to other RDs developing a practice in this area is to be sure that you have a strong referral network. Thanks to the attention focused on the efficacy of cholesterol lowering in recent years, few would argue with the benefits of nutrition counseling for these patients. The field is wide open. Go for it!

CONFIRMED HEART DISEASE

Cardiovascular disease remains a major cause of morbidity and mortality in the United States. Personalized nutrition counseling is vital for these patients. An intensive approach with a Step 2 diets defined by the NCEP and the AHA is required. Dietary cholesterol intake should be under 200 mg. daily and saturated fat less than seven percent of calories. A registered dietitian can individualize this strict prescription according to the patients' preferences, making it more palatable. Working one-on-one helps compliance. The dietitian must be patient and flexible, often working slowly to decrease the saturated fat and cholesterol content of the diet and achieve the above goal. These patients may be on a prescribed exercise program, and coordination between the dietitian, exercise therapist and cardiologist will achieve maximal results.

WHERE TO GET INFORMATION

Although the need for adequate initial training is emphasized above, equally important is keeping up with new information and materials. Included in this area are professional meetings, reading selected journals and networking with colleagues. Sports and Cardiovascular Nutritionist (SCAN) of the American Dietetic Association represents a broad group of Registered Dietitians who are working in this area. They publish a quarterly newsletter and hold an annual symposium.

American College of Sports Medicine, headquartered in Indianapolis, Indiana, represents over fifty different professions involved in sports, exercise and fitness. They also hold an annual meeting and publish a monthly journal. A suggested bibliography follows.

SUGGESTED BIBLIOGRAPHY

Nutrition and Cardiovascular Disease

Kris-Etherton PM (Ed). Cardiovascular Disease: Nutrition for Prevent Treatment. Sports and Cardiovascular Nutritionists Practice GI American Dietetic Association, Chicago, IL; 1990.

Sports Nutrition

Benardot D (Ed). Sports Nutrition: A Guide for the Professional Won With Active People, 2nd edition. Sports and Cardiovascular Nutritionists Practice Group, American Dietetic Association.

Berning J, Steen S. Nutrition for Sport and Exercise. Gaithersburg, MD: Aspen Pub.; 1998.

Clark N. Nancy Clark's Sports Nutrition Guidebook. Champaign, IL: Leisure Press; 1990.

Coleman E. Eating For Endurance. Palo Alto, CA: Bull Pub.; 1997.

McArdle W. Exercise Physiology: Energy, Nutrition and Human Performance. Philadelphia: Lea and Febiger; 2001.

Peterson M, Peterson K. Eat to Compete. Yearbook Med. Pub; 1996.

Smith N, Roberts BW. Food For Sport. Palo Alto, CA: Bull Pub.; 1989.

JOURNALS/NEWSLETTERS

Pulse, The newsletter of the Sports and Cardiovascular Nutrition Dietetic Practice Group, free with $20 annual membership, 4 issues per yr. Write for subscription to SCAN c/o ADA, 216 W. Jackson Blvd., Chicago, IL 60606-6995.

Sports Science Exchange, Gatorade Sports Science Institute, P. O. Box 9005, Chicago, IL 60604-9005.

Medicine and Science in Sports and Exercise, bimonthly, free with membership in the American College of Sports Medicine.

International Journal of Sports Nutrition, quarterly, Human Kinetics Publishers, Box 5076 ,Champaign, IL 61825-5076.

CONTINUING EDUCATION

Nutrition for Sport and Exercise. Book by Jackie Berning and Suzanne Nelson Steen. Course by Kathy King. Helm Publishing, toll-free (877) 560-6025. 25 CPE hours.

Chapter 30
The Wellness Movement
Kathy King, RD, Wendy Perkins, MSW, MPA

Wanting "wellness" and other self-help information is an ongoing trend of a large segment of American people and businesses. Many people are excited about taking more responsibility for their own health and lives, while others don't want to be bothered but are becoming more aware out of financial necessity.

Kindy Peaslee, RD, a wellness consultant in New York, shares that in 2000, as more businesses devoted increased money toward health care, only 5 percent was going to preventive health care-95 percent went to treat illness. In 2015, experts estimate 40 percent of the workforce will be 60 years of age or older, as compared to only 6.2 percent in 2000. Given these statistics, corporate executives are beginning to think differently about wellness. (1)

The research regularly offers proof that a person's cardiovascular fitness, stress management and general health can be improved through lifestyle changes made by the individual.

WHAT IS WELLNESS?

The term "wellness," although we consider it new and futuristic, is what many people have been saying for ages should be health care's major concern---prevention, or keeping well people (the majority of us) well. Wellness involves striving for a state of health that is not just absent from disease, but optimum. People get into wellness programs to be healthier, to enjoy their lives, spend more quality time with their families, and feel better.

Most wellness leaders assert that wellness is a multidisciplinary approach to health. It is not just exercise or nutrition or stopping smoking or handling stress or making better choices. It is all of these and more. What wellness programs offer depends upon variables such as client interests, financial support, availability of stimulating teachers, and the business' leadership. Typically, programs include encouraging physical fitness, good nutrition and healthy lifestyle choices. However, it is not uncommon for only one of these areas to be stressed more heavily, often to the exclusion of the other two.

Charles Sterling, Ed.D., Executive Director of Cooper's Institute for Aerobics Research in Dallas, Texas states, "Holistic is associated with treatments of all sorts used to attain good health. Wellness is a lifestyle approach to realizing your best potential for physical health, mental alertness and serenity. It is not about extending your life or curing disease." (2)

In his book, *High Level Wellness,* Dr. Don Ardell explains that traditional medicine usually stops treatment when a patient's disability or symptoms no longer exist. Wellness starts taking place when patients become educated about their bodies and good health, when they practice new health habits, and take responsibility for their own bodies by keeping them healthy. (3)

The Wellness Mind Set

For traditionally trained health professionals, the wellness concept may require a new mindset about their role as health providers. No longer does the medical professional do the work and make all of the decisions for a passive patient. Patients are taught the responsibility for their wellness is theirs.The health provider becomes teacher, friend and information specialist, as well as provider.

Wellness doesn't involve quick, curative measures, such as drugs and surgery; instead one works with something much more challenging---the human mind. The wellness-oriented medical specialist works with changing habits, giving guidance to people who may feel well, are energetic and are excited about life.

Health professionals who are not wellness-oriented have problems understanding how they are supposed to help this individual, since there isn't anything to cure. People must motivate themselves, but the professional can help by using the three components of successful behavior change:
1. Raise a person's awareness and assess stage of motivation or change, (use lifestyle questionnaires, stress tests, blood pressure, lab values, fitness testing, diet evaluation, and so on).
2. Provide skills and knowledge to facilitate behavior change.
3. Provide reinforcement, environmental and cultural changes (cafeteria alterations, bike tracks, follow-up visits, peer support, and so on).
Without these three factors change does not happen.

The biggest challenge that nutritionists have with wellness is learning about the normal individual and making normal nutrition exciting to the listener or reader. Good marketing is essential. Merely having fantastic handout information will not have people flocking to the door. The presentations must be interesting, fun, stimulating, creative, timely, and packaged well. For the first time in our nutritional careers, our effectiveness may depend 80 to 90 percent upon our personal skills, instead of our knowledge. Successful program directors are aware of that fact and are looking for nutritionists with unique skills in effective speaking, leadership, marketing, and public relations.

WHY WELLNESS NOW?

The wellness concept is growing and coming into its own now because of problems in our present medical system, and because statistics are being generated by reputable sources that show positive results of wellness programs.

The way medicine has been practiced, acute care with passive patients and too much managed care, has reached its limits in public acceptance. Many physicians believe that iatrogenic care (physician-induced problems) and misdiagnosis may cause far more discomfort to a patient than the flu or infection that precipitated the medical visit.

Many patients want good, prudent state of the art medical care from caring health professionals who involve their patients in the decision-making. After the symptoms disappear, growing numbers of patients want to know what they can do to keep the symptoms or illness from recurring. Patients and their families are usually scared and motivated at this time to adjust their life habits to help avoid problems later.

MEASURABLE RESULTS

Trying to measure the results of a wellness program is difficult. Some changes, such as attitude improvement and better quality of life, are so subjective they are not easily quantified. The indices used are aerobic fitness, absenteeism, medical claim costs, sick days, accidents on the job, and productivity. However, variables other than a wellness program may influence these indices.

Companies with employee wellness programs are becoming more plentiful. Pioneer programs have reported their preliminary results: Reduction in job-related accidents, reduced medical claims, lower absenteeism, reduction in lost work hours, and reduction in disability costs. The results are encouraging and indicate that altering one's lifestyle may produce measurable, as well as very personal, health improvements.

CORPORATE WELLNESS PROGRAMS ————————————

Businesses are understandably interested in the boost in productivity output and morale good lifestyle changes can produce. The financial savings produced by some companies are also very impressive, though other businesses have tried and failed to duplicate such reductions in costs.

When wellness programs are introduced into the workplace, it is imperative that employees are approached correctly, especially when unions are involved. The motives for encouraging wellness can be misinterpreted, or sometimes interpreted correctly, as coming from management for purely financial reasons (instead of their purported humanitarian ones).

Some companies have begun programs that spread some of the financial savings around. They offer bonus plans when fewer sick days are used, mental health days off, bonuses for exercise participation and stopping smoking, all in the hope of changing lifestyles. Some companies use peer teachers to train and encourage their colleagues, while others use competitions or private professional counseling.

Consulting nutritionists can perform a variety of services for a corporate program: counsel clients, adjust cafeteria menus, train other staff members, give speeches, write newsletters and brochures, make videos, and so on.

There are several interesting corporate wellness programs created by dietitians. One program described by Donna Israel, PhD, RD, president of Preferred Nutrition Therapists (7), is at Texas Instruments, Inc. in Dallas, Texas. PNT negotiated a service where nutrition therapy would be covered for its self-referred employees with nutrition-related medical problems. "The goal was to use MNT as a toll to prevent the progression of clients' diseases to states that require more costly treatments."(7)
(This full article can be downloaded at
www.eatright.org/images/gov/1999Israel.pdf).

Another corporate dietitian is Linda Welch, MS, RD who works as the Worksite Wellness Coordinator for Home Depot. "Welch organizes a variety of wellness programs-from quarterly mammogram screenings and lactation classes to annual golf and tennis tournaments. She provides one-on-one nutrition counseling for employees, coordinates lunchtime seminars, and has even conducted a healthy eating teleconference for 150,000

Home Depot employees nationwide." (8) Besides her nutrition training, Linda holds a certification as a health fitness instructor through the American College of Sports Medicine. (8)

WELLNESS IN HOSPITAL SYSTEMS

Hospital systems are interested in the wellness concept for several reasons. It offers public relations opportunities to improve the image of the hospital in the community. It may reduce health care costs for self-insured institutions or give premium breaks to those who have an outside insurer. It can offer a source of income by offering community and corporate outreach programs.

Creating an in-house wellness program presents many challenges for an institution. Obtaining financing is usually not as difficult as gaining consensus about programming, staffing and defining wellness. The most successful programs use an integrated approach to wellness, treating equally the importance of nourishment, being physically fit and making lifestyle choices.

Wellness Programs Come in Many Forms

Facilities for wellness programs vary from the very elaborate with exercise equipment, pool, masseuse or masseur, jogging track, and meeting room to only an office for one or two people to coordinate the programs for a staff of consultants in a variety of outlying locations.

Special events offered by wellness programs include sponsoring races, health fairs and wellness retreats, as well as 900 education phone lines and media spots on health topics. Classes and seminars cover topics such as:
- alcohol or smoking cessation,
- stress management and relaxation,
- all facets of recreational sports,
- prenatal care,
- parenting,
- healthful cooking,
- vegetarian diets,
- weight loss,
- aerobic and strength exercises,
- kick boxing, tai chi and
- flexibility exercises.

In a corporate setting, there are also programs on self-esteem, communication, team building, time management, and wellness as a whole person or whole organization effort.

WINNING A NUTRITION POSITION IN WELLNESS ———

Most wellness programs assume that nutrition is a necessary component of health. However, that assumption does not necessarily include programs or having a registered dietitian giving the nutrition information. Today, ethical information on basic nutrition is readily available. Dietitians face competition in wellness settings even in some hospitals from at least exercise instructors, health educators, nurses, exercise physiologists, and physicians. However, dietitians who distinguish themselves with exciting teaching skills, creative programs and marketing, and current nutrition knowledge will always have jobs-it just takes time.

Several years ago, a hospital in a Denver suburb decided to cut expenses at their wellness program and only keep the programs that were generating a profit. That left only the dietitian on staff. Eventually, she built up her staff and wielded much more professional weight because she had demonstrated fiscal profitability.

Wellness programs are looking for dietitians or dietetic technicians who are assertive leaders, while appreciating what other wellness professionals have to offer. Appreciation of the team approach is vital. It is also important we understand the "larger picture" of the organization, and contribute to financial goals.

Seeking Leads and Making Contacts

Hospitals and corporations are usually very good about advertising available positions on their staff. However, to be associated with a wellness program during its beginning developmental stages, contact should be made early. In other words, it will be necessary to "cold call" many institutions to establish your interest.

Promote yourself for the position with:
- a good resume written with emphasis on skills and experience useful in a wellness program,
- an impressive review of wellness research showing the cost savings of programming to improve diabetes control, weight loss and overall health,

- provide copies of published articles about you or your programs,
- booklets or teaching materials you've written,
- brochures or flyers promoting your programs or speaking and, finally,
- an oral or written proposal for their program.

If you do not have enough information to offer suggestions on the first visit, offer to write a simple proposal after you meet. Try to return the proposal within a week so they feel your work is timely and efficient.

Dietitians can be hired as employees (and acquire all of the benefits of a salaried person). They must be willing to accept the fact the institution owns the developed materials and programs (unless negotiated otherwise).

Wellness programs also hire consultant dietitians either individually or as part of a group of consultants. Consultants are often paid to bring expertise that is not easily found, or their passion to inspire a program. Usually the materials created belong to whoever paid for their development. Some consultants prefer to create them on their own time and then sell the materials or license the rights to an institution. These dietitians prefer to take more risk and the responsibility for their own vacations, insurance and continuing educations in return for more money and freedom.

Nutrition Services to Offer

Dietitians offer a variety of services to wellness programs. They include nutrition counseling one-on-one or conducting weight loss classes with an exercise specialist or psychologist. More dietitians are beginning to offer diabetes education classes, since diabetes is the most expensive chronic disease for medical insurers to cover. Others work with the cafeteria to change recipes and menu items to lower fat and sugar or "gourmet natural." Some wellness programs are also interested in dietitians who have media experience and can do media interviews, cable and video programs. Dietitians with writing skills and experience are in demand by programs to produce educational materials for sale. Computer expertise has opened doors for some dietitians when wellness programs wanted to produce their own educational software.

WHY WELLNESS PROGRAMS FAIL ————————————

Even wellness programs with good financing and staffs can have problems and eventually fail. In surveys conducted by Robert Allen, Ph.D., and reported in "The Corporate Health-Buying Spree: Boon or Boondoggle?" he found:

Six factors that contribute to failure:
1. Fragmentation of effort--timing, organization or marketing were off.
2. Overemphasis on initial motivation--lack of long-term effect or follow through.
3. Misdirected emphasis on illness--trying to motivate by avoiding disease, instead of encouraging the positive potential of a healthy lifestyle.
4. Appeal to individual heroics--there is a need for a supportive environment that is not competitive.
5. Overemphasis on activities as opposed to results--a successful program produces lifestyle changes, not just good attendance.
6. A "we will do it for you" approach, rather than a better "together we can do it for ourselves" attitude--avoid passive programs. (4)

MARKETING AND PROMOTION ARE MUSTS! ————————

Wellness programs must recognize early on that their competition is in the private sector. They do not have the luxury of a "captive audience." Unlike a hospitalized patient, wellness participants are not ill and do not require immediate treatment. Therefore, employees and the community have to be enticed and excited about the programs being offered or they will go elsewhere, if they go at all.

It will take a while for the image of a center to become established and for the staff, classes and programs to become known. More time and money must be spent up front to acquaint prospective clients with you and what you offer. It may be necessary to market your program with introductory "brown bag" talks to nurses on the patient floors or to employees at a bank, or give a pre-race seminar.

To promote an individual program, such as a new weight loss series, marketing tools could include: An easy to remember name and logo, colorful posters, brochures, and folders for handout materials, and a personal letter to all department heads or physicians promoting the classes. Display t-shirts that will be given out at the class. Use paycheck stuffers and newsletters to promote the program. Ads can be purchased in local newspapers. Public service announcements are effective through local media and, occasionally, a local newspaper will write an article and take photographs.

Marketing is so important and critical to the survival of your programs. Don't leave it to chance, and don't assume that someone else has it all under control. Stay on top of marketing!

REFERENCES

1. Peaslee K. On the Job Wellness. Today's Dietitian; September 2000.
2. Fitness Leadership Program Manual. Dallas, TX: Cooper Clinic Publisher; March 1983: 21-25.
3. Ardell D. High Level Wellness. New York, NY: Bantam; 1979: 1.
4. Allen RF. The Corporate Health Buying Spree: Boon or Boondoggle? New York: American Management Association;1980.
5. Fitness Leadership Program. Dallas, TX: Cooper Clinic; 1983: 21-25.
6. Kimberly-Clark Health Management Program Aimed at Prevention. Occupational Health and Safety. November/December 1977: 25.
7. Israel D, McCabe M. Using disease-state management as the key to promoting employer sponsorship of medical nutrition therapy. J Am Diet Assoc: 1999; 99:5.
8. Career Snapshots: Linda Welch, RD. ADA Courier. April 1999.

Chapter 31
Continued Competency

Our consumers often take it for granted that dietitians and dietetic technicians stay current with new advances in the field of nutrition. However, staying up-to-date is not a task that can be accomplished by attending a meeting or two a year and skimming a monthly journal.

The rate of change in nutrition and its related specialties is happening faster than we have ever experienced before, and it will continue that way for some time. Money is finally starting to be earmarked for research in nutrition, and "new" breakthroughs are regularly hitting the media. Government expectations are demanding changes in nutrition documentation and expected output. "Outside" competition to nutrition practice is growing. The use of high technology, the computer and Internet in particular, requires that we add new skills in our practice. New counseling techniques and human behavior skills from other disciplines need to be employed to make us more effective. The public expects us to take stands on the issues and provide better information than they can get from a television reporter. Maintaining the status quo will drop us behind.

New emerging fields of study like Functional Medicine started by Jeffrey Bland, PhD, has Functional Nutrition Therapy as a cornerstone of its philosophy. The therapy believes in reestablishing the normal function or balance of body function by balancing the nutrients needed for normal organ function and biochemical processes in the body. Normal function is influenced positively by certain nutrients or negatively by caffeine, alcohol; poor or imbalanced eating and other factors. Nutrition therapy on the cellular level will be one of the ways medicine is practiced in the future. We need training in Functional Nutrition Therapy.

Merely getting seventy-five hours of continuing education credit every five years will keep a dietitian registered but depending upon the quality of the programs and the subjects chosen to attend, a practitioner may or may not learn anything new. That is why the Commission on Dietetic Registration changed to the portfolio system to help practitioners determine what continuing education topics and methods of learning a person should pursue.

A practitioner's goal should not be to stay registered, but instead to become an expert in some area of dietetics and remain one.

As the marketplaces continue to change, especially for entrepreneurs, it is imperative that dietitians gain non-dietetic experience and attend other disciplines' seminars and educational training. Also, lay literature and world business/economy periodicals should be regularly reviewed. Nutrition can no longer be seen as a narrow field of study. It is an element of life intertwined and influenced by many other constituent parts.

In business, the practitioner is greatly affected by non-dietetic influences. The local and national economies, health care and consumer trends, insurance coverage, competition, and available financing are just a few of the concerns. The more knowledgeable an entrepreneur is about these topics, the more prepared the person will be to handle business life.

Educators tell us the mark of an educated person is one who knows where to look something up. If you subscribe to several newsletters and take the time to read the Periodical Reviews in the back of the Journal of the American Dietetic Association, scanning nutrition-related literature is relatively simple. It is not necessary to purchase all of the most expensive resource books, as long as you have several current ones available to you. World and economic news can be found encapsulated in the daily newspapers. Business news is found in magazines, trade journals, newspapers, and newsletters.

The following list of references is not meant to be a complete list or an endorsement. Practitioners have shared the names of references and resources that have been beneficial to them. You may have additional ones that fit your needs better. Before subscribing to the periodicals, buy a few issues at the newsstand, look up journals in the library, or try online literature searches. Take advantage of trial offers, and don't hesitate to stop publications that do not fit your needs or interests. Staying current can be costly, both in time and money, so evaluate your references carefully.

THE NEW DIETETICS

(Adapted from: Hospital Food Nutrition Focus, July 1985. Reprinted with permission of Aspen Publishers, Inc. Copyright 1985.)

For over 50 years, a few basic diet therapy regimens have consumed the majority of our labor hours. Calorie control, diabetes limitations, sodium, and fat modifications have taken the front seat in terms of interest and deployment of resources. Our menus are devised in accord with the premises of these diets; our very world has depended upon providing services to those patients--patients with diagnoses of obesity, heart disease, diabetes, renal disease, and many others.

In the last decade we have become more sophisticated in our provision of nutritional care. We now focus more closely on laboratory values, on protein (nitrogen) and calorie ratios, and on measuring the relative risk of malnutrition. But the content of the diets we provide has really not changed. There are still low sodium products, controlled fat products, and "magic" mixtures that emanate from the nourishment centers. The nutrients in favor may differ from setting to setting but our basic approach to treatment has been static.

America is in the bionic age. Artificial organs, transplants, and other such medical wonders are becoming commonplace in some settings. Few deny that soon the lifelong behavior modification requirements for diabetes mellitus clients will no longer be necessary---an artificial or transplanted pancreas will eliminate the need for diet control. Liberality in treatment of the aged and increasing knowledge of consumers concerning nutrition has altered the requirements for our services. Sodium modification is no longer universally viewed as the treatment of choice for hypertension and coronary artery disease. Our bread and butter theories are not held in high esteem in all medical circles.

The implications for our profession are clear. Recognizing that many of our staff possess insufficient current knowledge to bridge the gap from the old to the new dietetics, we have a responsibility to provide meaningful continuing education for the seasoned---not just the novice---practitioner.

If we bury our noses in current staffing configurations and fail to look to the future promised by new research, we will be poorly equipped to have a role in the new dietetics.

Certainly, our entire future does not rest on research in the nutrient-brain matrix, bio-engineering, or functional nutrition therapy, but how many of our dietitians have even heard of the research? How many of us have enough familiarity with these activities to respond to the questions of consumers or physicians? If we are acquainted with the research, are we discounting it as "not yet proven", rather than preparing ourselves for potential opportunities?

Are we ready and willing to look beyond our old realm, our old world? Are we prepared to adapt our entrepreneurial approach to the new reality of medical advances?

James C. Rose, R.D., DHCFA, LD Editor

BIBLIOGRAPHY AND REFERENCES

Books

Chenevert M. STA T: Special Techniques in Assertiveness Training for Women in Health Professions. St. Louis, MO: CV Mosby; 1983.

Covey S. The Seven Habits of Highly Effective People. New York: Simon & Schuster; 1989.

Holtz H. How to Succeed as an Independent Consultant. New York: John Wiley; 1993.

Kiyosaki RT. Rich Dad Poor Dad. New York: Warner Books;1998.

Mackay H. Swim With the Sharks Without Being Eaten Alive. New York: Wm. Morrow & Co.; 1996.

Matheson B. Asking For Money: The Entrepreneur's Guide to the Financing Process. Orlando, FL: Financial Systems Associates, Inc.; 1990.

McCormack Mark. What They Don't Teach You at Harvard Business School. New York: Bantam; 1988.

McCormack Mark. What They Still Don't Teach You at Harvard Business School. New York: Bantam; 1990.

Shook Robert. Why Didn't I Think of That! New York: New American Library; 1983.

Zemke R, Albrecht K. Service America! Homewood, IL: Dow-Jones Irwin; 2001.

Zemke R. The Service Edge. New York: New American Library; 1990.

Small Business

ACE (Active Corps Executives): Working business people who volunteer their time to consult with entrepreneurs and conduct seminars.

SCORE (Service Corps of Retired Executives): Retired business people who volunteer their time to consult with entrepreneurs.

SBI (Small Business Institute): Training and classes for entrepreneurs, plus publications.

Small Business Administration offices are located in each state. Look in the telephone book under "U.S. Government" and ask for the address and telephone number of the nearest office.

Newsletters and Journals

American Journal of Clinical Nutrition
Consumer Reports.
Environmental Nutrition
FDA Consumer
Harvard Medical School Health Letter (The)
Journal of American Dietetic Association
Journal of Nutrition Education
Journal of Nutrition for the Elderly
Kiplinger Washington Letter
Nutrition Action
Nutrition and Health, Institute of Human Nutrition, Columbia Univ.
Nutrition and the M.D
Healthy Weight Network
Today's Dietitian
Topics in Clinical Nutrition
Tufts University Diet & Nutrition Letter

Web Sites for Reliable Nutrition

www.arbor.com
www.nutritionucanuse.com
www.navigator.tufts.edu
www.mlm.nih.gov
www.amhrt.org
www.medscape.com
www.vrg.org

INDEX

Aaseng, Nathan, 29
Accountants, 152, 155
Accounting, 170-171, 194, 223
ADA (American Dietetic Association)
   CDR, 418
   and ethics, 62-62
   and marketing, 120
   and third party, 204
Advertising, 66,195, 252-257, 285
Advisors, professional, 149-155
Agreements, 135, 216
Appearance, 74-75
Ardell, Don, 408
Assertiveness, 76, 214
Attorneys, 151, 155
Balance sheet, 165
Bankers, 152, 155, 159-162
Banners, 247, 315
Barone, Orlando, 46-51
Beckwith, Harry, 103-104, 235-236
Berne, Eric, 45-46
Bids, 217
Bland, Jeffery, 417
Bookkeeping, 170-171, 194, 223
Brainstorming, 57-58
Brochures, 194, 246, 248-249
Budget, 171
Buffington, Perry, 55-57
Burge, Diana, 401
Business cards, 193, 242-243
Business closing, 42
Business concept (Executive summary), 96-97
Business consultant, 153-155
Business, failure, 16, 112-113
Business, fears, 4, 13
Business, mature, 39-40
Business plan, 95-100
Business strategies, 27, 30-31
Business success, 17, 27-29, 43, 78
By-line, 308, 371, 386
Cardiovascular nutrition, 397, 404
Careers, 3,8
CPA (Certified Public Accountants), 123, 170
Clark, Nancy, 402
Client-centered therapy, 81-92
Co-leasing, 188-189
Collection, 169
Computers, 221-224, 369-370
Confidentiality, 64, 136, 281-286, 292
Conflict of interest, 67
Consulting, 7, 179, 202, 333
Continuing education, 417-421
Contracts, 216-220, 341
Cooking school directors, 331
Copyrights, 136-142
Corporations, 123-133, 145
   C or "full", 123, 125, 130-133
   LLC   123, 125, 133
   S, 123,125, 133
Counseling, 8, 12, 81-92, 200-201, 398-399

On-line, 91-92, 287, 291
Creativity, 53-60, 74
Credibility, 45-51, 78
Credit cards, 168-169
Credit score, 162
Culinary, 343-365
Cummings, Merilyn, 37
Customer service, 28, 256-257, 273-274
DBA (Doing Business As) name, 124
Delegation, 35
Desk top publishing, 222, 369-370
Dietetic Technician, 331
Direct mail, 245
Dittoe, Alanna, 225
Dodd, Judith, 6
Dolins, Karen Reznick, 395, 403
Dorner, Becky, 42-43, 333
Drucker, Peter, 5
Edwards, Paul & Sarah, 59, 149-150
E-book, 378
E-commerce, 278
E-mail, 259-264, 267, 291, 307-310, 316
Employee, 40, 179, 191, 231
Entrepreneur, 11-24, 240
   Character, 12
   Experience, 22
   Lifestyle, 28
   Strengths, 20
   Weaknesses, 20
Entrepreneurship, 3-9, 11-23
Equipment, 194-195
Ethics, 61-71
Federal Identification number (SS-4), 124
Fees, 197, 228-229
Finances, 157-179
   Cash flow, 164-165, 167
   Loan package, 160-162
   managing, 163-179
   sources, 158
Fitness, 330
Form SS-4, 124
Franz, Marianne, 103, 198
Functional Nutrition Therapy, 3, 8, 417
Give-aways, 249
Global markets, 7
Hess, Mary Abbott, 343, 378
HMOs, 30, 169
Home-based business, 4, 6, 183
Home visits, 184
Image, 73-79, 273
Incorporation, 123-133, 145
IRA (Individual Retirement Account), 176
Information therapy, 261-264
Insurance, 144-145, 191-193
Integrative medicine, 3,8
Intellectual property, 135-138
IRS, Internal Revenue Service, 123
Internet/Web, 256, 259-270
Invention, selling, 114-116
Investment counselor, 155
Israel, Donna, 410

Job, leaving, 22-23
Job market, 2-4
Johnson, Spencer, 6
Kanter, Rosabeth Moss, 5
KEOGH (HR-10) pension plan, 79, 112
Kickback, 66
Laboratory tests, 65
Lambert, Paulette, 81-92
Leasing agreements, 186-189
Legal, 123, 135, 288, 385
Letterheads, 193
Letters
    of agreement, 218-219
    query, 371-373
    reference, 246
Levine, Mark, 5
Libel, 71
Licensing, 124, 288
Lifestyle entrepreneurs, 28
Literary agent, 374-375
Loans, 160-162
Logos, 240-241
Long term care, 333-341
Luros, Ellyn, 37, 221
Luther, John, 38-39
McManus, Jim, 38-39
Malpractice, 69-70, 290, 385
Management, 11, 27, 34-36, 223
Mancuso, Joseph, 97-98
Mangum, Karen, 374
Marketing, 7, 103-121, 409, 414
    products, 9, 37-39, 274
    plan, 116-119
    service, 113-114, 235-236
    social, 110-111
    strategies, 109-110, 274
Media, 8, 383-393
    for promotion, 250
    spokesperson, 12, 391
Medicine, practicing, 68
Mentoring, 13
National Assoc. of the Self-Employed, 4
Negotiation, 207-210
Networking, 7, 87
Newspapers, 254-255
Noncompete clause, 23, 220
Nondiet, 86
Nontraditional jobs, 7
Nurses, 329-330
Nutrient analysis, 221-222, 358-361
    assessment, 222
Nutrition,
    education in, 21, 53-54
Nutrition Entreprenurs DPG, 331
Nutrition Therapist, 3, 81-92
Nutrition Therapy, 81-92, 259-260
Office policy, 225-232
Offices, 182, 225-232
    Home, 4, 6, 183
    lease, 186-189
    rental, 182-189

sharing, 188-189
Partnerships, 123, 125, 128-130
Patents, 143-144
Permits, 124
Personal discretion, 136
Peters, Tom, 9
Physicians,
    contracts with, 329
    working with, 327-329
Pollan, Stephen, 5
Portfolio, 246
Posters, 247
Press release, 247, 311
Price fixing, 68
Private practice,
    buying/selling, 176-178
    commonalities in, 17-18
Product life cycle, 31-33
Product,
    based business, 9, 37-39
Profit and loss statement, 166
Promotion, 7, 237-257
    On-line, 314-317
Proposals,
    book, 373-374
    selling, 212-214
Proprietorships, 123, 125-128
Psychotherapeutic counseling, 12, 82-83
Public domain, 135
PSA Public service announcements, 250
Publicity, 251
Public relations, 150
Public relations expert, 153-155
Publishing,
    literary agent, 374-375
    self, 375-378
Query letter, 371-373
Radio, 255
Recipe development, 346-358
Recordkeeping, 172-174
Referrals, 64
Reimbursement, 204-206
Resume, 245
Retirement Plans, 176
Risk taking, 13-14, 16, 146
Rock, Arthur, 11
Rose, James C., 103, 419-420
Salk, Jonas, 54
Satterwhite, Olga, 149
SBA (Small Business Administration), 3,4, 159-160
SCAN (Sports & Cardiovascular Nutrition), 395, 404
SCORE (Service Corps of Retired Executives) 150
S Corporations, 123, 125, 133
Search engine, 265-267, 297
Secretary, 40, 179, 191, 231
Self-publishing, 364, 375-378
Selling, 210-212, 371
    Business, 176-178
    intangible products, 113-114, 235-236

      invention, 114-116
      product, 37-39, 114-116
      yourself, 87, 111, 240, 325, 387, 409, 412
Service,
      design, 37
      marketing, 113-114, 235-236
Service mark, 142
SEP(Simplified Employee Pension), 176
Shadix, Kyle, 156
Shenson, Howard, 7
Social marketing, 110-111
Software, 216-220, 224, 360
Sole proprietorship, 123, 125-128
Speaking, 9, 201, 239
Sports nutrition, 395-405
Spouses, 14
SS-4, 124
Start-up costs, 181-185
Sterling, Charles, 408
Strategic assumptions, 106
Strategic thinking, 35-36
Subcontracting, 40-42, 179
Subleasing, 188-189
Superbill, 169, 205
Supplements, selling, 65-66
Surveys, 261
SWOT, 108
Taxes, 174
      deductions, 174-176
Telephone, 190, 225-226, 326
      answering service, 191, 225
Television, 255
Third party reimbursement, 204-206
Tougas, Jane Grant, 343
Trademarks, 142-143
Trade secrets, 136
Venture capital, 11
Verbal agreement, 216
WWW World Wide Web, 256, 259-294
      Confidentiality, 281, 286, 292
      Deep, 265-266
      Domain name, 277
      Keywords, 297-302
      Links, 303, 311-312
      Meta tags, 297, 300-302
      Search engine, 265-267, 297-307
Web designer, 275-276
Web master, 293
Web page, 271-294
Website, 271-294, 297-321
Wellness, 86, 332, 407-415
Welch, Linda, 410
Williams, Sue Rodwell, 65
Woman-owned business, 4
Word processing, 222, 369-370
Working capital, 182
Worth, Randye, 37
Writing, 9, 242, 362-365, 367-382
X-Point, 7
Yancey, Jean, 7
Yellow pages, 253-254, 386